THIRD EDITION

Pharmacology Clear & Simple

A Guide to Drug Classifications and Dosage Calculations

Cynthia J. Watkins, RN, MSN, CPN
Pediatric Intensive Care Staff Nurse
Halifax Health
Daytona Beach, Florida

F.A. Davis Company • Philadelphia

F. A. Davis Company
1915 Arch Street
Philadelphia, PA 19103
www.fadavis.com

Copyright © 2018 by F. A. Davis Company

Printed in the United States of America

Last digit indicates print number: 10 9 8 7 6 5 4

Senior Acquisitions Editor: Melissa A. Duffield
Senior Developmental Editor, Health Professions: Dean W. DeChambeau
Director of Content Development, Health Professions: George W. Lang
Art and Design Manager: Carolyn O'Brien

As new scientific information becomes available through basic and clinical research, recommended treatments and drug therapies undergo changes. The author(s) and publisher have done everything possible to make this book accurate, up to date, and in accord with accepted standards at the time of publication. The authors, editors, and publisher are not responsible for errors or omissions or for consequences from application of the book, and make no warranty, expressed or implied, in regard to the contents of the book. Any practice described in this book should be applied by the reader in accordance with professional standards of care used in regard to the unique circumstances that may apply in each situation. The reader is advised always to check product information (package inserts) for changes and new information regarding dose and contraindications before administering any drug. Caution is especially urged when using new or infrequently ordered drugs.

Library of Congress Cataloging-in-Publication Data

Names: Watkins, Cynthia J., author.
Title: Pharmacology clear & simple : a guide to drug classifications and
    dosage calculations / Cynthia J. Watkins.
Other titles: Pharmacology clear and simple
Description: Third edition. | Philadelphia, PA : F.A. Davis Company, [2018] |
    Includes bibliographical references and index.
Identifiers: LCCN 2018006898 (print) | LCCN 2018007839 (ebook) | ISBN
    9780803677319 (epub) | ISBN 9780803666528 (pbk. : alk. paper)
Subjects: | MESH: Pharmaceutical Preparations—administration & dosage | Drug
    Dosage Calculations | Drug Administration Routes | Pharmaceutical
    Preparations—classification | Medication Errors—prevention & control |
    Problems and Exercises
Classification: LCC RM300 (ebook) | LCC RM300 (print) | NLM QV 18.2 | DDC
    615/.1—dc23
LC record available at https://lccn.loc.gov/2018006898

*I would like to dedicate this textbook
to the love of my life, Jeffrey Watkins,
who continues to be incredibly supportive of my venture
into the realm of being an author.*

Preface

In my 32 years as a nurse, I have been involved with direct patient care as well as taught a variety of students in nursing, medical assisting, surgical technology, and respiratory therapy. I have also taught those who may not deliver direct patient care, such as students of psychology and clinical lab science. There is always one constant challenge: to provide students with enough pharmacology knowledge so that they feel confident as they embark on their health profession careers but not so much that they are overwhelmed. For those students who will administer medication, pharmacology is critical; for others, it is a subject that will aid their understanding of the patient care relationship, although they may not be directly involved with the patient.

This edition of the book has been expanded in response to the requests of our reviewers. I've tried to build on the solid foundation of the second edition and to expand the coverage of drugs, keeping in mind always the suggestions we received from pharmacology faculty from around the nation. I hope you will be pleased with the results.

My goal for the third edition of this book is to continue to bring the most current information to pharmacology topics as well as continue to provide elemental concepts that will enable students to understand how medications work and how they are administered. These concepts include the health professionals' role in the process. This edition is divided into four units:

Unit 1: Introduction to Pharmacology discusses the fundamentals of pharmacology, including history, patient safety and regulations, and prescription labels. Each topic lays the foundation for the work ahead.

Unit 2: Calculations begins with Chapter 6, Review of Mathematics, which begins with a basic review of fractions and decimals and progresses to more advanced mathematical calculations. This review provides many testing opportunities for students to assess their knowledge through the Check Up exercises throughout the chapter. Chapter 7, Measurement Systems, addresses the various measurements systems and shows students how to convert among the metric, household, and apothecary systems. Chapter 8, Dosage Calculations, ends this unit by showing students how to calculate dosages. In this chapter, students have many opportunities to practice dosage calculations using a variety of examples to increase their knowledge and confidence in administering medications.

Unit 3: Administration of Medications includes Chapters 9 and 10, Enteral Medications and Administration and Parenteral Medications and Administration, respectively, which provide step-by-step instructions through Procedure Boxes with supporting images.

Unit 4: Classifications of Drugs addresses all major drug classifications by body system. Although individual drugs are mentioned, each chapter primarily focuses on key attributes of that particular body system. This focus allows the student to understand how a particular set of drugs works and how individual drugs within that set function the same way.

FEATURES

The following features are included to further facilitate students in their learning and to help them better retain pharmacological content.

- **Check Up** boxes have mathematical calculation exercises in Unit 2. Each Check Up appears following a math review section to test the student's knowledge and understanding of basic math concepts.

- **Fast Tip** boxes provide brief bits of useful information on various topics within the chapters.

- **A Closer Look** boxes examine special topics in each chapter.

- **Drug Spotlight** boxes highlight one or two drugs in each chapter and provide detailed information.

- **Critical Thinking** exercises encourage students to think beyond the chapter and apply their new knowledge to real-life scenarios.

- **Master the Essentials** tables cover indications, side effects, precautions, contraindications, interactions, and examples for each drug classification. They are perfect for study and review because all the drug classifications in the chapters are covered.

- **Chapter Review** questions in multiple formats appear at the end of each chapter to test student comprehension. **Internet Research** activities encourage students to use the Internet to research and locate important information on specific drugs, drug safety, and how to educate and instruct patients to use various medications.

ANCILLARY CONTENT

- Accompanying the text are online resources to help support both students and instructors. For the student, the eBook is available online at www.DavisPlus.com. For medical assisting educators and nursing educators, separate resources include test banks, instructor guides, teaching guides, and PowerPoint presentations. Medical assisting resources also include documentation exercises and a competencies checklist.

I hope this third edition of *Pharmacology Clear & Simple* meets all your teaching and learning needs.

Cynthia J. Watkins, RN, MSN, CPN

Reviewers

Kathi Gilmore, MA, AS, AHI
Medical Assistant Instructor
Allied Health
Tennessee College of Applied Technology
Nashville, Tennessee

Joseph M. Glass, BS, MS, RPh
Staff Pharmacist with Potomac Valley Pharmacy
Instructor, Co-coordinator of Pharmacy
Technician Program at Allegany College of Maryland
Cumberland, Maryland

Cheri Goretti, MT (ASCP), CMA (AAMA)
Professor and Coordinator
Medical Assisting and Allied Health
Quinebaug Valley Community College
Danielson, Connecticut

Tanya Gwin, RN, MSN
Nursing Instructor
Health Science
Copper Mountain College
Joshua Tree, California

Rachel M. Houston, BS, CMA (AAMA)
Program Director
Medical Assistant Program
Cabarrus College of Health Sciences
Concord, North Carolina

Dawn K. Kochara, RN, BSN, DHSc
Department Chair/Director, Nursing Programs
Health Sciences
Orange Technical College
Orlando, Florida

Naomi D. Lee, MSN, RN
Instructor
Applied Technology Services
Special School District of St. Louis County
St. Louis, Missouri

Mischelle Monagle, MSN, MBA, RN
Dean of College of Nursing & Health Professions
College of Nursing & Health Professions
Carl Sandburg College
Galesburg, Illinois

Lisa Ann Sailor, BS, CMA (AAMA)
Program Director/Instructor/Medical Assistant
Anoka Technical College
Anoka, Minnesota

Stephanie Stanley, RN, BSN, LNC
Program Head/Instructor
Nursing-CNA & LPN programs
Ridgeview High School/Technical Programs
Clintwood, Virginia

Pamela Michelle Thurman, BSBA, BSN, RN
Practical Nursing Program Coordinator/Pharmacology
Instructor
Practical Nursing Program
Franklin Technology Center
Joplin, Missouri

Ronald Lee Vestal, BSN, RN
PN Instructor
Nursing Department
Mid-Del Technology Center
Midwest City, Oklahoma

Acknowledgments

I thank Andy McPhee for recruiting me and having faith in my ability to complete this project. Thank you to Dean DeChambeau for all the assistance required to bring this work to publication. I want to acknowledge all the staff of F. A. Davis as well as the editors who have also had input on this project. Thanks to all!

Contents in Brief

Contents

Introduction to Pharmacology

History of Pharmacology

Medications, their origins, and their uses are older than any written records that we have. Many ancient cultures have contributed to the knowledge base and evolution of pharmacology, including Greek, Chinese, Egyptian, Persian, and Arabic. The healers were called by many names, but all shared an extensive knowledge of plants, minerals, and animal products. Pharmacology has evolved significantly from the days when these resources were used to cure the ill without understanding why they worked or did not work. Some ancient remedies are still valuable medicines today, whereas others have been discarded as worthless or dangerous. With the advent of scientific inquiry and technology, researchers around the world have created new and better medications. The ability to isolate pure substances and formulate drugs in a laboratory enables pharmaceutical companies to mass-produce needed medicines in a timely manner.

In this chapter, you will learn about the history of pharmacology and sources used for developing drugs; the acceptance of alternative medicine, and its place in medicine; and the six main categories of drugs and their uses.

LEARNING OUTCOMES

At the end of this chapter, you should be able to:

1.1 Define all key terms.
1.2 List three societies critical to the development and evolution of pharmacology.
1.3 List four sources of drugs.
1.4 List 10 drugs, and record their sources.

KEY TERMS

Al-Hawi	Diagnostic	Pharmakon
Alternative medicine	Drug/*droog*	Porcine
Antineoplastic	Ebers Papyrus	Prophylactic
Bovine	Palliative	Replacement drugs
Curative	Pharmacodynamics	Synthetic drugs
Destructive	Pharmacology	

■ HISTORY OF PHARMACOLOGY

The history of pharmacology helps us to understand that even though there have been huge advances in medications, scientists are coming to understand that by disregarding ancient practices, they have been missing a treasure trove of useful medications. Many practitioners are utilizing **alternative medicine** to maximize their patients' health, and scientists are looking to older remedies to see if and why they work and how to reproduce them in the modern world. We as practitioners also need to understand that many patients are using many different forms of self-medication, from home remedies to substances they learned about on an infomercial that promise to cure all types of problems; if these substances are not understood, they may interfere or counteract a prescribed pharmaceutical medication. In other words, we need a complete picture of every substance patients are taking in order to assist in their care.

The term **pharmacology** is of Greek origin from two words: **pharmakon,** meaning "medicine," and *ology,* meaning "the study of." Pharmakon also meant poison *and* remedy, poison because some of the early medicines were toxic enough to kill, and remedy because, at times, early medicines cured the illness. The word **drug** has a Dutch origin in which **droog** meant "dry" as in the use of dry herbs.

Most ancient societies had little knowledge about the human body and how it worked, so treating illness was often based on trial and error. Early records document that treatments consisted of plants, minerals, and animal products because no other sources were available. "Healers" were known as wise men, shamans, witch doctors, medicine men and women, and so on (Fig. 1-1), depending on the culture, and were chosen based on their knowledge of which plants or other substance to use, how to prepare it, and how much to give the patient.

Pharmacology in Ancient Times and Cultures

Early documentation of medicine and various remedies is evident in several cultures. For example, "The Yellow Emperors' Inner Classic," a Chinese document, was a very early discussion of yin-yang and acupuncture. The first Chinese manual on pharmacology was written in the first century A.D. and included 365 medicines, 252 of which were herbs. In Egypt, a medical document called the **Ebers Papyrus** was written circa 1550 B.C. and lists about 700 "recipes" for a host of illnesses, from crocodile bites to psychiatric illnesses. Another document, the **Al-Hawi,** is a large, 20-volume medical book written by the physician Al-Razi in ancient Persia (Iran). It was translated into Latin in the 13th century and greatly influenced medicine in medieval Europe.

The contributions from these cultures led to the advancement of pharmacology. When treatments for many conditions were discovered, the findings were recorded on papyrus or paper to pass on to future generations. Documenting this early information was extremely important, as belief systems changed over time. Without these earlier writings, traditional oral knowledge might have been lost or suppressed and much progress could not have been made.

During the 17th and 18th centuries, there was a real lack of knowledge in the use of medications and their dangers. A prime example of this is mercury, which was used for a variety of ailments from skin conditions to syphilis. Specifically, in the late 1700s a prominent physician, Dr. Benjamin Rush used a mercury compound in high doses to treat yellow fever patients. Of course, it has since been discovered that mercury is so harmful to humans that we no longer use mercury blood pressure cuffs or thermometers for fear of exposure.

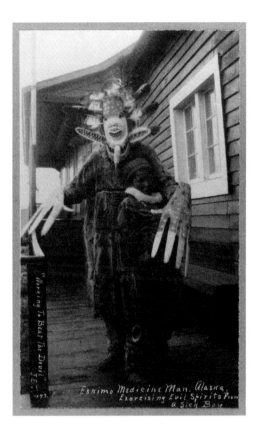

FIGURE 1-1: Eskimo medicine man. *(From the Library of Congress Prints and Photographs Division, Washington, D.C.)*

Pharmacological Advances Through the 19th and 20th Centuries

Over time, an increasingly scientific approach to the discovery and understanding of drugs was taken. During the 1800s, chemists were able to identify and then isolate the active ingredients (those pure chemicals in the plants that had the actual therapeutic properties). They were also able to determine how the drug acted on the body. This marked the beginning of modern pharmacology. Up until the early 1900s, preparing medicine was very labor-intensive; the pharmacist had to distill and prepare each medicine when it was ordered (Fig. 1-2). Not until World War II (1939 to 1945) did the mass-production of medicine begin (Fig. 1-3). More U.S. soldiers died in World War I from infection and accidents than from actual combat injuries; however, the mass-production of penicillin minimized the number of deaths from infection during World War II (Table 1-1). For instance, the death rate from pneumonia

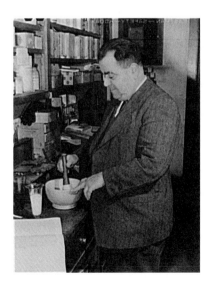

FIGURE 1-2: Pharmacist preparing a prescription, 1939. *(From the Library of Congress Prints and Photographs Division, Washington, D.C.)*

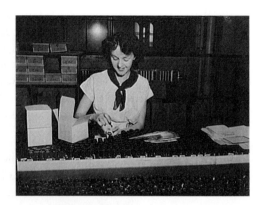

FIGURE 1-3: Mass-production of medication, 1944.
(From the Library of Congress Prints and Photographs Division, Washington, D.C.)

TABLE 1.1 U.S. Casualties in Major Wars

War	Number Serving	Battle Deaths	Disease and Accidents
Civil War	2,213,363	140,414	224,097
Spanish-American War	306,760	385	2,061
World War I	4,743,826	53,513	63,195
World War II	16,353,659	292,131	115,185

Source: U.S. Department of Justice

in the U.S. Army was 18% during World War I, decreasing to 1% during World War II. Death from combat injuries complicated by infections also decreased.

With the discoveries of new drugs like penicillin that could save millions of lives, the belief grew that new drugs must be better than old standard herbs and treatments, especially if created or refined in a scientific manner. Pharmacology therefore advanced rapidly in the second half of the 20th century as many new drugs were either discovered or developed. In an effort to discover possible new drugs, researchers studied plants, marine animals, and micro-organisms in soil, water, and air. Partially or totally synthesized medications were produced by combining two or more compounds or elements. Partially synthesized medications were made by adding a pure chemical to a natural substance. Totally synthesized medications were created by combing two or more pure chemicals to produce a new substance that could be used as a medication. One major breakthrough was the discovery of ways to create large amounts of viable drugs from a small amount of natural resources using genetic engineering. For example, human insulin can be mass-produced by adding the human insulin gene to a nonpathogenic strain of *Escherichia coli*.

Pharmacology in the 21st Century

In the 21st century science is booming. One of the most promising advances in the field of medications is that of pharmacogenetics, which is the "study of individual candidate genes as powerful tools to explain interindividual variability in drug response." In other words, the patient's genetic material is analyzed, and then in the case of cancer, the tumor's genetics are analyzed to figure out the best drug and what dosage will work best to combat the disease. Currently there are certain medications and doses used to treat conditions for every adult patient with that condition. Through these advances in pharmacogenetics, the ability to individualize drugs and their dosage is happening in the treatment of HIV and rheumatoid arthritis. In addition, the hope is that in the future we can specifically tailor drugs and dosages for opioids and antihypertensives among other medications.

■ SOURCES OF DRUGS

Although most drugs are now manufactured in laboratories, many agents are still derived from natural substances such as plants, animals, minerals, and toxins. Some are utilized by extracting active ingredients from animals or plants and using these ingredients to manufacture a medication. Other times the original or natural source serves as a template for creating a synthetic equivalent, which is especially useful if the natural source is a rare plant. Scientists are constantly researching natural sources (plants, animals, marine animals, and microbes) in the hope of finding new sources of medications. Some drugs are made by combining chemicals with natural products, such as hydrocodone, which combines natural opium in the form of codeine combined with acetaminophen (a man-made medication), whereas other drugs are synthesized in a laboratory. Barbiturates are an example of synthetic drugs because they are chemically derived from barbituric acid (itself an artificial compound of urea and malonic acid).

Plants

Today plants are rarely used as medications; instead the active component of the plant is extracted and utilized in the manufacturing of the drug. Digoxin (Lanoxin), a drug used to treat heart failure, is made from the foxglove plant and has been used for healing since the 1500s. Most estrogen hormone replacements come from yams. Procaine (Novocain), used as an anesthetic, is derived from the coca plant. Rose hips are a rich source of vitamin C and are sold as an ingredient in vitamin C supplements. Aspirin (acetylsalicylic acid) is a compound based on salicin, which is found in the bark of a white willow tree, and is used to relieve pain and to treat inflammation.

Unfortunately, as less land becomes available for growing plants, fewer plants will exist for making medications. For example, as the rain forest diminishes, the rare plants that are located only in this environment may become extinct. In this instance, these rare plants are used as a template to manufacture a medication instead of using the plants and depleting them.

 CRITICAL THINKING

If people rely on plants for medication, what effect does the increasing human population have on the potential supply of medications?

Animals

Domesticated animals are also a source of drugs. To ensure the purity of the drugs, donor animals are generally well cared for. Some examples include sheep, which provide lanolin, a topical skin medication that comes from the wool. Cows **(bovine)** and pigs **(porcine)** are good sources of hormone replacements. If a patient's body cannot manufacture a hormone, animal hormones can serve as a substitute. Horses provide humans with the replacement hormone conjugated estrogen (Premarin), which comes from a pregnant mare's urine. In addition, insulin is collected from the pancreases of cows or pigs. We obtain IGG (Immunoglobulin G) by injecting an antigen into animals (most commonly cows) and collecting the antibody that is formed. The drug heparin is extracted from porcine intestinal mucosa and bovine lungs.

 CRITICAL THINKING

Cows and pigs are good sources of hormones. Do you think animals may be a better hormone source than humans? Why or why not?

Minerals

When foods grown from rich soil are unavailable, calcium, iron, zinc, magnesium, copper, and selenium are some of the minerals that are offered as necessary supplements.

For patients taking certain medications, mineral replacement is critical. Diuretic drugs such as furosemide (Lasix) cause the body to lose excess water through the kidneys, and potassium, a vital mineral, is also excreted with the water. Potassium is needed for the heart to function normally, so supplemental potassium chloride is frequently prescribed in addition to the medication. Potassium is also contained in sweet potatoes, bananas, and oranges.

Minerals are also used to treat certain conditions. For example, gold is used in the treatment of arthritis, iodine is used to treat goiter, and magnesium sulfate is used for constipation and eclampsia.

Toxins

Toxins, by definition, are poisons. Despite this fact, chemical and biological toxins are commonly used in medicine. The key is in the dosage. For instance, certain radioactive chemicals are used to diagnose and treat illnesses. Radioactive iodine, for example, in small doses can help pinpoint problems in a patient's thyroid, a small gland in the neck. In higher doses, radioactive iodine is used to shrink thyroid tumors.

Biological toxins can also be used in medicine. Botulinum toxin (Botox), which comes from a bacterium called *Clostridium botulinum,* is used in patients with torticollis (a condition in which neck muscles contract causing the head to turn to one side), strabismus (eye misalignment), and migraines. It is used in tiny doses.

 CRITICAL THINKING

What are some of the dangers of using toxins as medicine?

Synthetic Medications

Synthetic drugs can be created by chemical processes, genetic engineering, or by altering animal cells. Often, drugs that are obtained from another source can be synthesized in the laboratory, thus preserving natural resources. For example, paclitaxel (Taxol), a drug for patients with cancer, was first made from the bark of the Pacific yew tree. Then a template or blueprint was developed to create a synthetic form of this drug, thus preserving the yew tree. Insulin can be obtained from pigs or cows, but a synthetic source is most commonly used. Human insulin is produced by using recombinant technology to add the insulin gene into a nonpathogenic strain of *E. coli.* This change occurred because of concern over the possible transmission of disease from animals to humans. In addition, there is a risk for immune reactions because of impurities found in the animal products. One additional advantage is that synthetic medications are usually more inexpensive because they are mass-produced.

Because scientists have been able to map the human genome, it is becoming possible to choose medications that are appropriate for individual patients, not patients as a whole. One area of uniqueness is the variation in the amount of drug-metabolizing enzymes each patient has and the effectiveness of these enzymes. The scientist can manipulate the DNA material of the medication source by changing it or combining it with DNA from another organism to target the patient's levels of the drug-metabolizing enzyme. Therefore, prescribers are able to choose drugs that work better for one population than for another. Research is also being conducted on the use of existing drugs in targeted populations. For example, BiDil is a combination of two generic drugs—hydralazine hydrochloride and isosorbide dinitrate—and is used to treat African American patients with heart failure.

 CRITICAL THINKING

What are some of the ethical issues of genetically engineered drugs?

■ CATEGORIZING MEDICATIONS

The term **pharmacodynamics** refers to the effect of a drug on the body, or more scientifically, the negative and positive biochemical or physiological changes that a drug creates. Drugs fall into six categories of desired effects (Table 1-2).

- ■ **Curative.** Some drugs restore normal physiological function, as in diuretics, which help the body rid itself of excess fluid.
- ■ **Prophylactic.** These drugs prevent diseases or disorders, as in antibiotics given before surgery to prevent infection.

TABLE 1.2   Drug Categories

Category	Main Action	Examples
Curative	Cures or treats a problem	• Penicillin to treat strep throat
Prophylactic	Prevents a problem	• Cefazolin (Ancef, Kefzol) to prevent infections from surgery • Vaccine to prevent measles, mumps, and rubella
Diagnostic	Helps diagnose a disease or condition	• Diatrizoate meglumine and diatrizoate sodium (Gastrografin) • Barium sulfate (Gastrografin and Barium sulfate are used for computed tomography scans)
Palliative	Treats symptoms to make the patient more comfortable	• Morphine to relieve the pain of cancer • Oxygen to make breathing more comfortable
Replacement	Replaces a missing substance	• Levothyroxine • Natural thyroid to treat hypothyroidism
Destructive	Destroys tumors and/or microbes	• Carbimazole to inhibit the production of thyroid hormone to treat hyperthyroidism

■ **Diagnostic.** Some drugs help diagnose a disease, such as barium that patients swallow to help highlight digestive problems on a radiograph.

■ **Palliative.** Other drugs, such as pain relievers, do not cure disease, but they make patients more comfortable.

■ **Replacement.** These drugs "replace" missing substances. Levothyroxine sodium (Synthroid), for example, is a drug that replaces a missing thyroid hormone.

■ **Destructive.** Some medications destroy tumors and microbes. **Antineoplastic** (anticancer) drugs are an example of destructive, toxic drugs.

Medications are used for various reasons during a patient's life span. As a health-care provider, you must know how the different categories of drugs may affect a patient. Understanding this information will help you provide effective counseling, patient care, and safe administration of drugs depending on your role and scope of practice.

 CRITICAL THINKING

Identify the following drugs as curative, prophylactic, diagnostic, palliative, replacement, or destructive.

• Synthroid
• Diuretic ("water pill")
• Flu vaccine
• Radiopaque dye
• Fever reducer
• Anticancer drug

THE ROLES OF THE LICENSED PRACTICAL NURSE, LICENSED VOCATIONAL NURSE, AND MEDICAL ASSISTANT IN THE ADMINISTRATION OF MEDICATIONS

All health-care providers must work within their scope of practice, which is a standardized set of health-care services providers can render and the extent they may do so independently. These functions are based on state laws and the provider's education, experience, and skills. Facilities may have their own additional policies. It is important to know your scope of practice in your state so that you can provide the best care possible to your patients while abiding by state regulations.

The individual State Boards of Nursing are the governing bodies that determine the scopes of practices for Licensed Practical Nurses (LPNs) and Licensed Vocational Nurses (LVNs). LPNs/LVNs generally administer oral, rectal, ophthalmic, otic, intradermal, subcutaneous, intradermal, and intravenous (IV) medications. In most states, LPNs may not give medications by rapid IV push. Many states additionally regulate if an LPN/LVN can start, discontinue, and/or monitor IV fluids. They also may not be allowed to administer or monitor IV medications and fluids via a central line (one that is in a large vein close to the patient's heart). LPNs/LVNs usually work under the direct supervision of a registered nurse.

Medical assistants may usually administer oral, intradermal, subcutaneous, and intramuscular medications as well as rectal, otic, and ophthalmic medications. In some states, they are allowed to have some involvement with IV fluids and medications after additional training once they receive their initial certification. Medical assistants generally work under direct supervision of a physician, physician assistant, or nurse practitioner.

● ● ● SUMMARY

- Ancient cultures have contributed to the knowledge base and evolution of pharmacology, including Greek, Chinese, Egyptian, Persian (Iranian), and Arabic. Examples of early documentation include the Egyptian Ebers papyrus (1550 B.C.) and the Persian Al-Hawi.

- The 19th and 20th centuries saw rapid advancement in organic chemistry and technology that enabled scientists to identify and isolate active ingredients in plants and allowed the creation of synthetic drugs.

- Advancements in the study of human physiology enabled a better understanding of pharmacodynamics, the study of the negative and positive biochemical or physiological changes that a drug creates in the body.

- Mass-production of medications began around 1939 to 1945, and genetic engineering produced large amounts of drugs from small amounts of natural resources.

- In the 21st century, the field of pharmacogenetics is developing as physicians use genetic testing to determine how a patient will respond to specific medications and thus individualize treatment for the patient and his or her disease.

- Sources of drugs include plants, animals, minerals, toxins, and synthetic creations.

- The six categories of a drug's effect on the body are curative, prophylactic, diagnostic, palliative, replacement, and destructive.

- Roles of the LPN/LVN and medical assistant in medication administration are governed by their scope of practice, which is established by state regulations and facility policies.

Activities

To make sure that you have learned the key points covered in this chapter, complete the following activities.

Multiple Choice

Choose the best answer for each question.

1. Which of the following is the source of lanolin?

    A. Animal

    B. Plant

    C. Mineral

    D. Human

    E. Synthesis

2. Which of the following is the source of potassium chloride?

    A. Animal

    B. Plant

    C. Mineral

    D. Human

    E. Synthesis

3. Which of the following is the source of digoxin (Lanoxin)?

    A. Animal

    B. Plant

    C. Mineral

    D. Human

    E. Synthesis

4. Which of the following is the source of barbiturates?

    A. Animal

    B. Plant

    C. Mineral

    D. Human

    E. Synthesis

5. Which of the following is the source of leukocytes?

    A. Animal

    B. Plant

    C. Mineral

    D. Human

    E. Synthesis

6. **During which war did mass-production of penicillin begin?**

   A. Civil War

   B. World War I

   C. World War II

   D. Korean War

   E. Vietnam War

7. **Genetic engineering is used to make what type of drugs?**

   A. Synthetic

   B. Homeopathic

   C. Natural

   D. None of the above

8. **What was the source of insulin prior to the synthetic production of medicine?**

   A. Cows

   B. Horses

   C. Pigs

   D. Both A and C

   E. All of the above

9. **Toxins are commonly used to treat what aging symptom?**

   A. Loss of hearing

   B. Diminished sight

   C. Wrinkling of skin

   D. Depression

10. **What drug used in the treatment of menopause is obtained from horses?**

    A. Estrogen

    B. Premarin

    C. Paxil

    D. None of the above

Short Answer Questions

1. Are animals a good source for drugs? Explain your answer. _____

   _____

   _____

2. What source of drugs is in danger of disappearing? _____

   _____

   _____

3. What was the catalyst to begin mass-production of medicine? _____

   _____

   _____

4. Discuss alternative medicine and what role it should play (in your opinion) in patient care.

_____

_____

Application Exercises
Respond to the following scenarios.

1. Muhammed A. is a devout Muslim. He does not eat pork. What is the best choice of insulin for him? Explain your rationale for this choice. _____

_____

_____

2. Mary L. is adamantly against stem cell research and is refusing to use Humulin insulin. What do you think? How is Humulin insulin created? Explain how Humulin insulin is okay to be used, or not used based on Mary's beliefs. _____

_____

_____

3. Harold P. comes to the office complaining of sinus pressure and pain. In the intake interview, you discover that he has been utilizing aromatherapy for the past 3 weeks. What do you do? _____

_____

_____

4. Raymond H. comes to his cardiologist with complaints of an irregular heartbeat and dizziness. In further talking with him, you discover he has been seeing a homeopathic healer and has been drinking foxglove tea to improve his circulation. What do you say? _____

_____

_____

Internet Research
1. Use the keywords "cultures contributing to pharmacology" to research cultures that were not discussed in this chapter. Pick one culture, and write a synopsis of that culture's contribution.

2. Use the keywords "the future of pharmacology" to research possible directions that pharmacology is headed. Select and describe one specific area of future development that you find.

3. Use your search engine to discover sources of drugs used now and possibly in the future. Use the keywords "medication sources past, present, and future." Pick one source that was not discussed in this chapter, and write about it to share with your class.

4. Use the keywords "medications made using recombinant DNA" to locate information on recombinant DNA. Pick one medication that you find, and write about how recombinant DNA is used to make it.

Basics of Pharmacology

Pharmacology is studied to discover the most effective medications that cause the least amount of problems for patients. The drug cycle consists of four phases: absorption, distribution, metabolism, and excretion. Each phase has implications for the health-care worker. Health-care professionals must know how best to administer medications for optimal absorption into the bloodstream. For effective care and education of the patient, they must also know where the medications will be distributed and any possible negative side effects. Health-care professionals must be vigilant about knowing how a drug is metabolized and what symptoms or laboratory test results to watch for that may indicate a potential issue. Finally, understanding how drugs are excreted and being aware of potential issues related to drug cumulation are critical. Health-care professionals are the patient's best advocate.

Chapter 1 discusses the history and evolution of pharmacology. In this chapter, we look at the science of pharmacology, how medications affect the body, how they interact with each other to produce either a positive or negative effect on the body, and why it is important as a prescriber to understand these effects and interactions. We begin by looking at **pharmacokinetics,** *which is the study of how the body absorbs, distributes, and excretes drugs (the drug cycle). We learn what happens once medications are ingested, injected, or applied.*

LEARNING OUTCOMES

At the end of this chapter, you should be able to:

2.1 Define key terms.

2.2 List the four steps in the drug cycle and their effects on the body.

2.3 Differentiate between the therapeutic level and potency of a drug.

2.4 Describe how drugs can interact.

2.5 Differentiate between a side effect and an adverse reaction.

2.6 Compare and contrast the usefulness of different drug resources.

KEY TERMS

Absorption	Distribution	Side effects
Adverse reaction	Excretion	Synergism
Agonist	Half-life	Teratogenic
Antagonist	Idiosyncratic	Toxic
Bioavailability	Pharmacokinetics	
Biotransformation/Metabolism	Receptors	

WHAT IS PHARMACOLOGY?

What is pharmacology, and why is it studied? Pharmacology is the exploration of substances that are used to heal and comfort the sick and in other ways help us to live longer and healthier lives. Do you ever wonder who first thought that placing maggots on a black necrotic wound was a good idea and would lead to healthy, clean tissue, or who decided that brewing a tea out of the beautiful, but poisonous foxglove plant should be used to help with heart failure? These pioneering individuals were extremely brave because they would likely have been banished or killed if they had guessed wrong. They were the first pharmacologists. These courageous men and women and their followers began the journey that led to the wonderful discoveries of the modern era. The advances have enabled us to increase life expectancy by eradicating most childhood illnesses and by producing antibiotics to cure many infections. The science of pharmacology has allowed us to research and produce potential medications while minimizing danger to the patient in the process.

THE DRUG CYCLE

When a medication is ingested, applied, or injected, it enters the bloodstream and begins the drug cycle. This cycle has four main phases: absorption (how the medication enters our bloodstream), distribution (how the medication travels to the appropriate site), metabolism or biotransformation (how our body breaks the medication down into usable components and waste products), and excretion (how our body eliminates the extra medication and waste products) (Fig. 2-1).

Factors influencing the time it takes to complete the drug cycle include the drug itself, the route of administration, and the health of the patient's organs. For example, medication given by mouth takes much longer to enter the bloodstream and to reach the site where it is needed than does medication given directly into the circulatory system. Some medications take longer to break down than others, and the effects of these drugs are prolonged. The estimated time for the cycle to be completed ranges from 15 minutes to days.

Absorption

Absorption is the process by which a substance moves into the bloodstream from the site where it was administered. A drug can be administered in one of two ways: (1) enterally, which means the drug is given directly into the gastrointestinal (GI) system orally, rectally, or through a tube entering this system; or (2) parenterally, by all other routes that do not touch the GI system.

How quickly a medication is absorbed depends on how it is administered and whether it is topical or systemic. **Topical drugs act locally; systemic drugs act on one or more body systems.**

A topical medication is applied directly to the site of concern and can work quickly. Examples include Desitin and Balmex to treat diaper rash. Another example is EMLA cream, which is applied as a local anesthetic prior to blood draws or IV insertions in small children to numb the area prior to the needlestick. Lidocaine can be injected into an area of tissue to provide numbing prior to placement of sutures after an injury. Systemic medications are taken by mouth or are administered intravenously, intramuscularly, or as a patch applied to the skin, to circulate throughout the body. A medication the patient takes by mouth must be transferred through the stomach or intestinal mucosa into the circulating blood. Liquid medications act faster than pills because pills must first be broken down to be

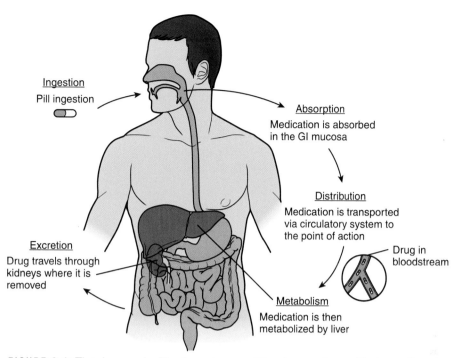

FIGURE 2-1: The drug cycle. The four phases of the drug cycle are (1) absorption via the gastrointestinal mucosa, (2) distribution via the circulatory system, (3) metabolism via the liver, and finally (4) excretion via the kidneys.

absorbed. Intramuscular injections provide fairly quick absorption because muscles have a rich supply of blood to provide rapid entry into the circulation. Intravenous (IV) injection is the fastest way to the blood supply because the drug is injected directly into a vein.

As a health-care professional, you can take steps to facilitate drug absorption. For instance, when administering an ointment for a rash, you can make sure that the skin is clean and dry. If a prescriber orders an intramuscular injection, you will choose which muscle to use for best absorption. A tattooed arm could possibly hinder absorption because of decreased blood flow caused by scar tissue and tattoo paint. You would choose a muscle that is free of any lesions. Conversely, you must be careful when giving IV medications so that they are not absorbed too rapidly. For example, if morphine is given too rapidly, a patient may become severely hypotensive and stop breathing.

Other factors that may vary the absorption rate and **bioavailability** (how much of the drug is absorbed for use) of medications include:

- *Fat or lipid solubility:* The more soluble a medication is in fat or lipids, the more easily it is dissolved and absorbed through the stomach into the bloodstream.

- *pH:* Medications with a low pH (acidic) are easily absorbed in the stomach, whereas those with a higher pH (alkalotic) are less likely to be absorbed effectively.

- *Concentration of the medication:* The higher the medication concentration is, the more easily the medication is absorbed.

- *Length of contact:* The longer a topical medication remains on the skin or mucosa, the greater the absorption will be. If a patient sucks on a lozenge until it dissolves, more medication is released in the mouth than if the patient chews and swallows the lozenge.

- *Age:* Both children and older patients absorb more medication through the skin than do healthy adults, so topical medication is usually applied in a very thin layer.

- *Food:* A large amount of food slows the absorption of systemic medications. Stomach acid facilitates absorption of systemic medications; therefore, medication is absorbed faster when acid in the stomach is increased.

■ *Depth of breathing:* For inhalants, the more deeply patients breathe, the more medication they inhale. For example, ask patients to inhale deeply to receive maximum benefit during treatment for asthma.

 CRITICAL THINKING

Explain how to overcome the following issue to increase absorption and bioavailability of an inhaled drug.

A patient who is taking shallow breaths and who is unable to follow directions to "breath deeply."

Distribution

The second phase in the drug cycle is **distribution,** which is the delivery of a drug to the appropriate site after the drug has been absorbed into the bloodstream. Once the medication is in the bloodstream, it is rapidly distributed throughout the body. Initially, well-perfused organs such as the brain, heart, kidneys, and lungs receive the majority of the medication. The lesser perfused organs such as the skin, muscles, and fat receive the medication at a slower rate.

Tissues in the body are either permeable or nonpermeable, meaning that substances can or cannot pass through them. A drug's ability to pass through tissue depends on whether it is a lipid-soluble or non–lipid-soluble drug. Lipid-soluble drugs can easily pass through the lipid layer of membranes due to their small molecular size, while non–lipid-soluble (water-soluble) drugs have a very difficult time passing through these tissues.

Certain tissues have specialized physiological "barriers," such as densely packed cells that allow nutrients and certain chemicals, but not other substances, including medications, to pass from the blood through the tissue. Examples of these densely packed cells include the blood-brain barrier, the blood-testicular barrier, and the blood-placental barrier.

The blood-placental barrier helps to filter drugs and other substances passing from mother to fetus and thereby protects the fetus. However, alcohol, cocaine, and even some over-the-counter drugs can cross this barrier easily and cause harm. Most lipid-soluble drugs readily cross this barrier, but water-soluble drugs do not. Many drugs, such as psychotropic (mind-altering) drugs, can cross the blood-brain barrier, although some antibiotics and other drugs that are easily absorbed in the stomach cannot cross. The blood-testicular barrier protects the male reproductive organs from toxins that could damage sperm. This barrier also makes certain male reproductive diseases difficult to treat because very little is allowed through it except for substances directly involved in functioning of the testes. Many psychotropic drugs have negative sexual effects, such as decreased libido, because they cross both the blood-brain barrier and the blood-testicular barrier.

 CRITICAL THINKING

Why do drugs that cross the blood-brain barrier tend to have strong negative effects?

 CRITICAL THINKING

Why should a woman actively trying to become pregnant consult her physician before taking an over-the-counter medication?

Metabolism

In the phase following distribution, the drug is metabolized by the liver, kidneys, and intestines. **Metabolism** or **biotransformation** means that the medication is chemically transformed to a less active or inactive form, called a *metabolite*. A medication is a foreign substance that the body does not normally require. Metabolism is necessary to break this foreign substance down into a form that no longer affects the body and can be effectively removed. The liver, kidneys, and intestines metabolize drugs. The liver does most of the work of drug metabolism by means of its enzymes.

This biotransformation may actually determine the route of administration because metabolism may transform the medication into a useless form too quickly. For example, insulin given by mouth is virtually useless; stomach acid breaks down insulin to an inactive form before it can be absorbed into the bloodstream.

In some instances, a drug's metabolite is the desired medication; therefore, the drug is administered in its inactive form to become activated through metabolism. This category of drugs is known as *prodrugs*. An example of a prodrug is fosamprenavir (Lexiva) used in the fight against HIV.

Like absorption, drug metabolism can be affected by the patient's age, genetics, disease state, and other factors. For example, blood flow to the liver is decreased in the elderly and therefore metabolism is slower. Genetics, which determine how much of certain enzymes that we each have, also determine how fast we metabolize a medication. Specific diseases, such as those that affect the liver, may cause slower metabolism. In all of these situations, medications may build up in the body to toxic levels as the patient may continue to receive more and more doses of the medication with it not being broken down into harmless metabolites.

 CRITICAL THINKING

David M. is a chronic alcoholic. How could that damage affect the way his body metabolizes drugs?

Excretion

Once a medication has acted in the body, it is excreted. This process occurs mainly through the kidneys, although some medications are released as a gas by the lungs, and a few are excreted through bile. Saliva and sweat glands excrete a small amount of drugs, and some medications are excreted through breast milk.

Excretion is necessary because it ensures that drugs and their transformed products are removed and do not build up in the body (called *cumulation*). If buildup occurs, the patient may become very ill. For example, if morphine is not excreted because a patient has decreased kidney or liver function, the buildup may cause diminished or absent respiration. Even seemingly harmless medications such as acetaminophen (Tylenol) or ibuprofen (e.g., Advil, Motrin) can cause a cumulative effect and damage the liver or kidneys. Aspirin can cause bleeding problems.

Excretion is an important factor to consider because of the specific time frame needed for exposure to a drug. A medication may not produce the desired effect if it is left in the system too long. A prime example of this is methotrexate (e.g. Rheumatrex, Trexall, Otrexup) when used in high does for certain types of cancer including leukemia. Methotrexate starves the cancer cell of folic acid; however, if the drug is left in the system too long it causes a lack of folic acid in all of the body's healthy cells too. Therefore, leucovorin is used as an antidote or rescue drug to stop methotrexate's effects at a specified interval after it is administered. Conversely, if a medication is metabolized too quickly, it may not have time to affect the body before its metabolites are excreted. Scientists work very hard to discover and develop medications in the correct format and strength to provide precise treatment before these drugs are metabolized and excreted.

ISSUES AFFECTING THE DRUG CYCLE

Therapeutic level, potency, and interactions with other medications affect the drug cycle. The therapeutic level of a medication refers to the point at which the drug has the optimum desired effect. Too little medication renders it less than effective; too much can be **toxic,** or poisonous, to the patient. The prescriber therefore routinely orders drugs at the lowest dose possible to obtain therapeutic levels. To be sure the drug level is in the therapeutic range, a patient's blood levels may need to be monitored. In addition, if a prescriber orders a drug with known toxic effects, the patient must be monitored for toxicity. An example is gentamicin (e.g., Garamycin, Cidomycin), which is known to be both nephrotoxic (toxic to the kidneys) and ototoxic (toxic to the ears). Thus, kidney function and hearing would be monitored closely in a patient taking this drug.

A drug's strength or ability to provide the desired effect is called its *potency*. The more potent a medication is, the smaller the amount is required to obtain the desired effect (Fast Tip 2.1). Taking multiple drugs at the same time can affect the potency of each drug taken. Some drugs potentiate (strengthen) the effects of other drugs, and some weaken them. A drug is called an **agonist** when it is taken with another drug so the two can work together. The drug combination provides a more potent effect **(synergism)** than when each drug is taken separately. Common examples of synergistic combinations are acetaminophen with codeine, used for pain relief, and codeine with a cough syrup to diminish the cough reflex and promote rest. **Antagonist** drugs do the opposite by rendering another drug less effective. For example, birth control pills can become less effective when they are taken with certain antibiotics or minor tranquilizers. Another example is the antibiotic tetracycline (e.g., Periostat, Vibramycin), which becomes ineffective when it is taken with penicillin. If a patient is taking several drugs, dosage adjustments may need to be made for each drug.

The therapeutic level of a drug can be affected by other drugs, age, nutritional factors, body size, environmental factors, gender, and culture. We discuss these factors in Chapter 3.

Natural and herbal remedies can also interact with drugs and affect dosing. Always ask the patient whether he or she is taking natural or herbal remedies. Whenever a combination of drugs is ordered, you must check your drug handbook to verify whether the drugs can be given together.

■ THE IMPORTANCE OF SIDE EFFECTS

Every medication carries a risk for side effects. The health-care professional must understand these effects and help the patient to prevent, minimize, or manage them. In addition, it is important to educate the patient about the distinction between side effects that he or she should try to manage and those that should be reported to the health-care provider immediately.

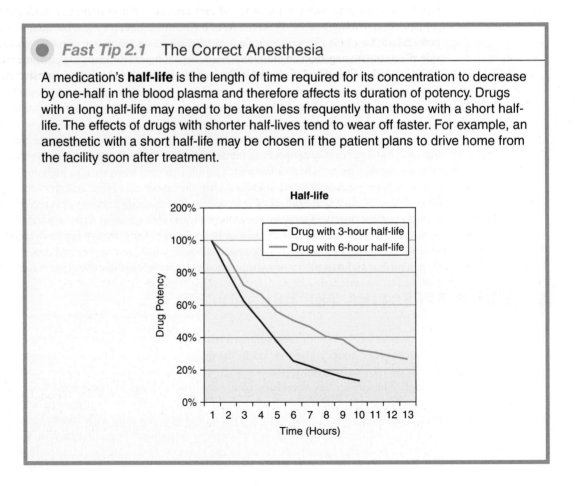

● *Fast Tip 2.1*   The Correct Anesthesia

A medication's **half-life** is the length of time required for its concentration to decrease by one-half in the blood plasma and therefore affects its duration of potency. Drugs with a long half-life may need to be taken less frequently than those with a short half-life. The effects of drugs with shorter half-lives tend to wear off faster. For example, an anesthetic with a short half-life may be chosen if the patient plans to drive home from the facility soon after treatment.

Half-life

Drug with 3-hour half-life
Drug with 6-hour half-life

Drug Potency

Time (Hours)

Side effects are usually mild, such as nausea, constipation, or sensitivity to light. Often, the patient can continue to take the medication and manage its side effects by taking the drug with food or by some other intervention such as taking care when rising from a sitting or lying position. An **adverse reaction** is a severe side effect that can cause severe harm or death, such as hallucinations, hypotension, or anaphylactic shock. An example is airway swelling, which can lead to suffocation and death if it is not treated immediately. Adverse reactions would likely cause the prescriber to change a medication.

A topical drug has fewer side effects than a systemic one. For example, applying an anti-inflammatory drug such as diphenhydramine (Benadryl) directly to itchy skin reduces the chance of systemic side effects. However, when this drug is taken by mouth to treat the inflammation systemically, it can cause side effects such as drowsiness.

Side effects happen because medications can affect the activity of nontargeted cells. All cells have numerous **receptors** that are activated or blocked by messengers to produce an effect. Think of a receptor as a lock and the messenger—in this case the medication—a key. The medication can either unlock the receptor and activate an effect, or it can be like a broken key in the lock. The stuck key prevents any other messenger from activating the effect. Most prescribed medications are intended for a single therapeutic effect, such as medications that destroy cancer cells in a tumor. Because cancer medications are targeting a specific type of cell (fast-dividing cells), other fast-dividing cells are affected. In this example, hair follicles and intestinal mucosa are affected, leading to the unwanted side effects of alopecia, anorexia, nausea, and vomiting.

Side effects are usually classified by body system or organ. Drugs can cause side effects of the central nervous system that include agitation, hallucinations, confusion, delirium, disorientation, depression, drowsiness, sedation, decreased respiration and circulation, dizziness, and coma. Muscle relaxants such as Flexeril (cyclobenzaprine) cause dizziness and drowsiness along with their intended actions.

As mentioned earlier, the liver is one of the main organs to metabolize medications, and it can be permanently damaged if drugs accumulate in it. Alcohol, acetaminophen, isoniazid, and aspirin can cause liver damage. Early side effects are detected by the presence of high liver enzyme levels in the blood. Jaundice (yellowing of the skin and eye) can occur if liver damage is undetected.

The GI system may suffer the most from medications because the most common side effects occur here. Examples of GI side effects include anorexia, nausea, vomiting, constipation, and diarrhea. The side effects are managed on an individual basis, depending on the medication. Some medications require ingestion with milk or food. For certain drugs, adding yogurt to the diet is suggested to prevent diarrhea, and others drugs may require the addition of a high-fiber laxative to the diet to prevent constipation.

Patients who take medications such as nonsteroidal anti-inflammatory drugs on a long-term basis run the risk for developing ulcers or colitis (inflammation of the intestines). The smallest effective dose is given to try to avoid this adverse effect. In addition, the synthetic prostaglandin misoprostol (Cytotec) may be given because it appears to prevent the development of ulcers. These patients are also urged to stop smoking to reduce the risk for ulcers.

As mentioned previously, the kidneys excrete most medications. Certain kinds of drugs (e.g., ibuprofen and other nonsteroidal anti-inflammatory medications) can damage kidney function because these drugs are primarily metabolized through the kidneys instead of the liver. This is especially true for patients with preexisting kidney disease. Impaired kidneys cannot effectively metabolize medications processed in the kidneys or excrete most metabolites from all medications. The result is toxic buildup of medications in the body. Patients may experience symptoms that include fluid and electrolyte imbalance and abnormally high potassium levels. If kidney damage or impairment is suspected, blood urea nitrogen (BUN) levels may be monitored to evaluate kidney functioning.

Some medications, such as certain types of antibiotics and anticancer drugs, can cause ototoxicity, with resulting loss of hearing or balance. An example of this type of drug is vancomycin (Vancocin). If vancomycin levels are not monitored closely, toxicity can cause permanent hearing loss and tinnitus. Another serious problem is the use of oxygen in premature infants. At high doses, oxygen is very damaging to the eyes. For this reason, oxygen is now used at the lowest therapeutic dose possible for all age groups.

Certain drugs can cause problems such as poor coagulation of the blood, bleeding, clotting, and immunosuppression. Anticancer drugs are especially toxic to bone marrow. Bone marrow produces all the blood supply, including the cells responsible for the immune system. Patients who lose large numbers of white blood cells have a high risk for infection. If their red blood cells are decreased, these patients will become anemic, leading to weakness, fatigue, and more difficulty in fighting illness. Finally, when the platelets are depleted, control of bleeding becomes very challenging. Thus, any patient receiving chemotherapy requires close supervision of the hematological system to prevent serious complications. Any patient taking an anticoagulant such as warfarin (Coumadin) to decrease clotting should be carefully monitored for signs of bleeding, including dark, tarry stool. Warfarin levels should be monitored to ensure that the drug level is therapeutic but not toxic.

As a health-care professional, you should always check a drug resource guide for the side effects of the medications your patient is taking so you can be aware of them and counsel the patient accordingly. Even though a side effect may not be listed, a patient can have a unique, or **idiosyncratic,** reaction to any drug. The effect may not have occurred in clinical trials because it is so rare, but it must be managed.

■ DRUG RESOURCES FOR INFORMATION

Several medication resources are available to health-care professionals to help with safe administration of drugs to patients. These resources are divided into two categories: comprehensive and clinical. Both types are available in print and online.

Comprehensive Resources

Comprehensive resources cover medications in depth and are usually available only in print. The government produces two major comprehensive resources:

■ *United States Pharmacopoeia/National Formulary (USP/NF)*

■ *United States Pharmacopoeia/Dispensing Information (USP/DI)*

The *USP/NF* is the official source of medication information for drugs approved by the U.S. Food and Drug Administration (FDA). It is updated every 5 years, with frequent supplements. This publication provides standards for identification, quality, strength, and purity of substances. The *USP/DI* has two volumes; the first is written primarily for the prescriber, and the second is written in lay terms to make it easy for patients to understand.

A more widely used comprehensive resource is the *Physicians' Desk Reference (PDR),* which is available in most health-care settings. This text contains information about thousands of drugs and is indexed by trade name, generic name, classification, and manufacturer. Color photographs of most common drugs are included to help identify medications when patients are unsure about what they are taking.

A CLOSER LOOK: Organization of the *Physicians' Desk Reference (PDR)*

The *PDR* is organized as follows:

• Section 1 (white): Manufacturer's Index. This is an alphabetical listing of manufacturers with their addresses and phone numbers.
• Section 2 (pink): Brand and Generic Name Index. This is an alphabetical listing of medications by generic and trade names.
• Section 3 (blue): Classification Index. This section lists drugs by classification (e.g., antibiotics, analgesics).
• Section 4 (gray): Product Identification Guide. Manufacturers display photographs of medications. The drugs are listed by manufacturer.
• Section 5 (white): Product Information Section. This section contains the detailed information you would find on package inserts, alphabetized by manufacturer and then product.
• Section 6 (white): This is a catch-all section that includes the following: controlled substances categories; FDA use-in-pregnancy ratings; FDA telephone directory; poison control centers; drug information centers; and look-alike/sound-alike drug names.

Fast Tip 2.2 Drug Handbook Features

Be sure you can easily find all these features when looking up a drug:

• Classifications of drugs
• Pregnancy categories
• Available forms
• Uses of drugs
• Action and therapeutic effects
• Contraindications and cautious use
• Route and dosage
• Administration
• Adverse effects
• Diagnostic test interference
• Interactions
• Pharmacokinetics
• Clinical implications

 CRITICAL THINKING

What are the advantages and disadvantages of comprehensive books such as the *PDR*?

Clinically-Based Resources

In the daily clinical setting, the health-care professional turns to more user-friendly resources than the comprehensive sources discussed earlier. A pocket guide, or drug handbook, is optimal for easy access and often includes information in terms a patient can understand. Ideally, that handbook will indicate routes of drug administration, list appropriate doses, identify indications and contraindications, and explain how best to educate the patient regarding the medication (Fast Tip 2.2). Sometimes a book is supplemented with a CD-ROM or digital downloads for your cell phone or other handheld device.

Another clinically based resource is the manufacturer's package insert, which accompanies all drugs. The patient receives the same information from the pharmacy. It is good to have this information on hand in case the patient has any questions. The pharmacist, whether hospital or community based, is also a valuable resource. Pharmacists often can answer questions for both health-care professionals and patients when the answers cannot be found elsewhere.

●●● SUMMARY

■ The drug cycle has four main phases: Absorption, distribution, metabolism, and excretion.

■ Absorption occurs as the medication passes into the bloodstream from the site where it was administered. A drug can be administered enterally or parenterally. Topical drugs act locally; systemic drugs act on one or more body systems. Many factors vary the absorption rate and bioavailability.

■ Distribution occurs when the medication travels through the body. Once the medication is in the bloodstream, it is rapidly distributed to the intended tissue, organ, or body system. A drug's ability to pass through tissue depends on whether it is a lipid-soluble or non–lipid-soluble drug. The blood-brain barrier, the blood-testicular barrier, and the blood-placental barrier limit the movement of water-soluble drugs.

■ Metabolism, or biotransformation, is the breakdown of a medication into usable components and waste products. The liver, kidneys, and intestines metabolize drugs. Drug metabolism can be affected by the patient's age, genetics, disease state, and other factors.

■ Excretion occurs when the extra medication and waste products are eliminated from the body. This process occurs mainly through the kidneys. Excretion ensures that drugs and their transformed products do not build up in the body (cumulation).

■ Factors influencing the time it takes to complete the drug cycle include the drug itself (therapeutic level, potency, and interactions with other medications), the route of administration, and the health of the patient's organs.

■ The therapeutic level refers to the point at which the drug has the optimum desired effect. Too little of the drug can be less than effective; too much can be toxic, or poisonous. Drugs are usually administered at the lowest dose possible to obtain therapeutic levels.

■ The more potent a medication is, the smaller the amount is required to obtain the desired effect.

■ Drugs can interact. Synergism occurs when a drug combination provides a more potent effect than when each drug is taken separately. Antagonist drugs render another drug less effective.

■ Every medication carries a risk for side effects and adverse reactions. Side effects are usually mild. An adverse reaction is a severe side effect. An idiosyncratic reaction is a reaction unique to a single patient. Side effects and adverse reactions happen because medications can affect the activity of nontargeted cells. Side effects are usually classified by body system or organ.

■ Several medication resources are available to health-care professionals to help with safe administration of drugs to patients: The *United States Pharmacopoeial National Formulary (USP/NF)*, the *United States Pharmacopoeial Dispensing Information (USP/DI)*, the *Physicians' Desk Reference (PDR)*, clinically-based pocket guides or drug handbooks, the manufacturer's package insert, or the pharmacist.

Activities

To make sure that you have learned the key points covered in this chapter, complete the following activities.

True or False

Write true if the statement is true. Beside the false statements, write false and correct the statement to make it true.

1. Cumulation means a drug causes disease. _____

_____

2. An antagonist blocks a drug from being effective. _____

_____

3. A drug's half-life is the time needed to decrease the drug's plasma concentration by 50%.

_____

4. Psychotropic drugs can cross the blood-brain barrier. _____

_____

5. Anticancer drugs do not cross the blood-placental barrier. _____

_____

6. Ototoxicity can damage the eyes. _____

_____

7. Idiosyncratic means safe for children. _____

_____

8. The primary organ of metabolism is the kidneys. _____

_____

9. A package insert is a valuable source of information about medications. _____

_____

10. BUN is a blood test looking at the function of the kidneys. _____

_____

Multiple Choice

Choose the best answer for each question.

1. Which term means leaving the body?
   A. Absorption
   B. Biotransformation
   C. Distribution
   D. Excretion
   E. Metabolism

2. Which term means moving through membranes?

    A. Absorption

    B. Biotransformation

    C. Distribution

    D. Excretion

    E. Metabolism

3. Which term means chemical alteration to another substance in the body?

    A. Absorption

    B. Biotransformation

    C. Distribution

    D. Excretion

4. Which term means moving of the medication from the site of administration to the target organ?

    A. Absorption

    B. Biotransformation

    C. Distribution

    D. Excretion

5. Where does ototoxicity occur?

    A. Eyes

    B. Ears

    C. Liver

    D. Kidneys

    E. Brain

6. Where does nephrotoxicity occur?

    A. Eyes

    B. Ears

    C. Liver

    D. Kidneys

    E. Brain

7. Which of the following are sources of information about medications?

    A. *PDR (Physicians' Desk Reference)*

    B. *USP/DI*

    C. *USP/NF*

    D. Package insert

    E. All of the above

8. Which term means the point at which a medication has the optimal desired effect?

A. Therapeutic level

B. Therapeutic range

C. Toxic level

D. None of the above

9. Agonists are taken together to:

A. Interact with or counteract each other

B. Work together

C. Cause great pain

D. Relieve great pain

10. The section of the *PDR* that is a product identification guide is the:

A. White section

B. Pink section

C. Blue section

D. Gray section

Short Answer Questions

Answer these questions in the space provided.

1. Why would the physician order you to give an antagonist? _____

_____

_____

2. Why can a drug be toxic to a fetus without hurting the mother? _____

_____

_____

3. Why should a patient abstain from operating heavy equipment if he or she is given a

narcotic for nausea and vomiting? _____

_____

_____

4. Why would a physician give two different drugs at subtherapeutic levels? _____

_____

_____

5. The cabinet with all the drug resources is locked, and the key cannot be found. Where can

you find out about an ordered medication before administering it? _____

_____

_____

Respond to the following situations in the space provided.

1. Mary is taking a blood thinner. She does not understand why she needs to have blood drawn monthly. How would you educate her?

   _____

   _____

   _____

2. Daniel has cirrhosis of the liver. How may this affect his metabolism of drugs?

   _____

   _____

   _____

3. Butler is coming in for a flu shot into the muscle. He insists that he wants the injection in his arm, not his buttocks. Both his arms are covered in tattoos. What would you do?

   _____

   _____

   _____

4. Rose has diabetes. Because of her diabetes, she has increased blood pressure and kidney problems. How does this affect the distribution and elimination of drugs from her body?

   _____

   _____

   _____

5. Jerry, an older patient, comes in with a paper bag containing assorted pills. He is not sure which he is supposed to be taking. What would you do?

   _____

   _____

   _____

6. You draw blood from Gary to check compliance with drug therapy, but laboratory results show none of that drug in his blood. What could be happening? What would you do?

   _____

   _____

   _____

7. Vera complains that she hears ringing in her ears ever since starting a new drug. What is this called, and what could be causing this?

   _____

   _____

   _____

1. Use your search engine to research *lithium*. Make sure you are using a reputable website such as the FDA, the NIH, or a medical institution such as the Mayo Clinic. Wikipedia and WebMD are not acceptable sources. Some examples are: Why is it important to obtain frequent blood specimens from patients who take lithium?

2. Visit www.fda.gov, and enter "drug safety communications" into the search box on the upper-right side of the page. List and discuss at least two current drug safety issues.

4. Visit www.nih.gov. Research and list the adverse effects of too much vitamin A (beta carotene, retinol).

5. Visit http://nlm.nih.gov/medlineplus/, and find the side effects of:
   Coumadin
   Ritalin
   Valproic acid
   Lithium
   OxyContin
   Methotrexate

6. Use your search engine to research *fetal alcohol syndrome*. What are the **teratogenic** (interferes with normal fetal development) effects of alcohol ingestion during pregnancy?

3

Patient Safety in Medication Administration

*T*his chapter discusses the basics of safe medication administration by identifying the right patient, using the right medication, measuring the right dose, administering the medication at the right time, using the right route, using the right technique, and documenting the right procedure in the right manner. Ethical issues pertaining to the administration of medication are discussed. In addition, this chapter introduces abbreviations used in prescribers' orders and recounts how to respond to allergic reactions and poisoning incidents. Finally, special considerations of which the health-care professional must be aware in practice are addressed.

LEARNING OUTCOMES

At the end of this chapter, you should be able to:

3.1   Define all key terms.
3.2   List the seven rights of medication administration.
3.3   Explain the various considerations of medication administration.
3.4   Identify common abbreviations used in medicine administration.
3.5   Outline special considerations when administering medications to the elderly and to children.
3.6   Discuss cultural effects on drug use.
3.7   Name the actions taken during an emergency with a patient.

KEY TERMS

Anaphylaxis
Antihypertensive
Geriatric
Health Insurance
   Portability and
   Accountability Act
   (HIPAA)

Lavage
Occupational Safety and
   Health Administration
   (OSHA)
Pediatric
Polypharmacy

Seven rights of
   medication
   administration
Teratogen
Thrombolytic
Urticaria

■ PATIENT RIGHTS FOR SAFETY

Health-care professionals play a key role in ensuring that the patient safely receives a medication. When patients come to a medical facility, they may be in pain, grieving, depressed, frightened, or not at their mental or physical best. Therefore, you must take care when explaining and administering medications to patients.

To help you safely administer drugs, follow the **seven rights of medication administration.**

1. Right patient. Know the patient to whom you are administering the medication.
2. Right drug. Know the correct medication to be administered.
3. Right dose. Know the correct dose to give the patient.
4. Right time. Know the correct time the medication should be given, and inform the patient.
5. Right route. Know the correct route of administration by which the drug should be given.
6. Right technique. Know the correct method for administering the medication.
7. Right documentation. Know how to complete a patient's chart accurately, with all pertinent information.

The Right Patient, Drug, and Documentation

Before you administer any medication, be sure that you have the right patient by asking the patient to verify his or her full name and birth date. Next, verify that you have the correct medication for that patient. In a hospital, the patient's name is on the medicine container, which is then sent to the nursing unit. In an office or a clinic setting, you will likely be the one to select the medication from a medication closet or cabinet, and the patient's name will not appear on the container. In either case, be sure to select the correct drug by using the following steps:

1. Check the label before you take the bottle from the shelf.
2. Check the label before you pour the drug out.
3. Check the label before you put the bottle back on the shelf.

Drug cabinets in medical offices are arranged with both convenience and safety in mind. Arrange medications by classifications or manufacturer. In a hospital, scanning a bar code to double-check a medication with a computer system may help reduce medication errors.

 CRITICAL THINKING

You enter the reception area of a medical office to look for the patient whose name is on the medication container. How can you be certain of giving the medication to the right patient? Because patients are sometimes confused or hard of hearing, how can you be certain that the patient who responds is the right one?

The Right Dose

Once you have the right medication, you must ensure that the patient receives the right dose. If you suspect that a prescriber may have ordered an inappropriate dose, do not give the drug until you confirm it. The health-care professional must instruct patients and their caregivers in safe dosing and medication storage (Fast Tips 3.1 and 3.2), as well as emphasize that patients adhere to the exact prescription and avoid self-medication. What works for one patient may not for another. For example, if the patient is elderly or has liver or kidney problems, even a "normal" dose may be too much because the drug may not clear the body well and could accumulate to toxic levels.

The Right Time

Administering the medication at the right time is also critical. When a patient is in the hospital, medications are given according to hospital policy at a time that is convenient to staff members. At home, patients take their medications at a time that suits them. Morning medications, such as allergy pills, are usually taken with breakfast. Evening drugs, such as seizure medications, are taken at dinner. Drugs

Fast Tip 3.1   Safe Medication Storage

Most people know that medications should be safely locked away from young children, but they fail to think about others in the household. This negligence can have tragic consequences when individuals lack knowledge about drug safety. For example, teenagers can abuse vitamin pills, cough syrup, cold medications, and inhalable drugs. Older people who are confused may take medications that are left, for example, on the counter. Emphasize to patients the need to store medications safely no matter what the age of others in the household.

 Fast Tip 3.2   Age, Size, and Dosage

Babies and young children require lower dosages because their bodies are small and process drugs faster. A dosage that works on a 150-pound adult is not appropriate for a 75-pound child. Many institutions have a policy requiring you to double-check your calculations with a coworker before administering a dose to a child.

that help patients sleep at home are taken at the patient's usual bedtime, whereas drugs that help patients sleep in the hospital may be given at a set time. Some medications, such as antibiotics and antiseizure medications, need to be given a standard number of hours apart around the clock to maintain a consistent blood level.

The health-care professional may need to help the patient develop a schedule for taking medications at home. Sometimes, it is helpful to write a clear schedule on a chart for the patient to put on a wall at home (Fig. 3-1).

Prescribers may order that a drug *not* be given for a period of time or that a drug be discontinued. If a patient is having a test the next day that requires the gastrointestinal system to be clear, either for better diagnostic imaging or to prevent aspiration (inhaling into the lungs) of vomitus, the prescriber may want the patient to take nothing by mouth (abbreviated NPO) after midnight. Patients with diabetes who are NPO usually should not be given insulin because no food is available to interact with the insulin.

The physician may also order a medication to be discontinued because the patient does not need it anymore, or the prescriber wants to change the medication. You must tell the patient *not* to take the medication. For example, when a patient is taking a medication to lower blood pressure and the physician decides to change to a different medication with the same effect, the patient's blood pressure may become dangerously low if both medications are taken. Instruct the patient to throw out old prescription medications that have been discontinued, to prevent inadvertent ingestion.

 CRITICAL THINKING

Rachael S. has been told to be NPO after midnight before an x-ray series of her bowels. She calls to see whether she should take her morning dose of insulin. An office assistant says that she should take it because insulin is not given by mouth. If you had taken her call, what would you have said or done? Explain your answer.

 CRITICAL THINKING

Imagine that you gave Cecile M. 0.5 mL of a flu shot in the left deltoid muscle. You took the vaccine from a container that said lot no. 1234567, which expires on 12/01. How would you document this procedure?

Your name __Chester Earl__

Weekly Medicine Record			Week of __August 1, 20xx__						
Name of Medicine and Dose	**Shape, Size, and Color of Pill**	**When to Take**	**Place an X after taking each dose**						
			Sun	**Mon**	**Tues**	**Wed**	**Thurs**	**Fri**	**Sat**
1. Digoxin 0.125 mg	Round, 1/4 diameter, white	Daily	X	X	*Need refill*				
2. Coumadin 3–4 mg	Round, 5/16 diameter, blue	Daily	X	X	X				
3. Furosemide 40 mg (Lasix)	Round, 5/16 diameter, white	Daily (morning)	X	X	X				
4. Nitroglycerin 0.4 mg (transdermal system)	Patch	Daily (12-14 hs)	X	X	X				
5. Monopril 20 mg	Elongated, 3/8 diameter, white	Daily							
6. Oyster shell calcium 1500 mg	Round, 1/2 diameter, gray	Daily (morning)	X	X	X				
7. Potassium (K-Dur 20 mEq tablet SA Sch)	Large 13/16 x 3/16 x 3/16, white	Daily (morning)	X	X	X				
8. Tylenol 650 mg caplets	Caplet	As needed for headache		X					
9. Chlorpheniramine maleate (allergy tablets) 4 mg	Round tablet, 3/16 diameter, yellow	As needed for sleeplessness	X		X				

FIGURE 3-1: Sample medication schedule for the patient's use at home.

■ THE RIGHT ROUTE AND TECHNIQUE

Knowing where to administer the medication is also important. Most often, medications are given by mouth (PO). Sometimes drugs are given directly into other areas such as the ears, eyes, nose, vagina, or rectum. At other times, drugs are injected into a vein (intravenous [IV]), a muscle (intramuscular [IM]), skin (intradermal [ID]), or fat (subcutaneous [SC]). The pharmacist dispensing the medication may not know the patient or his or her special needs. For example, a liquid formulation may be necessary if the drug must be given through a feeding tube. In such cases, you need to alert the person dispensing the medication to your patient's individual needs.

Knowing the proper way to administer a medication by these various routes is important. For example, if an oral medication is given improperly, a patient could aspirate the medication into the lungs, thus causing a possible infection or other adverse reaction. If an injection is given at the wrong depth, angle, or site, possible nerve or bone damage could occur. Written procedure manuals are available for every procedure performed in the agency in which the patient is located. These manuals should be consulted whenever the health-care provider is unsure of the technique required.

Finally, be sure to document all pertinent information and know how to document a patient's chart accurately. Although a medical office can be busy, you must take the time for proper documentation whenever you give a medication. Be sure to document not only the medication but also the time and date of administration, dose, route (including site if injection), lot number of the drug, and expiration date of the drug. In addition, if there any adverse reactions to the medication, make sure to follow your agency procedures for documentation of that reaction.

CRITICAL THINKING

What kinds of drugs are usually prescribed to be given at equal intervals throughout the day? Explain why these drugs must be given at exact intervals. What could happen if doses are missed?

MEDICATION NAMES AND ABBREVIATIONS

As a health-care professional, it is your responsibility to be sure that medications are administered safely. This involves learning the many abbreviations used on prescription orders and medicine containers, making sure that the medication schedule is appropriate for the patient's needs while taking into consideration the patient's other medications, and accounting for individual factors such as nutrition, weight, gender, and age.

Many drugs have similar spellings or pronunciations. These drugs, known as "look-alike/sound-alike names," are responsible for some of the most common medication errors. The Institute for Safe Medication Practices (ISMP) publishes the "List of Confused Drug Names." The Joint Commission also publishes a list of commonly confused look-alike/sound-alike drug names and requires that all accredited health-care agencies create a list for use in the institution (Table 3-1).

Abbreviations abound in medicine, and they are especially important during medication administration (Fast Tip 3.3). Many of these abbreviations are similar but have very different meanings. It is therefore very important to keep a list of abbreviations approved for your agency close at hand for reference. If you are in doubt about an abbreviation, spell out the entire word, look it up, or ask the person who wrote it to explain what was meant.

Sometimes, drugs are taken to coat the stomach before a meal or are taken on a full stomach to reduce the chance of nausea. If a drug is to be given before meals, the prescriber may write a.c. (ante cibum). For after-meal administration, the prescription is written p.c. (post cibum). Some medications can be taken as needed (abbreviated prn). Table 3-2 summarizes common abbreviations related to medication administration. Some of these abbreviations are based on Latin words.

A CLOSER LOOK: Sinister and Dexter

Latin terms can seem daunting unless you can relate them to something familiar or interesting. Here is a story that can help you learn some abbreviations. In many cultures, people usually designate their left (in Latin, *sinister*) hand as their "evil" hand. They use the left hand for dirty activities and the right (in Latin, *dexter*) hand for courtesies such as shaking hands or eating food from a communal bowl. When shaking hands, it would be considered rude to extend the left hand because that is considered by many cultures to be the dirty hand. The abbreviation in Latin for ear is a. and for eye is o. Therefore, if a prescriber writes a.s., it means left (sinister) ear; o.s. means left eye.

TABLE 3.1 Sample List of Confused Drug Names

Drug Name	Confused Drug Name	Drug Name	Confused Drug Name
Adderall	Inderal	heparin	Hespan
Advair	Advicor	Klonopin	clonidine
Amicar	Omacor	Leukeran	leucovorin calcium
Benadryl	benazepril	OxyContin	Oxycodone
Celebrex	Cerebyx	Retrovir	ritonavir
Cozaar	Zocor		

> **Fast Tip 3.3**   Memory Joggers for Frequency of Drug Administration
>
> - *Bi*cycles have two wheels, so *bid* means twice a day.
> - *Tri*cycles have three wheels, so *tid* means three times a day.
> - *Quad*rangles have four sides, so *qid* means four times a day.

TABLE 3.2   Abbreviations for Drug Administration

a.c.	Before meals	o.d.	Right eye
a.d.	Right ear	o.s.	Left eye
a.s.	Left ear	o.u.	Both eyes
a.u.	Both ears	p.c.	After meals
bid	Two times a day	PO	By mouth (orally)
c̄	With	PRN	As needed
ID	Intradermally (into the skin)	qid	Four times a day
IM	Intramuscularly (into a muscle)	s̄	Without
IV	Intravenously (into a vein)	SC	Subcutaneously (into fat)
NPO	Nothing by mouth	tid	Three times a day

The Joint Commission stated that certain abbreviations are particularly likely to be confused and should not be used (Table 3-3). Any abbreviation not on the official "Do Not Use" list published by the Joint Commission may be used in an institution as long as the abbreviation is included on an official abbreviation list posted in the agency's policy manual and updated annually.

TABLE 3.3   Abbreviations to Avoid

Do Not Use	Potential Problem	Preferred Term
U (for unit)	Mistaken for zero, four, or cc	Write "unit"
IU (for international unit)	Mistaken for IV (intravenous) or 10 (ten)	Write "international unit"
q.d. and q.o.d.	Mistaken for each other; the period after the "q" can be mistaken for "I"; the "o" can be mistaken for "I"	Write "daily" and "every other day"
Trailing zero (x.0 mg); lack of leading zero (.x mg)	Decimal point is missed	Never write a zero by itself after a decimal point, and always use a zero before a decimal point (0.5 mg)
MS, MSO_4, $MgSO_4$	Confused for one another; can mean morphine sulfate or magnesium sulfate	Write "morphine sulfate" or "magnesium sulfate"
Avoid Using		
μg (for microgram)	Mistaken for mg (milligrams, resulting in 1,000-fold dosing overdose)	Write "mcg" or "micrograms"
> (greater than)	Misinterpreted as the number 7 (seven) or the letter L	Write "greater than"
< (less than)		Write "less than"
@	Mistaken for the number 2 (two)	Write "at"
cc	Mistaken for U (units) when poorly written	Write "mL" or "milliliters"

■ FACTORS AFFECTING MEDICATION ADMINISTRATION

When administering medications, certain factors must be considered to ensure that, as a health-care professional, you are following the seven rights. These factors include the following: nutrition and physical activity; age, gender, and culture; environment; pregnancy; and organ dysfunction.

Nutrition and Physical Activity Factors

Nutrition can affect how well a drug is absorbed. Some nutrients are needed for absorption, and some block absorption. For instance, administering tetracycline (an antibiotic) with calcium prevents the absorption of tetracycline. Most antibiotics work best when taken on an empty stomach. Food high in vitamin B_6 can impair the actions of drugs used to treat Parkinson's disease. Grapefruit juice inhibits the effectiveness of some drugs (fexofenadine), while potentiating or increasing the drug in the bloodstream (certain statins and blood pressure medications) if both are ingested at the same time. A patient who is dehydrated may have a medication blood level that is higher than normal. Consult your drug reference for any food interactions that the patient should be made aware of before a new medication is begun.

Exercise can influence metabolism and cause medications to be absorbed more quickly. Exercise also decreases the need for insulin and is used to control blood glucose concentrations in patients with diabetes. Chewing gum increases saliva, which enhances food breakdown and absorption.

Drug dosing is usually based on total body weight. Normal doses are based on an average adult body weight of 70 kg (about 150 lb). However, size and distribution of fat in the patient can change the way the drug is processed. If a drug that does not penetrate fatty tissues is used in obese patients, the dose may have to be higher than usual.

Similarly, underweight patients may need smaller amounts of drugs because of their lower body weight. Patients with amputated limbs also require lower doses because of lower body weight.

Age

In general, drug administration guidelines are based on the average adult patient. However, a health-care professional must consider two distinctive populations when administering medications: the elderly, or **geriatric,** population and the young, or **pediatric,** population.

Geriatric Patients

In patients older than 55 years of age, decreased absorption results from diminished gastrointestinal function and congestion of abdominal blood vessels. Distribution can also be altered by low plasma protein levels, particularly if the patient is malnourished. When plasma proteins are decreased, a larger amount of unbound drug increases the drug's action. Thus, elderly patients can have toxic drug levels, even at normal doses. The aging process also alters liver and kidney function and leads to accumulation of medications. Body composition changes as we age. Elderly patients have increased fatty tissue and decreased skeletal muscle and water. All these age-related changes slow drug absorption and distribution.

Because of these factors, doses may need to be adjusted for elderly patients and may vary greatly among older individuals. Of special concern are sedative-hypnotics, anticoagulants, nonsteroidal antiinflammatory drugs (NSAIDs), **antihypertensives** (drugs that lower blood pressure), and **thrombolytics** (drugs that break up blood clots). These medications are most commonly associated with adverse drug events. For example, sedative-hypnotics may be used to calm a patient, but they can worsen agitation and exacerbate dementia.

Another concern for geriatric patients is **polypharmacy,** defined as taking medications for more than one problem. Multiple medications increase the risk for drug interactions and side effects. The health-care professional must spend more time educating elderly patients because their treatment regimens are often more complex, and it may take these patients more time to understand the specifics of each medication.

Pediatric patients constitute a unique population. Children have a higher metabolism but lower weight than adults and therefore require less medication. Dose amounts and administration vary, depending on the age of the child.

A neonate or premature infant has special needs. Because the renal system and some endocrine systems of these infants are not mature at birth, drug metabolism and excretion are impaired. The nervous system and blood-brain barrier of these children are also not mature at birth; thus, the central nervous system is more susceptible to the effects of medications. In addition, because these infants are so small, any dosage miscalculation could be devastating. Medications such as digoxin and certain antibiotics that are used in older infants may therefore be much trickier to use in the newborn. The prescriber must be extremely meticulous in determining the proper dose for infants younger than 1 month of age. Drugs that are ototoxic and nephrotoxic are not given or are given very cautiously in the newborn. Premature infants have developed both hearing loss and kidney disease from some of these drugs, but the alternative is death from infection. The gastric pH and gastrointestinal motility of neonates and premature infants differ from those of an older child or an adult. Because weight changes rapidly in infants, frequent dose adjustments must be made.

Infants also have poorly developed arm muscles. Therefore, medications that must be given intramuscularly are injected into the infant's thigh because it has more muscle. The blood vessels of infants and children are more fragile than adult blood vessels, and these patients can easily become overhydrated if intravenous therapy is not carefully monitored. Children are frequently afraid of injections and other interventions, so age-appropriate explanations about the procedures to these patients may be necessary.

Most drugs are not tested on pediatric patients, and a drug tested in adults may not act the same way in a child (Table 3-4). Be especially alert to side effects, and fill out a MedWatch form if the child has an adverse reaction.

CRITICAL THINKING

A premature infant in your care is on the medication gentamicin, which you know is ototoxic. What are some ways to minimize the danger to this infant's hearing?

Gender and Culture

Gender must also be considered when administering medication. Men typically have more muscle than fat, as compared with women. Therefore, medications are absorbed and distributed in the body more quickly in men than in women. Other gender differences are body water content, metabolic rate, and

TABLE 3.4 Pharmacology in Neonates, Infants, and Young Children*

Developmental Factor	Effect
Gastric pH is higher in neonates and infants; adult levels at 20–30 months	Decreased absorption in younger patients
Irregular emptying time for stomach; adult functioning at 6–8 months	Unpredictable absorption
Decreased lipase secretion in infants	Poor absorption of lipid-formulated drugs
Thin stratum cornea in infants	Increased absorption of topical medications applied in the eye
Rectally administered drugs absorbed more	Increased absorption possibly leading to toxicity quickly in infants
Variable blood flow to muscles of neonates	Unpredictable absorption of drugs injected into muscle
Larger percentage of extracellular and total water in the body in neonates and infants	Wider distribution of drugs
Higher ratio of water to lipid in neonates and young adults in adipose tissue	Lower level of drug in bloodstream

*Because children's bodies are not fully developed, it is especially important to monitor drug effects in these age groups.

gonadal hormone variations. Men tend to respond to different antidepressants than women because of the hormones found in each.

A person's culture can also affect the use of medications. Some cultural beliefs are grounded in scientific research, and people in these cultures find comfort in knowing that medications have been rigorously tested before approval. These patients are more likely to depend on their primary health-care provider to choose drugs for them.

Conversely, more holistic cultures believe that imbalances in a person's life cause disease. People with a holistic outlook may be less likely to use conventional drugs and more inclined toward herbal remedies. Other cultures believe that illness comes from evil spirits who hurt people if taboos (rules) are broken. People in these cultures may search for alternative healers and may or may not continue to take medications prescribed by their primary health-care provider.

 CRITICAL THINKING

Seth E. comes to the office with a wound that does not seem to be healing. As he is leaving he states: "I am going to see my herbalist. Your drugs can't help me!" What would you do or say?

Environmental Factors

Environmental hazards may affect drug absorption and metabolism. Smoking cigarettes induces liver enzymes to metabolize drugs more rapidly. This may also be true for all other forms of smoking that contain nicotine, but research is not available to either support or disprove this supposition. Patients who smoke cigarettes may need larger doses of liver-metabolized drugs than do nonsmokers. The effects of active and secondhand smoke may persist for months. Many occupational exposures may also cause a change in metabolism of medications. For example, many industries use organic solvents, which can cause hepatic injuries. Once the liver is damaged, the metabolism is slowed down causing medications to accumulate in the body.

Pregnancy

Pregnancy is another consideration when administering medications. Drugs affect not only the mother, but also the fetus she is carrying. The blood-placental barrier protects the fetus from the effects of certain medications. Water-soluble medications such as heparin are kept from crossing this barrier, although fat-soluble medications are more like to cross it. **Teratogens** are drugs and other agents that cause abnormal fetal development. Severe malformations or death of the fetus can occur if a teratogenic drug crosses the placenta.

The fetus is especially vulnerable to medications during the first trimester, when vital organs are forming, and the last trimester, when the baby is prone to accumulating drugs before birth. The Food and Drug Administration (FDA) previously classified drugs according to their safety during pregnancy. In 2015, this was replaced with new requirements for pregnancy and lactation labeling requiring labeling to contain a summary of the risks when using each drug during both pregnancy and lactation. The labeling must include research data supporting the summary that will allow the health-care provider to make educated decisions when prescribing medications in these situations.

 CRITICAL THINKING

If an obstetric patient calls and asks what over-the-counter drugs she can take for a cold, where would you find that information? How would you explain your responses?

Patients with Organ Dysfunction

As discussed in Chapter 2, great care must be taken when medications are administered to patients with organ dysfunction because drugs can easily build up to undesirable levels. Pay close attention to the kidneys, liver, and heart, the organs most affected by systemic drug accumulation. The liver and kidneys metabolize and excrete medications, and the heart may change how quickly and effectively a medication is distributed throughout the circulatory system.

Because the liver metabolizes drugs, poor functioning of this organ leads to an accumulation of drugs and to toxic effects. Patients who abuse alcohol on a long-term basis may have destroyed much of their liver's ability to function. Decreased serum protein levels can alter the capacity of a drug to bond. More unbound medication is therefore available, and this can lead to side effects. Unfortunately, no laboratory test adequately predicts appropriate doses when the liver is not working properly.

 CRITICAL THINKING

How does liver disease affect the accumulation of drugs in the body?

Drugs that have passed unmetabolized through the liver put patients with kidney disease at risk for accumulating toxic amounts of drugs. These drugs can also destroy the kidneys. To determine proper doses of drugs in patients with kidney disease, blood specimens are drawn for laboratory tests, such as blood urea nitrogen (BUN) and creatinine clearance (CrCl).

In patients with heart failure, the heart fails to pump blood adequately. This condition can cause congestion of blood vessels in the gastrointestinal tract that decreases drug absorption and drug delivery to the liver. Kidney function is also compromised by the congestion, with resulting delayed excretion and thus drug accumulation in the patient. For these reasons, patients with heart failure usually take lower doses of medications.

■ PROTECTING THE PATIENT: ETHICAL AND SAFETY CONSIDERATIONS

As a health-care professional, it is your responsibility to see that medications are administered safely and ensure that the patient's rights, consent, and privacy are equally protected. You also have the responsibility of responding quickly, safely, and ethically should a patient have a medication emergency such as accidental ingestion of too much medication or an acute allergic reaction.

Patient Information

Patients have a right to participate in their treatment. Thus, it is important to teach patients about their medications in terms they can understand. Although you may understand medical terminology, the patient most likely does not. Misunderstandings can lead to injury, overdose, or subtherapeutic treatment. For example, patients may believe that taking more pain medication will relieve pain better or faster. If a patient is told to take a narcotic every 6 hours as needed for pain, he or she may take it more often and may not know that this could cause confusion, respiratory depression, or death. It is your responsibility as a health-care professional to educate the patient about the risks associated with taking more than the prescribed dose. All adults are vulnerable to making mistakes, such as combining over-the-counter medications with prescription drugs and not realizing that both contain the same or similar drug. A frequent example of this is a person suffering from a cold or flu taking a combination cold medication containing ibuprofen, and then taking a prescribed medication for arthritis containing another NSAID. Therefore, it is very important for the patient to tell the physician about any over-the-counter medication he or she is taking. Conversely, it is important to educate patients about the prescriptions they are taking and what over-the-counter drugs they should avoid. In addition, encourage patients to talk with the pharmacist about warning labels to make sure they understand the precautions of a new medication.

One way to ensure that patients receive enough information is to teach them to ask the questions in Box 3-1 whenever they start a new medication.

Patient Consent

Patients have the right to refuse treatment, including medications. If patients do not understand why they are required to take a medication, you should first give them the appropriate information. If they are still reluctant to take a medication, inform the prescriber. Giving a medication to someone who refuses to take it can be considered assault and battery.

BOX 3.1 What You Need to Know About Prescription Medicines

As a health-care professional, you should encourage patients to discuss their medication regimens with their health-care providers. When a new medicine is prescribed, patients can refer to the following list of questions to ask the prescriber or pharmacist.

- What are alternative names for this medication?
- What is it supposed to do?
- Is there a less expensive alternative?
- Why am I taking it?
- How and when do I take the medication and for how long?
- Should I store it in the refrigerator or the cabinet?
- Should I take it with water, food, or with another medication?
- What should I do if I miss or forget a dose?
- What food, drinks, other medications, dietary supplements, or activities should I avoid while taking this medication?
- Will any tests or monitoring be required while I am taking this medication? Do I need to come to the office with a certain frequency?
- What are the possible side effects, and what should I do if they happen?
- When should I expect the medication to start working, and how will I know if it is working?

A disoriented patient may not understand the treatment plan. Therefore, you may need to advocate for the patient. If the patient is frightened or confused, he or she may refuse an injection or to swallow a medication; educating the patient may facilitate understanding.

A patient who is taking an experimental drug has the right to informed consent, which means understanding the treatment, its effects, alternative treatments, and the possible outcome if the treatment is declined. It is essential to document informed consent. Ensure that the patient is comfortable with the decision and that the informed consent is documented correctly. If the patient seems reluctant to sign the consent form, notify the physician of your observation.

Patient Privacy

Patients have rights to privacy. The **Health Insurance Portability and Accountability Act (HIPAA)** Privacy Rule holds health-care professionals accountable to the government to protect the privacy of the patient. Medication records, like all items in the patient's medical record, are to be kept confidential, except for release to pharmacists and other professionals involved in the care of the patient. HIPAA standards also allow patients access to their own medical records and offer them more control over how the information in their records is shared. All health-care providers must supply patients with a notice alerting them to their rights and that medical information cannot be revealed to other people without the patient's consent. For more information on HIPAA, visit https://www.hhs.gov/.

Health-care professionals should take the steps necessary to ensure that all communications are confidential. For instance, to call a colleague across a waiting room to announce that a drug is ready for a patient whose name has been called out loud is illegal as well as unprofessional. Patients also have a right to receive medications in a quiet, private place.

 CRITICAL THINKING

When a patient arrives for an appointment in a clinic or physician's office, what are some ways that they can check in that will maintain their confidentiality?

Patient Emergencies

If a patient comes to your office or facility and presents with signs of accidental or deliberate medication overdose, you must respond quickly. Refer to office or facility protocols, but usually the first step is to notify the physician immediately and begin the ordered treatment.

If you receive a call from a patient who has ingested a toxic substance, call 911 or ask the patient to do so immediately. Usually, when you activate the emergency response system, the dispatcher will connect you to a poison control center. Experts at poison control hotlines are trained to manage toxic substance emergencies and have access to the latest research and recommended treatments. If possible, identify the substance so the staff can better diagnose and treat the problem.

The staff members at a poison control center may ask you to do any of the following, depending on the type of toxin:

- Administer activated charcoal, which will bind with the poison. Activated charcoal is usually administered by emergency medical personnel in the field or in emergency departments. This treatment is usually administered after **lavage** (pumping) of the patient's stomach to remove the toxin. If the toxin is caustic, lavage is not done because of the damage caused on ingestion: removing the substance may cause further harm.
- Have the patient drink a large amount of water to dilute the poison.
- Have the patient drink milk to reduce acidity.
- Monitor the patient for symptoms such as changes in vital signs (heart rate, respiratory rate, blood pressure, and temperature), seizures, and altered level of consciousness.

Follow the directions of the experts carefully. Immediate treatment of a toxin overdose can save the patient considerable discomfort and harm. Most poison control centers no longer suggest that vomiting be induced with syrup of ipecac because it is not completely effective and can cause complications. There has been some discussion of taking syrup of ipecac off the market.

In an emergency, ask the patient whether he or she has any allergies to medications *before* giving another medication. An allergic reaction may include **urticaria** (hives), in which the skin becomes red and itchy. Notify the physician immediately if this occurs.

A severe allergic reaction is called **anaphylaxis.** It is especially dangerous if swelling occurs in the neck because the swelling can constrict the trachea and cause death from suffocation. Patients experiencing anaphylaxis have difficulty breathing and may have other symptoms, such as itching, wheezing, anxiety, and lightheadedness. The physician may order you to give a medication to reverse the anaphylaxis, such as epinephrine or diphenhydramine (Benadryl). It is safe and best practice to observe a patient for 15 minutes following an injection, an antibiotic, or an allergy shot to be sure that an allergic reaction is not missed. Document your observation period, such as in the following example: "Patient observed for 15 minutes after allergy shot. No signs of anaphylaxis noted."

PROTECTING THE HEALTH-CARE WORKER

The **Occupational Safety and Health Administration (OSHA)** is a branch of the Department of Labor that helps ensure that all workers are not exposed to unnecessary job-related risks, such as electrical cords placed where workers could fall over them or a lack of portable fire extinguishers. Health-care workers, for example, have the right to be protected from patients' diseases. In turn, you must take steps to protect yourself. The following are some of OSHA's regulations for protecting yourself on the job:

- Hand washing is required before any patient is handled.
- Medications should not be touched unless the health-care worker is wearing gloves.
- Gloves should be worn in case of exposure to blood or other bodily fluids.
- Sharp objects (e.g., needles) should be disposed of in specialized sharps-disposal containers.

To ensure that health-care employees practice safe work habits, OSHA requires that all employees who may have access to blood-borne pathogens undergo annual training in workplace safety practices and the use of personal protective equipment (e.g., gloves, face shield). OSHA requires that employers provide safe supplies for workers, such as safety needles to avoid accidental needle sticks while drawing blood. Every practice setting must also have protective supplies, such as sharps-disposal containers, gloves, masks, and eyewash solutions, readily available.

Occupational injuries, such as being stuck with a dirty needle and falls, must be reported to OSHA. Further training may be required for organizations that report several occupational injuries. Because OSHA is a regulatory agency, its representatives can inspect a medical organization at any time to ensure adherence to regulations. Organizations that are not compliant may be fined.

SUMMARY

- As a health-care professional, you are responsible for the safe administration of medications.

- The seven rights of medication administration are the right drug, in the right dose, at the right time, by the right route, to the right patient, using the right technique, and then documenting the administration correctly.

- To administer medications safely, you need to know the acceptable abbreviations used to understand the medication order.

- Medication administration is affected by many variables, such as the patient's nutritional status and physical activity, as well as his or her size, age, and gender.

  - In geriatric patients, the changes in physiology affect drug distribution, absorption, and accumulation. Patients are at higher risk for drug interactions and side effects from polypharmacy.

  - Pediatric patients have a higher metabolism but lower weight than adults and therefore require less medication. A neonate or premature infant's central nervous system is more susceptible to the effects of medications. Drug metabolism and excretion are impaired.

  - The prescriber must be extremely meticulous in determining the proper dose for infants younger than 1 month of age.

  - The blood-placental barrier protects the fetus from the effects of certain medications. Water-soluble medications cannot cross this barrier, but fat-soluble medications are more likely to cross it.

  - Teratogens are drugs and other agents that cause abnormal fetal development. The fetus is especially vulnerable to medications during the first trimester and the last trimester.

- Medication administration is regulated for the public's safety.

- Health-care professionals must respect patients' rights to receive accurate information, obtain informed consent, and refuse treatment.

- Health-care professionals must protect patients' privacy.

- The Health Insurance Portability and Accountability Act (HIPAA) Privacy Rule holds health-care professionals accountable to the government to protect the privacy of the patient.

- The Occupational Safety and Health Administration (OSHA) helps ensure that all workers are not exposed to unnecessary job-related risks. Health-care professionals must take steps to protect themselves.

Activities

To make sure that you have learned the key points covered in this chapter, complete the following activities.

True or False

Write true if the statement is true. Beside the false statements, write false and correct the statement to make it true.

1. In patients more than 55 years of age, decreased absorption occurs because of diminished gastrointestinal function and congestion of abdominal blood vessels.

   _____

2. If a patient is NPO, he or she takes the medication only as needed.

   _____

3. Drugs that are given a.d. are given in the right eye.

   _____

4. There are five rights to medication administration.

   _____

5. You should compare the order with the bottle at least three times.

   _____

6. In case of anaphylaxis, administer syrup of ipecac.

   _____

7. Patients have the right to refuse treatment.

   _____

8. HIPAA refers to standards holding health-care professionals accountable to protect the privacy of patients.

   _____

9. Patients should be discouraged from discussing their prescriptions with the physician.

   _____

10. Lavage refers to the use of a large tube place through a patient's nose to the stomach to remove remnants of poisons.

   _____

Multiple Choice

Choose the best answer for each question.

1. Which of the following is a sign of anaphylaxis?
   A. Hallucinations
   B. Bleeding nose
   C. Fixed pupils
   D. Wheezing

2. Which abbreviation means "before meals"?

A. a.c.

B. a.d.

C. a.m.

D. a.s.

E. a.u.

3. In an examination room in a medical office, which of the following is the best way to identify a patient?

A. Check the patient's wrist identification band.

B. Call the patient by name.

C. Ask the patient his or her name.

D. Compare the photograph in the patient's chart with the patient.

E. Ask one of your coworkers who the patient is.

4. What does teratogenic refer to?

A. Causing birth defects in the unborn fetus

B. Endangering the health of the mother

C. Endangering the elderly

D. None of the above

5. Which of the following is NOT one of the seven rights of medication administration?

A. Right patient

B. Right route

C. Right time

D. Right place

E. Right documentation

6. Why should you have a patient remain seated in the examination room for 15 minutes after receiving an injection, antibiotic, or allergy shot?

A. This gives you time to chart and clean up.

B. The purpose is to watch for allergic reaction symptoms.

C. It gives the physician time to write any required prescriptions.

D. The patient does not have to wait and can leave immediately.

7. If a patient presents in your office and states that he has ingested a poisonous substance, what should you monitor while awaiting arrival of the emergency medical service?

A. Changes in vital signs (heart rate, blood pressure, respiratory rate, temperature)

B. Seizures

C. Level of consciousness

D. All of the above

8. What are some of the possible instructions that poison control may give you for the patient who has overdosed or ingested poison?

A. Administer activated charcoal.

B. Have the patient drink large amounts of water to dilute the poison or medication.

C. Have the patient drink milk to decrease the acidity of the poison.

D. Any of the above

9. Which of the following abbreviations means to administer three times a day?

A. bid

B. tid

C. qid

D. None of the above

10. Documenting drug administration correctly would include documenting which of the following?

A. Time

B. Dose

C. Route

D. Signature

E. All of the above

Short Answer Questions

1. What are the three steps to confirm you have the right drug? _____

_____

_____

2. What precautions should be taken in a medical office to ensure the safe dispensing of medications? What precautions are taken in a hospital setting? _____

_____

_____

3. What should you do if a patient begins itching after you give an immunization? _____

_____

_____

4. What factors affect drug absorption? _____

_____

_____

5. What information should you have ready when you call a poison control center? _____

_____

_____

Respond to the following scenarios.

1. In a closet, the office stores drug samples from drug company representatives. What would be the most efficient way to store these samples: by classification, company, or expiration date? Explain your answer. _____

   _____

   _____

2. You inject measles, mumps, and rubella vaccine into baby Brian's left leg. The drug was from lot no. 2468, expiration date 03/1/XX. After you give the injection, he begins to cry. How would you document this medication administration in baby Brian's chart?_____

   _____

   _____

3. You pull the chart for Walter Roberts, and you notice that five patients named Walter Roberts are seen at this practice. What information would you need to find the correct chart?

   _____

   _____

4. Inger frequently forgets to take her medications. She is 77 years of age and claims that she cannot remember well. What would you do to help her learn her medication schedule?

   _____

   _____

5. Derrick is a diabetic patient who lives with his daughter, who also has diabetes and wonders why they do not take the same dose of insulin. What would be your response? _____

   _____

   _____

6. Mrs. Valenzuela does not understand English well, but her son, who does understand English, is with her. How can you be sure that she understands how and when to take her medications?

   _____

   _____

7. Elaine is receiving an experimental drug. Write how you would document her informed consent. _____

   _____

   _____

8. Beth is pregnant. She calls the office to see what drugs she can use for cold symptoms. Where would you look to find out which drugs are safe for her? _____

_____

_____

9. Mickie is a diabetic patient with impaired vision. How should a health-care professional make sure Mickie can take his medication safely? _____

_____

_____

10. Valentina wants to know why she needs less of a medication as she ages. Because her liver is becoming more impaired, she insists that she should be taking more medication, not less. What would you say to her? _____

_____

_____

Abbreviation Study

Take a few minutes to study the abbreviations you have learned in this chapter. Then, test yourself. How did you do? If you missed any, you may want to make flash cards to help you learn. Put the abbreviation on one side of a 3-by-5–inch index card, and write its definition on the other side. Take these cards with you, and study whenever you get a chance. You will be able to learn the abbreviations quickly.

a.u. _____	a.d. _____	IM _____
IV _____	SC _____	tid _____
bid _____	p.c. _____	a.s. _____
prn _____	o.d. _____	o.u. _____
NPO _____	ID _____	o.s. _____

Matching

1. bid _____after meals

2. o.s. _____as needed

3. tid _____both ears

4. prn _____left eye

5. a.u. _____right eye

6. a.c. _____three times a day

7. p.c. _____twice a day

8. o.d. _____before meals

1. Visit http://drugtopics.com, and find the top 50 drugs most frequently associated with medication errors. List the top 10.

2. Visit http://ismp.org (Institute for Safe Medication Practices), and click on "Tools" and then "DO NOT CRUSH List." Pick a drug, and explain why it should not be crushed.

3. Visit http://aapcc.org (American Association of Poison Control Centers), and find which drug most commonly poisons patients. You will find the information in the National Poison Data System's Current Annual Report.

4. Visit http://osha.gov/ (Occupational Safety and Health Administration), and find out where your regional office is located. Discover how you can report violations of OSHA regulations.

Regulations

To ensure public safety, the U.S. government enacts and enforces laws and regulations related to drugs. The Food and Drug Administration (FDA), the Drug Enforcement Administration (DEA), and other government agencies safeguard the public by protecting workers, approving drugs, and enforcing drug laws. This chapter reviews the roles of these agencies, the process for developing new drugs to be sold in the United States, the way in which drugs are classified, and the illegal use of drugs. Many medications require a prescription from a licensed health-care provider. The health-care worker has a professional responsibility to know the main laws and regulations related to medications. Although drugs can be helpful, they can harm people if they are used inappropriately. The health-care professional must be alert to signs of addiction in both patients and colleagues.

LEARNING OUTCOMES

At the end of this chapter, you should be able to:

4.1 Define all key terms.

4.2 Describe the roles of the FDA and DEA in patient safety.

4.3 Discuss how drugs are developed.

4.4 Distinguish among brand, generic, and trade names.

4.5 Know the slang names for illegal street drugs.

4.6 Discuss why some drugs are controlled more strictly than others.

4.7 Give an example of a drug from each controlled substances schedule, and explain its classification.

4.8 Discuss the role of health-care professionals in recognizing and reporting impaired patients and professionals.

KEY TERMS		
Addiction	Double-blind	Investigational New
Chemical name	Drug Enforcement	Drug (IND)
Clinical trials	Administration (DEA)	New drug application (NDA)
Compassionate use	Food and Drug	Patent medicine
Control group	Administration	Placebo
Controlled Substances	(FDA)	Substance abuse
Act	Generic name	

HISTORY OF DRUG REGULATIONS

In the early 1900s, many adults in the United States were addicted to drugs in large part because of legal **patent medicines.** An early definition of patent medicine referred to remedies of questionable value that had the potential to cause intentional or accidental harm. Patent medicines were often called "tonics," "elixirs," or "therapeutic agents." Manufacturers sold their patent medicines to unsuspecting people, with exaggerated claims of cures for their ailments. More addictive than curative, these toxic substances contained alcohol, morphine, heroin, or opium. They provided temporary euphoria and therefore relief from pain, but they also caused many deaths from overdoses, especially in children. Even Coca-Cola, developed in the late 1800s, was rumored to use coca leaves, from which cocaine is produced.

The roots of the **Food and Drug Administration (FDA)** can be traced back to Abraham Lincoln, who created the Bureau of Chemistry in 1862. The office was formed to evaluate agricultural products. This bureau had a difficult time passing many resolutions until new and serious concerns arose regarding public food consumption and its safety. During the Spanish-American War, it was rumored that soldiers were fed "embalmed beef," which caused serious illness. As a result of these concerns and the patent medicine problems, Congress passed the first federal drug law: The Pure Food and Drug Act of 1906 (Box 4-1). This bill required accurate labeling of drugs to prevent substitution or mislabeled ingredients.

In 1927 the Bureau of Chemistry was divided into the Food, Drug and Insecticide Bureau, which dealt with regulatory functions and the Bureau of Chemistry and Soils, which dealt with nonregulatory functions. In 1930 the Food, Drug and Insecticide Bureau was shortened to the Food and Drug Administration, or the FDA.

The Food, Drug, and Cosmetic Act of 1938 (Box 4-2) replaced the previous law with more specific regulations including holding the drug developer responsible for drug safety, which oversees the safe

---

BOX 4.1 The Pure Food and Drug Act of 1906

- States are outlawed from buying and selling food, drinks, and drugs that have been mislabeled and/or tainted.
- Ingredients now must be clearly labeled by quantity or percentage.
- Imitation of popular items is banned.
- False or misleading claims are banned, including claims about contents of the labeled item.
- Habit-forming drugs must now have a warning label.

BOX 4.2 The Food, Drug, and Cosmetic Act of 1938

- Placed cosmetics and medical devices under government control
- Required preapproval of all new drugs after manufacture proved safety to the FDA
- Prohibited false advertising about medication therapeutic properties
- Required correction of deficiencies in food quality and packaging
- Authorized manufacturing inspections

development of new drugs. With the passage of the Pure Food and Drug Act of 1906, this office took on its familiar role in regulating medications.

The Durham-Humphrey Amendment (1951) defined prescription drugs as drugs that must be administered under the supervision of a physician. In 1962, the Kefauver-Harris Amendment (Box 4-3) was enacted in response to thalidomide use during pregnancy and the drug's direct link to birth defects. This act requires drug manufacturers to show product effectiveness and safety, to report adverse events to the FDA, and to ensure that any advertisements to physicians disclose a product's risks and benefits.

The **Controlled Substances Act** of 1970 established the **Drug Enforcement Administration (DEA).** This law provided the legal foundation for preventing abuse of drugs and other substances. The DEA regulates the manufacture and distribution of controlled drugs (narcotics, stimulants, depressants, hallucinogens, and anabolic steroids) as well as the substances used in their production.)

The Orphan Drug Act of 1983 was established to facilitate the development of drugs for rare diseases (i.e., diseases that affect fewer than 1 in 200,000 people). Pharmaceutical manufacturers had been reluctant to produce these drugs because of poor return on investment. In addition, these drugs were often expensive for patients. The Orphan Drug Act encouraged the development of these "orphan" drugs by guaranteeing marketing exclusivity, tax credits, and waiver of other fees.

■ THE FDA AND DRUG DEVELOPMENT

The FDA was created to maintain public safety by establishing guidelines and regulations for food quality and drug development and distribution. The FDA evaluates premarket drugs through its Center for Drug Evaluation and Research (CDER). The Center's goals are to ensure that beneficial drug products are safe, available, and labeled with information on risks and benefits. The FDA approves a drug when it deems that the benefits of the drug outweigh the risks for the intended population and use. Once a drug is approved by the FDA, it is added to the *United States Pharmacopoeial/National Formulary,* or *USP/NF,* which is a comprehensive listing of all approved drugs in the United States.

All drugs must be proven safe and effective before they can be approved and marketed. This means that the drugs must perform the indicated action without causing unacceptable harm. For example, one medication may work to eliminate lung cancer; however, it may also cause many patients to suffer cardiac arrest. The benefit is therefore not worth the risk.

The FDA requires that drugs be scientifically researched. The FDA insists on high standards of scientific research, so it may take 8 years or longer for a company to gain approval of a drug, even if that drug is approved and sold in another country. Each drug must go through extensive development and clinical trials. Since 1997, however, the FDA has had the authority to accelerate their review and approval process (to as quickly as 6 months) for drugs needed by patients who are in a critical or life-threatening stage of illness.

 CRITICAL THINKING

Mr. Dupee is upset that he is unable to obtain a drug in the United States. He knows of a website from which he can order the medication from Mexico. What are the potential dangers of ordering a drug from another country? How would you discuss this with him?

BOX 4.3 Amendments to the Food, Drug, and Cosmetic Act of 1938

Durham-Humphrey Amendment of 1951
- Defines which types of drugs cannot be used without medical supervision
- Limits sale of these drugs to prescription only by a medical professional
- All other drugs available without prescription

Kefauver-Harris Drug Amendments
- Requires drug makers to prove their drug works before approval for sale
- The Advisory Committee on Investigation Drugs advises the FDA on product approval and policy making

Drug Development

Drug development begins after researchers discover, identify, or create agents that show promising effects against a disease or disorder. These agents must pass through many stages of development and exploration and meet strict regulatory requirements before they can be tested on humans.

A major part of drug development requires that developers conduct clinical trials or studies. After testing in laboratories and/or on animals, a drug must be carefully tested in humans. Researchers use clinical trials with human subjects to test the effects of a drug with the goal of determining effectiveness, side effects, toxicity, and interactions. During the study or trial, the effect of the active drug is compared with a **placebo.** A placebo is an inactive (inert) substance that is sometimes given to participants in clinical trials to compare the response the patient has with an inert substance with the response they have to an active substance. The study drug may also be compared with a drug already on the market. For example, ibuprofen was possibly compared with other, well-known pain relievers such as aspirin or acetaminophen (Tylenol).

Study participants are randomly assigned to one of at least two groups (Fig. 4-1). One group is the placebo or **control group;** the other group receives the active study drug or drugs. Because the participants do not know whether they are receiving the active or inactive drug, they are prevented from invalidating the study by reporting effects they were not truly experiencing. Similarly, if the clinician conducting the study knew which patients were taking the active drug, the scientist could change the results, consciously or subconsciously. Therefore, to be sure the results of the drug trials are uncompromised, most studies are **double-blind,** meaning that neither the participants nor the clinicians know

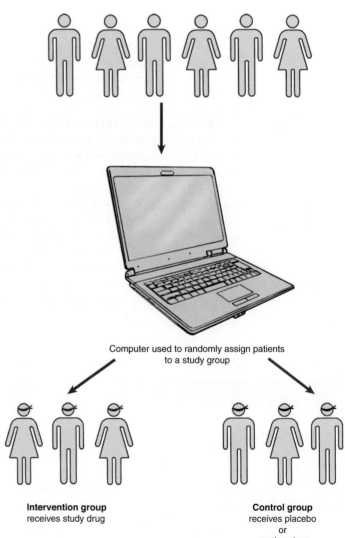

Computer used to randomly assign patients to a study group

Intervention group
receives study drug

Control group
receives placebo
or
another drug

FIGURE 4-1: Double-blind clinical trial. In a randomized, double-blind clinical trial, neither patients nor clinicians know who is receiving the drug or placebo.

who is receiving the active drug. Computers are used to generate random numbers to assign to patients, and the study drug and placebo look alike.

To encourage volunteers, treatment is usually free. Volunteers also may be paid for participating or may receive funds to cover transportation costs to and from the trial facilities. These volunteers must sign a detailed consent form.

Human clinical trials are conducted in several phases (Table 4-1). The goal of phase I trials is to determine safety. A few healthy participants take a drug for several months to measure any harmful effects. For example, a drug may cause diarrhea or may negatively affect vital signs. If the drug causes significant harmful effects, the trial stops. Usually, the participants are men because of concern over giving experimental drugs to women who could become pregnant. One disadvantage of this practice is that researchers may not become aware of any harmful effects that occur only in women until a later research phase.

Phase II clinical trials involve hundreds of patients (all of whom have the disease targeted by the drug) for longer periods of time. Although safety is important, the main goal of these trials is to see whether a drug works as desired (efficacy). For example, if a drug is meant to lower cholesterol, samples of participants' blood are checked to see whether blood cholesterol levels are lower while participants are taking the medication.

Phase III trials are for drugs that have been proven to be safe and effective. These trials involve hundreds to thousands of participants and can last 1 to 4 years. Frequently, phase III trials are conducted in several facilities (e.g., hospitals, physicians' offices, clinics), each of which enrolls hundreds of patients. The manufacturer is testing for safety, effectiveness, and dosage. The therapeutic (best) dose is evaluated during this phase; the goal is to give the least amount of drug possible to gain the necessary effect.

 CRITICAL THINKING

Not all people who volunteer for clinical trials are acceptable for the research. What do you think could eliminate a patient from clinical trials?

During the first three phases of clinical trials, the drug is known as an **investigational new drug (IND)**, and its use is limited to persons who meet specific criteria for inclusion in the trial. If the drug is being developed to help critically ill patients, special exceptions can be made. The FDA allows some physicians the **compassionate use** of INDs before approval. If a patient is suffering greatly and may die without the drug, a physician can prescribe it before FDA approval. However, most Health Maintenance Organizations (HMOs) and other private or public insurers do not cover the costs of experimental drugs because these drugs are expensive to obtain if you are not participating in the research.

If the clinical trials show that the drug is safe and effective, and a therapeutic dose is established, the manufacturer next applies to the FDA for approval. The manufacturer submits a **new drug application (NDA),** with the results of the scientific testing. Depending on the drug, the approval process can take 6 months to several years, and up to 12 years may pass from preclinical trails to approval. Because the process of drug approval is long and expensive, only about 1 drug is marketed for every

TABLE 4.1   Clinical Trial Phases

Phase	Number of Patients	Length	Purpose
I	20–100	Several months	Safety—Does the drug do harm?
II	Up to several hundred	Several months–2 years	Efficacy—Does the drug help the patient? Also looks at safety
III	Several hundred to thousands	1–4 years	Also looks at safety and efficacy
IV (postmarketing trials)	Thousands	Ongoing	Continuing evaluation through MedWatch

5,000 to 10,000 compounds tested. The manufacturer usually receives a 17- to 20-year patent to recover the cost and make a profit.

Once approved by the FDA, a drug can be marketed and distributed outside clinical trial groups. Additional research may also be conducted. These activities are referred to as postmarketing (or phase IV) trials.

CRITICAL THINKING

Canadians are protected by the Health Protection Branch (HPB) of the Department of Health and Welfare. Why would it be important for countries to cooperate in drug research?

Drug Monitoring

After a drug is on the market and available for use, it is continually monitored and evaluated for its benefits and risks, not only by the FDA, but also by health-care providers and patients taking the drugs. The FDA holds annual public meetings to hear comments from patients, pharmaceutical manufacturers, and health-care professionals about the safety and effectiveness of drugs. Figure 4-2 demonstrates the FDA's role in risk management.

Surveillance for any problems not previously identified continues through the FDA's MedWatch program. Although the reporting of these problems is voluntary, it helps the FDA track trends. If a drug has multiple reports of adverse reactions or a serious event such as death, the manufacturer may voluntarily recall a drug, or the FDA may order a recall. In a recall, the manufacturer of the drug must stop distributing it and must contact customers to inform them of the product name, size, lot number, code or serial number, reason for recall, and instructions on how to proceed. Recalled drugs are listed in a weekly FDA Enforcement Report, available on the FDA website (www.fda.gov/).

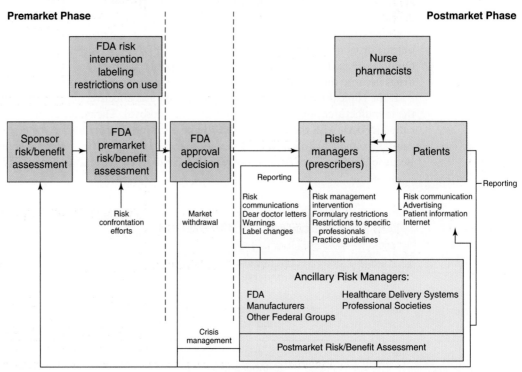

FIGURE 4-2: Role of the Food and Drug Administration in risk management of approved drugs. *(Reprinted from U.S. Department of Health and Human Services, Food and Drug Administration. Retrieved June 22, 2011, from http://fda.gov.)*

It is your responsibility as a health-care professional to report an adverse reaction to a medication to MedWatch. Guidelines for what and how to report are available on the FDA website (www.fda.gov. Search for Medwatch). You can post reports on the Internet or by telephone. The appropriate form is available on the website (Fig. 4-3). If the adverse event was caused by a vaccine, online reporting is encouraged, but the Vaccine Adverse Event Form shown in Figure 4-4 can be used if necessary.

U.S. Department of Health and Human Services

Form Approved: OMB No. 0910-0291
See OMB statement on reverse.

MEDWATCH
The FDA Safety Information and Adverse Event Reporting Program

For VOLUNTARY reporting of adverse events, product problems and product use errors

Page 1 of ____

FDA USE ONLY
Triage unit sequence #

PLEASE TYPE OR USE BLACK INK

A. PATIENT INFORMATION

1. **Patient Identifier** — In confidence
2. **Age at Time of Event or Date of Birth:**
3. **Sex** — ☐ Female ☐ Male
4. **Weight** — ______ lb or ______ kg

B. ADVERSE EVENT, PRODUCT PROBLEM OR ERROR

Check all that apply:
1. ☐ **Adverse Event** ☐ **Product Problem** *(e.g., defects/malfunctions)*
☐ **Product Use Error** ☐ **Problem with Different Manufacturer of Same Medicine**

2. **Outcomes Attributed to Adverse Event** *(Check all that apply)*
☐ Death: ______________ *(mm/dd/yyyy)*
☐ Disability or Permanent Damage
☐ Life-threatening
☐ Congenital Anomaly/Birth Defect
☐ Hospitalization - initial or prolonged
☐ Other Serious (Important Medical Events)
☐ Required intervention to Prevent Permanent Impairment/Damage (Devices)

3. **Date of Event** *(mm/dd/yyyy)*
4. **Date of this Report** *(mm/dd/yyyy)*
5. **Describe Event, Problem or Product Use Error**
6. **Relevant Tests/Laboratory Data, Including Dates**
7. **Other Relevant History, Including Preexisting Medical Conditions** *(e.g., allergies, race, pregnancy, smoking and alcohol use, liver/kidney problems, etc.)*

C. PRODUCT AVAILABILITY

Product Available for Evaluation? *(Do not send product to FDA)*
☐ Yes ☐ No ☐ Returned to Manufacturer on: ______________ *(mm/dd/yyyy)*

D. SUSPECT PRODUCT(S)

1. **Name, Strength, Manufacturer** *(from product label)*
#1 Name:
Strength:
Manufacturer:
#2 Name:
Strength:
Manufacturer:

2. **Dose or Amount** / **Frequency** / **Route**
#1
#2

3. **Date of Use** *(if unknown, give duration) from/to (or best estimate)*
#1
#2

4. **Diagnosis or Reason for Use** *(Indication)*
#1
#2

5. **Event Abated After Use Stopped or Dose Reduced?**
#1 ☐ Yes ☐ No ☐ Doesn't Apply
#2 ☐ Yes ☐ No ☐ Doesn't Apply

6. **Lot #**
#1
#2

7. **Expiration Date**
#1
#2

8. **Event Reappeared After Reintroduction?**
#1 ☐ Yes ☐ No ☐ Doesn't Apply
#2 ☐ Yes ☐ No ☐ Doesn't Apply

9. **NDC # or Unique ID**

E. SUSPECT MEDICAL DEVICE

1. **Brand Name**
2. **Common Device Name**
3. **Manufacturer Name, City and State**
4. **Model #** / **Lot #** / **Catalog #** / **Expiration Date** *(mm/dd/yyyy)* / **Serial #** / **Other #**
5. **Operator of Device**
☐ Health Professional
☐ Lay User/Patient
☐ Other:
6. **If Implanted, Give Date** *(mm/dd/yyyy)*
7. **If Explanted, Give Date** *(mm/dd/yyyy)*
8. **Is this a Single-use Device that was Reprocessed and Reused on a Patient?**
☐ Yes ☐ No
9. **If Yes to Item No. 8, Enter Name and Address of Reprocessor**

F. OTHER (CONCOMITANT) MEDICAL PRODUCTS

Product names and therapy dates *(exclude treatment of event)*

G. REPORTER *(See confidentiality section on back)*

1. **Name and Address**
Name:
Address:
City: State: Zip:
Phone # **E-mail**
2. **Health Professional?** ☐ Yes ☐ No
3. **Occupation**
4. **Also Reported to:**
☐ Manufacturer
☐ User Facility
☐ Distributor/Importer
5. **If you do NOT want your identity disclosed to the manufacturer, place an "X" in this box:** ☐

FORM FDA 3500 (1/09) Submission of a report does not constitute an admission that medical personnel or the product caused or contributed to the event.

FIGURE 4-3: MedWatch form. An electronic form containing similar information is completed online to report serious adverse events that result from drug administration. *(Reprinted from U.S. Department of Health and Human Services, Food and Drug Administration. Retrieved June 22, 2011, from https://www.fda.gov/downloads/AboutFDA/ReportsManualsForms/Forms/UCM163919.pdf.)*

VAERS Vaccine Adverse Event Reporting System
www.vaers.hhs.gov

Adverse events are possible reactions or problems that occur during or after vaccination. Items 2, 3, 4, 5, 6, 17, 18 and 21 are **ESSENTIAL** and should be completed. Patient identity is kept confidential. Instructions are provided on the last two pages.

INFORMATION ABOUT THE PATIENT WHO RECEIVED THE VACCINE (Use Continuation Page if needed).

1. Patient name: (first) ______ (last) ______
Street address: ______
City: ______ State: ______ County: ______
ZIP code: ______ Phone: ( ) ______ Email: ______

2. Date of birth: (mm/dd/yyyy) ______ 3. Sex: ☐ Male ☐ Female ☐ Unknown

4. Date and time of vaccination: (mm/dd/yyyy) ______ Time: hh:mm ☐AM ☐PM

5. Date and time adverse event started: (mm/dd/yyyy) ______ Time: hh:mm ☐AM ☐PM

6. Age at vaccination: ___ Years ___ Months 7. Today's date: (mm/dd/yyyy) ______

8. Is the report about vaccine(s) given to a pregnant woman?: ☐ No ☐ Unknown ☐ Yes
(If yes, describe the event, any pregnancy complications, and estimated due date if known in item 18).

9. Prescriptions, over-the-counter medications, dietary supplements, or herbal remedies being taken at the time of vaccination:

10. Allergies to medications, food, or other products:

11. Other illnesses at the time of vaccination and up to one month prior:

12. Chronic or long-standing health conditions:

INFORMATION ABOUT THE PERSON COMPLETING THIS FORM

13. Form completed by: (name) ______
Relation to patient: ☐ Healthcare professional/staff ☐ Patient (yourself) ☐ Parent/guardian/caregiver ☐ Other: ______
Street address: ______ ☐ Check if same as item 1.
City: ______ State: ______ ZIP code: ______
Phone: ( ) ______ Email: ______

14. Best doctor/healthcare professional to contact about the adverse event: Name: ______ Phone: ( ) ______ Ext: ______

INFORMATION ABOUT THE FACILITY WHERE VACCINE WAS GIVEN

15. Facility/clinic name: ______
Fax: ( ) ______
Street address: ______ ☐ Check if same as item 13.
City: ______
State: ______ ZIP code: ______
Phone: ( ) ______

16. Type of facility: (Check one).
☐ Doctor's office or hospital
☐ Pharmacy or drug store
☐ Workplace clinic
☐ Public health clinic
☐ Nursing home or senior living facility
☐ School/student health clinic
☐ Other: ______
☐ Unknown

WHICH VACCINES WERE GIVEN? WHAT HAPPENED TO THE PATIENT?

17. Enter all vaccines given on the date listed in item 4: (Route is HOW vaccine was given, Body site is WHERE vaccine was given). Use **Continuation Page** if needed.

Vaccine (type and brand name)	Manufacturer	Lot number	Route	Body site	Dose no. in series
select			select	select	select
select			select	select	select
select			select	select	select
select			select	select	select

18. Describe the adverse event(s), treatment, and outcome(s), if any: (symptoms, signs, time course, etc.)
Use **Continuation Page** if needed.

19. Medical tests and laboratory results related to the adverse event(s): (include dates)
Use **Continuation Page** if needed.

20. Has the patient recovered from the adverse event(s)?: ☐ Yes ☐ No ☐ Unknown

21. Result or outcome of adverse event(s): (Check all that apply).
☐ Doctor or other healthcare professional office/clinic visit
☐ Emergency room or emergency department visit
☐ Hospitalization: Number of days (if known) ______
Hospital name: ______
City: ______ State: ______
☐ Prolongation of existing hospitalization (vaccine received during existing hospitalization)
☐ Life threatening illness (immediate risk of death from the event)
☐ Disability or permanent damage
☐ Patient died: Date of death ______ (mm/dd/yyyy)
☐ Congenital anomaly or birth defect
☐ None of the above

ADDITIONAL INFORMATION (Use Continuation Page if needed).

22. Any other vaccines received within one month prior to the date listed in item 4:

Vaccine (type and brand name)	Manufacturer	Lot number	Route	Body site	Dose no. in series
select			select	select	select
select			select	select	select

23. Has the patient ever had an adverse event following any previous vaccine?: (If yes, describe adverse event, patient age at vaccination, vaccination dates, vaccine type, and brand name).
☐ No ☐ Unknown ☐ Yes ______

24. Patient's race: (Check all that apply). ☐ American Indian or Alaska Native ☐ Asian ☐ Black or African American ☐ Native Hawaiian or Other Pacific Islander ☐ White ☐ Unknown ☐ Other: ______

25. Patient's ethnicity: ☐ Hispanic or Latino ☐ Not Hispanic or Latino ☐ Unknown 26. Immuniz. proj. report no.: (Health Dept use only). ______

COMPLETE ONLY FOR U.S. MILITARY/DEPARTMENT OF DEFENSE (DoD) RELATED REPORTS

27. Status at vaccination: ☐ Active duty ☐ Reserve ☐ National Guard ☐ Beneficiary ☐ Other: ______ 28. Vaccinated at Military/DoD site: ☐ Yes ☐ No

FORM FDA VAERS-2.0 (6/17) SAVE

FIGURE 4-4: Vaccine Adverse Event Reporting System. If an adverse event results from a vaccine, the health-care professional must complete the Vaccine Adverse Event Reporting System form. *(Reprinted from U.S. Department of Health and Human Services, Food and Drug Administration. Retrieved November 7, 2017, from https://vaers.hhs.gov/reportevent.html.)*

Naming Drugs

Part of the process of developing drugs and taking them through FDA approval involves assigning names. When a drug is first developed, it is known by its mix of chemicals. The **chemical name** and structure is meaningful to researchers and to those companies who want to copy a successful drug, but it means little to others. For example, the chemical name of aspirin is 2-acetyloxybenzoic acid, and morphine's chemical name is (5.alpha., 6.alpha.)-7,8-didehydro-4,5-epoxy-17-methylmorphinan-3,6-diol. Complicated chemical names would be difficult for the health-care professional to memorize.

Once a drug clears phases I to III of clinical trials, it is ready to be put on the market and is given a **brand** or **trade name** (also sometimes called a *proprietary name*), to which the company owns the rights. Because the brand name is used in advertising, the company selects a name that is easy to remember and may indicate the drug's purposes. For example, Restoril® helps patients sleep. Another example is Aleve®, which helps relieve pain. The initial letters of brand names are capitalized. A brand name is usually followed by the letters R or TM with circles around them, to signify that the name is a registered trademark and no other manufacturer can use that name during the patent period.

Once a drug's patent period has ended, the drug's trademark status is not protected, so other companies may produce the drug under its common or **generic name** (Table 4-2). No one except the manufacturer holding the trademark status can use the brand name, but other companies can manufacture the drug. Because these other companies did not do the research or spend as much on marketing, they can produce the medication much more cheaply than the original manufacturer.

 CRITICAL THINKING

Drug names can reflect their treatment effect. Try to determine what the drugs listed here could be used for, and then check a drug reference book to see how close you were.

Azmacort	Lipitor
Bronkaid	NasalCrom
Elimite	Nicoderm
Flexeril	Pepcid
Glucotrol	Rythmol

How did you do?

TABLE 4.2   Sample Drug Names

Chemical Name and Structure	Generic Name	Brand Name(s)
N-acetyl-p-aminophenol $C_8H_9NO_2$	acetaminophen	Tylenol Paracetamol Mapap Panadol
N[2-[[[5-[(dimethylamino)methyl]-2furanyl]methyl]thio]ethyl]-N′-methyl-2-nitro-1,1-ethenediamine, HCl $C_{13}H_{22}N_4O_3S$	ranitidine hydrochloride	Zantac Deprizine
L-3,3′,5,5′-tetraiodothyronine sodium salt $C_{15}H_{11}I_4NO_4$	levothyroxine	Synthroid Levoxyl Tirosint Levothroid
4-[2-(tert-butylamino)-1-hydroxyethyl]-2-(hydroxymethyl)phenol $C_{13}H_{21}NO_3$	albuterol	Ventolin Proventil
Calcium;(E,3R,5S)-7-[4-(4-fluorophenyl)-2-[methyl(methylsulfonyl)amino]-6-propan-2-ylpyrimidin-5-yl]-3,5-dihydroxyhept-6-enoate $C_{44}H_{54}CaF_2N_6O_{12}S_2$	rosuvastatin	Crestor
Magnesium; 5-methoxy-2-[(4-methoxy-3,5-dimethylpyridin-2-yl)methylsulfinyl]benzimidazol-1-ide;trihydrate $C_{34}H_{42}MGN_6O_9S_2$	esomeprazole	Nexium

The FDA has specific requirements for manufacturers of generic drugs (Box 4-4). If the company uses the generic name, the drug must have the active ingredient the generic name specifies, but different fillers can be used. In some patients, the drug is more effective in the brand name form than in the generic form, but most adapt well to a generic brand. Because the generic drug is less expensive, HMOs often require that patients and prescribers use it or forfeit reimbursement.

Unlike the brand name, the first letter of the generic name is capitalized only if it begins a sentence. The generic name can also provide a clue to a drug's class (type) (see Fast Tip 4.1). The generic name becomes the official name of the drug.

The prescriber may use shortened generic names. If the chemical is followed by the terms *carbonate, citrate, gluconate, hydrochloride, hydroxide, phosphate, sodium,* or *sulfate,* the prescriber assumes that the pharmacist understands the generic name without the second term. For example, potassium chloride is often ordered as potassium, although the drug label should contain the complete name. If you have any doubt about the correct name, check with the pharmacist or prescriber.

The generic drug may have a different shape and/or color from the trade drug. A change in the appearance of medications can confuse patients. Encourage patients to contact the pharmacy if they are unsure of a change in drugs. The pharmacy may have purchased the drug from a different manufacturer, but the change may also be an error.

■ DRUG CONTROL

The Drug Enforcement Administration (DEA) was established in 1973. The purpose of the DEA is to enforce the controlled substances laws and regulations for the United States. This includes the provisions of the Controlled Substances Act as they pertain to the manufacture, distribution, and dispensing of legally produced controlled substances. Controlled substances are those that must be tracked or tightly controlled (narcotics, stimulants, depressants, hallucinogens, and anabolic steroids). Most of these

---

BOX 4.4 Food and Drug Administration Requirements for Generic Drugs

- An FDA-approved brand name drug must be the reference for the proposed generic. The generic drug must have the same active ingredient or ingredients and the same labeled strength as this reference product. It must have the same dosage form: tablets, patches, and liquids are examples of dosage forms. It must be administered in the same way (e.g., swallowed as a pill or given as an injection).
- The manufacturer must show the generic drug is "bioequivalent" to the brand name drug. This means that the generic version delivers the same amount of active ingredients into a patient's bloodstream in the same amount as the brand name drug.
- The generic drug's labeling must be essentially the same as that of the approved drug.
- The firm must fully document the generic drug's chemistry, manufacturing steps, and quality control measures. Each step of the process must be detailed for FDA review.
- The firm must assure the FDA that the raw materials and the finished product meet USP specifications, if these have been set. The USP is the nonprofit scientific body chartered by Congress to set standards for drug purity in the United States.
- Before the generic drug can be sold, the manufacturing firm must show that the drug maintains stability as labeled. Once the drug is on the market, the firm must continue to monitor the drug's stability. The firm must show that the container and its closure system will not interact with the drug. Firms making sterile drugs must submit sterility assurance data showing microbiologic integrity of these products.
- The firm must provide a full description of the facilities it uses to manufacture, process, test, package, label, and control the drug. It must certify that it complies with federal regulations about current good manufacturing practices and must undergo FDA inspection of the manufacturing facility to ensure compliance.
- Before the FDA approves a generic drug, it usually conducts an inspection at the proposed manufacturing site to make sure the firm is capable of meeting its application commitments and to ensure the firm can manufacture the product consistently.
- FDA, Food and Drug Administration; USP, United States Pharmacopoeia. Source: U.S. Food and Drug Administration.

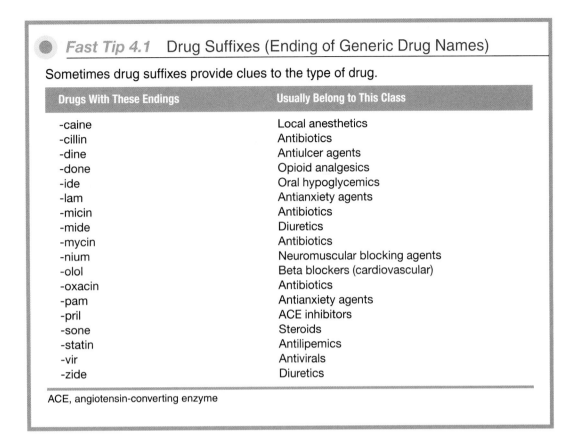

Fast Tip 4.1   Drug Suffixes (Ending of Generic Drug Names)

Sometimes drug suffixes provide clues to the type of drug.

Drugs With These Endings	Usually Belong to This Class
-caine	Local anesthetics
-cillin	Antibiotics
-dine	Antiulcer agents
-done	Opioid analgesics
-ide	Oral hypoglycemics
-lam	Antianxiety agents
-micin	Antibiotics
-mide	Diuretics
-mycin	Antibiotics
-nium	Neuromuscular blocking agents
-olol	Beta blockers (cardiovascular)
-oxacin	Antibiotics
-pam	Antianxiety agents
-pril	ACE inhibitors
-sone	Steroids
-statin	Antilipemics
-vir	Antivirals
-zide	Diuretics

ACE, angiotensin-converting enzyme

drugs are available by prescription only. The Combat Methamphetamine Epidemic Act of 2005 was passed to regulate over-the-counter drugs that contain ephedrine, pseudoephedrine, or phenylpropanolamine, which are ingredients used in the production of crystal meth, an illegal street drug. The OTC drugs do not require a prescription, but the purchaser must present a valid ID at the pharmacy and sign for the drug. This protocol may vary from state to state. Some discussion has suggested adding these drugs to the controlled substances list, which would make them at least schedule V drugs.

Although the FDA determines which drugs are available only by prescription, the DEA decides which drugs are controlled and assigns the drugs to a schedule, or category, based on their abuse potential.

Drug Schedules

Controlled substances are assigned one of five schedules designated by the Roman numerals I to V according to their potential for addiction and abuse. The most highly controlled drugs are Schedule I drugs, and the least controlled are Schedule V drugs (Table 4-3). It is not necessary to memorize all these drugs, but knowing the categories is important to understand the effects of each type of drug on the patient.

Schedule I drugs are considered to be highly addictive, both physically and psychologically, and they have no medical use. Heroin is considered a Schedule I drug. These drugs are considered so dangerous that they are illegal to process, distribute, and use. Schedule I drugs are not prescribed except in carefully controlled research facilities in which patients are closely monitored, such as the study of the street drug ecstasy in the treatment of post-traumatic stress disorder. Marijuana is a schedule I drug, but as more and more states are legalizing marijuana for medical use, this may change. Healthcare professionals should never possess these drugs because criminal prosecution may result.

Schedule II drugs have a high potential for physical and psychological addiction. The use of these drugs is heavily restricted because they are popular with addicts. These drugs are dispensed through written prescription only; an office assistant cannot call in the prescription to the pharmacy. Additionally, no refills are permitted. This does not mean that patients cannot have more of the medication, but they must have a written prescription for each new supply. The office staff may fax the prescription

TABLE 4.3 Drug Enforcement Administration Controlled Substance Schedules

Schedule	Abuse Potential	Medications	Examples
I	High	No accepted medical use in the United States	Heroin, marijuana, LSD, methaqualone
II	High; may lead to severe dependence (psychological or physical)	Has a currently accepted medical use; may have severe restrictions	Cocaine, hydrocodone, methadone, methamphetamine, morphine, PCP, OxyContin, Ritalin
III	Less than drugs and substances in Schedules I and II; may lead to moderate or low physical dependence or high psychological dependence	Has a currently accepted medical use	Anabolic steroids, codeine with aspirin or Tylenol, ketamine, testosterone
IV	Low relative to substances in Schedule III; may lead to limited dependence	Has a currently accepted medical use	Ambien, Ativan, Tramadol, Valium, Xanax
V	Low, relative to substances in Schedule IV; may lead to limited dependence (psychological or physical)	Has a currently accepted medical use	Cough medicine with codeine, Lomotil

Source: http://usdoj.gov/dea/pubs/abuse/1-csa.htm

to the pharmacy, but the patient must also give a handwritten prescription to the pharmacist to receive the medicine. In an emergency, the prescriber may phone in an order to a nurse (e.g., if the patient is in the hospital), but a handwritten copy of the prescription must be submitted within 72 hours. This category includes drugs that suppress the central nervous system such as morphine, as well as amphetamines, which stimulate it. Examples include cocaine, PCP, methylphenidate (Ritalin), hydrocodone (Hydrocet), and oxycodone (OxyContin).

Schedule III drugs are moderately addictive and may lead to limited dependence. Refills are allowed up to five times in 6 months. This category includes combination drugs that contain a small amount of a narcotic with a less-addictive medication, such as acetaminophen or aspirin. The patient absorbs less of the narcotic dose in each tablet, but the drug is still powerful. Examples are anabolic steroids, ketamine, testosterone, and Tylenol with codeine. Health-care professionals may write the prescription for the drug, but the prescriber must sign it.

Schedule IV drugs have lower abuse potential but are still controlled. As with Schedule III drugs, health-care professionals may write the prescription (e.g., name, route, dosage), but the prescriber must sign it. A health-care professional can fax or phone in these orders to the pharmacy or facility. Refills of drugs in this category are allowed up to five times in 6 months. Examples include lorazepam (Ativan), diazepam (Valium), and alprazolam (Xanax).

Schedule V drugs have the lowest potential for abuse. They include OTC cough suppressants to which a small amount of codeine has been added, as well as preparations for diarrhea, such as paregoric and opium tincture. Because the cough syrup is thick, overdose is difficult. However, small children like the taste of syrup, so advise parents to store the medicine away from children. Examples are diphenoxylate hydrochloride and atropine sulfate preparations (Lomotil), Robitussin A-C, and Children's Tylenol 3.

Drugs may be described in more than one schedule. For example, full-strength codeine is a Schedule II drug because it is a highly addictive narcotic. If a manufacturer adds more acetaminophen or aspirin so that only a small amount of the narcotic is present in the medication, it can be classified as a Schedule III drug. If the manufacturer adds a small amount of narcotic to a large amount of syrup, the medication can be classified as Schedule V (e.g., Children's Tylenol® with Codeine syrup) because the narcotic is less addictive when taken in such a small quantity.

Legal and illegal drugs often have *street* or slang names. Although you may not know the names of illegal drugs used on the street, your patients may use these terms; therefore, you should be familiar with them. Box 4-5 provides common street names for drugs that are frequently used.

BOX 4.5 Street Names for Commonly Abused Drugs

Cannabinoids

Hashish—boom, chronic, gangster, hash, hash oil, hemp

Marijuana—blunt, bud, dope, ganja, grass, green, herb, joints, Mary Jane, pot, reefer, sinsemilla, skunk, smoke, trees, wacky weed, weed, widow

Synthetic cannabinoids—K2, Spice, black mamba, bliss, Bombay, blue, fake weed, fire, genie, moon, rocks, skunk, smacked, Yucatan, Zohai

Depressants

Barbiturates—barbs, phennies, reds, red birds, tooies, yellows, yellow jackets

Benzodiazepines—candy, downers, sleeping pills, tranks

Flunitrazepam—forget-me pill, Mexican Valium, mind eraser, R2, roach, Roche, roofies, roofinol, rope, rophies, trip and fall, wolfies

GHB—G, Georgia home boy, grievous bodily harm, liquid ecstasy, Liquid X, Soap, Scoop

Methaqualone—ludes, mandrex, quad, quay

Sleep medications—A-minus, zombie pills

Dissociative Anesthetics

Ketamine—cat Valium, K, special K, vitamin K

PCP and analogs—angel dust, boat, hog, love boat, peace pill

Salvia—magic mint, Maria Pastora, Slly-D, Shepherdess's Herb, Diviner's sage

Hallucinogens

Ayahuasca—Aya, Yage, Hoasca

LSD—acid, blotter, blue heaven, cubes, microdot, red/green dragon, yellow sunshine

Mescaline—buttons, cactus, mesc, peyote

Psilocybin—little smoke, magic mushroom, purple passion, shrooms

Opioids and Morphine Derivatives

Codeine—Captain Cody, Cody, lean, schoolboy, sizzurp, doors and fours, loads, pancakes and syrup

Fentanyl—Apache, China girl, China white, dance fever, friend, goodfella, jackpot, murder 8, TNT, Tango and cash

Heroin—Brown sugar, China White, Doper, H, Horse, Junk, Skag, Skunk, Smack, Cheese

Hydrocodone—Vike, Watson-387

Hydromorphone (Dilaudid)—D, Dillies, Footballs, Juick, Smack

Meperidine (Demerol)—Demmies, Pain killer

Methadone—Amidone

Morphine—M, Miss Emma, monkey, white stuff

Opium—big O, black stuff, block, gum, hop

Oxycodone—O.C, Oxycet, Oxycotton, hillbilly heroin percs

Oxymorphone—biscuits, blue heaven blues, Mrs. O, O, bomb, octagons, stop signs

Stimulants

Amphetamines—bennies, black beauties, crosses, hearts, LA turnaround, speed, truck drivers, uppers

Bath Salts—Bloom, cloud nine, cosmic blast, flakka, ivory wave, lunar wave, scarface, vanilla sky, white lightning

Cocaine—blow, bump, C, candy, Charlie, coke, crack, flake, rock, snow, toot

Methamphetamine—chalk, crank, crystal, fire, glass, go fast, ice, meth, speed

Methylphenidate—JIF, MPH, R-ball, Skippy, the smart drug, Vitamin R

Other

Anabolic steroids—gym candy, juice, pumpers, roids

Ecstasy—Adam, Clarity, Eve, Lover's Speed, Peace, Uppers

Inhalants—poppers, snappers, whippets, laughing gas

Over the counter cough/cold medicines (Dextromethorphan or DXM)—Robotripping, Robo, Triple C

Controlled Substances Management

Whether you work in an office, hospital, or other health-care facility, if there are controlled substances utilized, there will be policies and procedures for the handling and storing these controlled substances. Legally they must be accounted for, and if you have access to them you are responsible for them. An inventory log will be required to document when you receive certain controlled medications and to whom you dispense them. Be sure to follow your agency's policies in regard to signing off regarding which patient received what dosage along with your signature. Some agencies will have a computerized system in place for this documentation, and others will have a paper document that needs to be signed. In both instances, a witness will be required for any controlled substances wasted. In other words, if you do not administer a full dose, break a vial, or drop a pill, you need a witness to this event.

Sign your name to the drug count only if you have counted the drugs to show that the actual controlled substances on hand match what the computer or paper log say should be on hand. Be aware of agency policy mandating the timing of a narcotic count. The count may be performed as often as once per day, once per shift, or once per week depending on the type of facility. In a narcotic count, two professionals count the controlled substances on hand. One person counts the actual medications, and one compares that count with the narcotics log to verify that the numbers match.

Notify the physician or supervisor immediately if the controlled drug count is not as recorded. For example, if the log shows eight remaining Demerol tablets but only five tablets are present in the narcotics cabinet, you would immediately notify the physician or supervisor. These records must be kept for 2 years. See the DEA website for complete information. In the hospital setting, nurses usually count and log out the controlled substances. These drugs should be kept double-locked in a safe place whenever they are not in your sight. Patients should not know where these drugs are stored. Be suspicious of a patient who asks you for this information. If controlled substances are stolen or lost, the prescriber who has a DEA number must file DEA Form 106, Theft or Loss of Controlled Substances, which is also available on the DEA website. Theft of a significant amount should be reported to the local police department.

If you need to dispose of a controlled medication, you must have someone witness the disposal, and the medication must be destroyed beyond any possible reuse. Many states require that you return unused medications to a pharmacy or state police facility for incineration, to ensure complete disposal. Controlled substances must be clearly marked as controlled. The label on the medication bottle shows a "C" for controlled substances. Do not put controlled substances in unmarked containers.

■ SUBSTANCE ABUSE

Substance abuse is a maladaptive pattern of behavior marked by the use of chemical agents. The key to substance abuse is that the patient does not adapt well under the influence of the substance.

Each year, numerous deaths in the United States result from substance abuse. Some substances are commonly and legally used, such as nicotine and alcohol (EtOH). Others are illegal drugs. Still others, such as steroids, are seen as a way to enhance athletic performance (Fast Tip 4-2). Any drug can be

---

 Fast Tip 4.2 Steroid Abuse

The National Institute on Drug Abuse (NIDA) reports that anabolic steroids are frequently abused by people who want to build muscles, reduce body fat, and improve sports performance. Abuse is estimated to be high among competitive body builders and athletes. Men usually abuse steroids to become larger and more muscular, whereas women abuse steroids to become lean and muscular. Doses taken by abusers can be up to 100 times greater than doses used for treating medical conditions, such as the muscle wasting seen in AIDS. Anabolic steroids can cause hormonal system disruptions, musculoskeletal system effects, infections, cardiovascular diseases, liver and skin dysfunction, and behavioral effects. (Source: National Institute of Drug Abuse: NIDA Notes 15[3], 2000.)

abused if it is used improperly. For example, a person obsessed with losing weight may choose to use laxatives as aids but may harm himself or herself in the process. Health-care professionals may see patients who show signs of substance abuse, including tremors (shaking), poor judgment, or slurred speech. Because these signs can also reflect disease states, include all the facts when documenting such signs in the medical record.

Some drugs are particularly addictive. **Addiction** means being compulsively driven to take a drug, often to the exclusion of all other activities. Most patients do not start taking a drug with the thought of becoming addicted, but over time they may become dependent on the drug and crave it either psychologically or physically. For example, a patient experiencing pain after an injury may take an increasing amount of pain medication. Soon more of the drug is needed to produce the same effect because the person has developed a **tolerance** to it.

Other people become **habituated** to drugs. This means they are psychologically dependent on the drug. They may not physically need the drug but believe that they cannot live without it. For example, a patient may be prescribed an antianxiety medication to help her cope with stressful work situation, but she begins to enjoy the way the drug makes her feel. She may take more of the medication to cope with perceived anxiety. Soon she takes increasing amounts of the drug because she has developed a tolerance to it. Having the drug in her system becomes "normal." Those who stop taking a medication suddenly may experience symptoms of **withdrawal,** such as tremors, emotional distress, and hallucinations.

It is vital to keep patients free from pain when they are in the acute stage of a disease or are recovering from surgery. However, prescribers are typically reluctant to increase dosages over the long term. If patients engage in drug-seeking behavior (i.e., requesting more medication out of proportion to physiological needs), the prescriber may reduce the amount of medication allowed and refer the patient for psychological counseling. Chronic pain is a particular challenge, especially in patients who are terminally ill (dying). These patients may experience increasing, not decreasing, pain as the disease worsens. The health-care provider may prescribe more painkillers as time goes on but must be careful not to overprescribe drugs that can injure the patient by suppressing respiration.

 CRITICAL THINKING

A patient calls frequently and begs for more pain medication. The doctor and staff are frustrated by the repeated requests and attribute them to drug-seeking behavior. How would you handle this situation?

Preventing Substance Abuse

One of the best ways to mitigate behavior that may lead to tolerance or habituation is education. Frequently, patients do not understand the purpose of the medication or the reason for adhering to the ordered dose. You can help educate patients by teaching them about side effects and cautionary situations (e.g., do not take during pregnancy).

Perhaps a more difficult situation is learning that a member of your office staff is abusing substances. If a health-care provider is impaired (not fully functional mentally or physically) when caring for patients, the consequences can be deadly. The provider, under the influence of alcohol or other substances, may prescribe a wrong drug or be unable to perform minor surgery safely. An addicted staff member may steal drugs from the health-care provider's stock, a facility's medication cart, or even patients. Persons suffering from an addiction go to extreme lengths to obtain their drugs of choice and often lie to cover their behavior. This is the major reason that health-care professionals must be vigilant in maintaining the security of controlled substances. These substances should be locked in a cabinet with two locking doors. Only one person should have responsibility for the key, and the controlled substances should be frequently inventoried. Strict security can prevent the use of an agency's drugs for addictive purposes.

Signs of Substance Abuse

Substance abuse is sometimes extremely difficult to detect until the abuse has become chronic. Many individuals have learned to function adequately under the influence of drugs and/or alcohol and appear normal. Not until you notice the physical changes in their appearance and the deterioration of their work do you begin to suspect that something is wrong. If the person is someone you have worked with for a long time, substance abuse may be the farthest thing from your mind as you try to discover the cause of these changes. Abuse of drugs and/or alcohol can affect most organs of the body. In addition to the physical signs caused by damage done to the liver, kidneys, and other organs, certain behaviors can signal substance abuse. Some of the most common physical symptoms are as follows:

- Changes in sleep habits (either too much or too little energy alters sleep patterns)
- Excessive weight change
- Excessive sweating
- Excessive tremors
- Confusion
- Poor coordination or slow reflexes
- Jaundice
- Dilated or constricted pupils
- Needle marks

Some behaviors signaling substance abuse are as follows:

- Poor work performance
- Sloppy work and frequent mistakes
- Moodiness, including restlessness, irritability, withdrawal, defensiveness, and violent temper outbursts
- Forgetfulness
- Change in personal hygiene (e.g., clothes, bathing)

Additional possible signs and symptoms of substance abuse in a health-care coworker are summarized in Box 4-6.

These signs may not positively indicate drug or alcohol abuse, but they should trigger an investigation into the cause of these changes to protect patients and coworkers, as well as the employee. Typically, people who are addicted may deny substance abuse or minimize the effects of their habit. If you have noticed that someone is impaired, you must focus on ensuring that the person receives treatment.

Treating Substance Abuse

Follow your agency's protocol on referral of impaired employees for substance abuse treatment. Many employers have employee assistance programs or support groups organized through the human resources department. If a patient or family member is suspected of substance abuse, again follow your agency's protocol. Usually, the issue is discussed with the physician before any action is taken.

Be familiar with local resources for treatment, so you can help your colleague or patient by suggesting community resources. Patients and/or families may also come to you for advice about helping a loved one. Having these resources on hand will help them, too.

BOX 4.6 Signs of Possible Substance Abuse in a Coworker

Is frequently late or absent from work because of "illness"

Spends an inappropriate time away from patients and makes strange excuses for the absences

Documents poorly

Does not keep scheduled appointments

Has difficulty working with many staff members

Relates to patients unprofessionally

You must set boundaries and not accommodate the substance abuse by covering up inappropriate behavior. Abusers sometimes lose their families and jobs before they receive help. As a health-care professional, you have the knowledge and ability to help these people obtain the assistance they need.

Substance Abuse and Legal Issues

If any of your colleagues is impaired, report the behavior to your supervisor or office manager immediately. If the impaired colleague has a license, your supervisor should report the behavior to the state Board of Medicine, Board of Nursing, or another board, depending on the license. Most licensing boards will not take away a person's license to practice permanently unless that person has caused serious harm while impaired. The board may limit this colleague's practice for a period of time or indefinitely. For example, a nurse who is having an addiction problem may be barred from working in a facility with controlled substances on the premises. If you fail to report this colleague and he or she harms a patient, coworker, or himself or herself, you could be held responsible because you could have prevented the situation.

If you suspect any other member of the community (e.g., patients, their families, clergy) of being impaired, you need to follow your agency policy regarding the steps to take to handle the situation appropriately. If no one is in danger from the impairment, following your agency policies should protect you legally from any repercussions of your actions.

SUMMARY

- Drug regulations are instituted to protect the public from the use, sale, and consumption of worthless or dangerous medications.
- The FDA approves drugs for sale in the United States, determining which will be available over the counter and which will require a prescription.
- All drugs must be proven safe and effective before they can be approved and marketed. Each drug must go through extensive development and clinical trials.
- Researchers use several phases of clinical trials to test the effects of a drug with the goal of determining effectiveness, side effects, toxicity, and interactions.
- The pharmaceutical company submits a new drug application (NDA) to the FDA, with the results of the scientific testing, for approval.
- The pharmaceutical company gives a new drug a trade name, also known as a brand or proprietary name, for marketing purposes. No other company can use that name.
- The generic name is the official, nonproprietary name for a drug.
- The DEA ensures that addictive drugs are carefully controlled.
- Controlled substances are assigned to one of five schedules according to their potential for addiction and abuse. Schedule I drugs are the most highly addictive and are therefore most controlled.
- Coworkers or patients addicted to drugs need recognition of the addiction and interventions to assist in treatment.

Activities

To make sure that you have learned the key points covered in this chapter, complete the following activities.

True or False

Write true if the statement is true. Beside the false statements, write false and correct the statement to make it true.

1. The DEA approves drugs for dispensing in the United States. _____

_____

2. Schedule II drugs are highly addictive. _____

_____

3. MedWatch is a way of reporting adverse reactions. _____

_____

4. The DEA is a part of the Department of Justice. _____

_____

5. Clinical trials in drug development have two phases. _____

_____

6. Phase IV clinical trials happen after the drug is released to the public. _____

_____

7. In a double-blind clinical trial, neither patients nor clinicians know who is receiving a drug

or a placebo. _____

_____

_____

8. Generic drugs are trademark protected. _____

_____

9. The drug suffix -cillin is closely associated with antibiotics. _____

_____

Multiple Choice

Choose the best answer for each question.

1. Which governmental department enforces the Controlled Substances Act?

   A. DEA

   B. DOJ

   C. FDA

   D. DHHS

2. What is a drug known as during the first three phases of clinical trials?

A. Experimental new drug

B. Investigational new drug

C. Orphan drug

D. Generic drug

E. Chemical drug

3. The goal of phase I drug trials is to test:

A. Toxicity

B. Dosage

C. Control groups

D. Efficacy

4. Once a drug clears the first three phases of clinical trials, it is given a _____ name:

A. Generic

B. Trade

C. Brand

D. Chemical

E. B or C

5. The most addictive schedule of drugs, with no accepted medical use, is:

A. Schedule I

B. Schedule II

C. Schedule III

D. Schedule IV

E. Schedule V

6. An example of a Schedule II drug is:

A. Ritalin

B. Valium

C. Tylenol with codeine

D. Cocaine

7. A damaged controlled substance should be disposed by:

A. Flushing it down the toilet

B. Throwing it in the garbage

C. Destroying it beyond any possible use in the presence of a witness

D. None of the above

8. What schedule includes anabolic steroids?

A. Schedule I

B. Schedule II

C. Schedule III

D. Schedule IV

E. Schedule V

9. **Symptoms of substance abuse include:**

   A. Tremors

   B. Poor judgment

   C. Slurred speech

   D. Changes in behavior

   E. All of the above

10. **The Orphan Drug Act:**

   A. Facilitates the development of drugs for rare diseases

   B. Facilitates the development of drugs for children

   C. Facilitates the development of drugs for almost eradicated diseases

   D. None of the above

Application Exercises

Respond to the following scenarios.

1. You just started a new job in Dr. Johnson's office. When you ask about safety needles for injections, you are told that the office is using nonsafety needles. Is this a problem? What would you do? _____

_____

2. You have a patient diagnosed with a rare form of leukemia. She is thinking of entering clinical trials for a new drug and wants your opinion. What would you say to her? _____

_____

_____

3. At the end of the day, you are counting the scheduled drugs in the locked cabinet and discover that an entire box of morphine is missing. What do you do?_____

_____

_____

4. You are administering an antibiotic injection to a patient. Five minutes after the injection, he has a grand mal seizure. The patient has never had a seizure before, and the physician thinks it may be related to the medication. What do you do, and to whom do you report this? _____

_____

_____

5. You are the office manager in a busy family practice. You have a medical assistant who has incurred a dirty needlestick four times this month. What should you do? _____

_____

_____

1. Visit http://www.accessdata.fda.gov/scripts/opdlisting/oopd/index.cfm, and find two orphan drugs under current research and their orphan designation.

2. Check out the FDA's website at https://www.fda.gov/. Search for and download MedWatch Form 3500. Fill it out as though you were reporting adverse effects of a medication.

3. Visit http://deadiversion.usdoj.gov. According to the DEA controlled substances schedules list, under which schedule is each of the following classified?
Marinol
Kaolin Pectin PG
Meperidine
Midazolam

4. The following website offers information on drug misuse: http://www.dea.gov. Find out how to obtain information on teaching children not to abuse drugs.

5. Visit the Association for Addiction Professionals at http://naadac.org, and find a list of clinicians who treat impaired professionals in your area.

6. Go to your favorite search engine, and search for your state's board of medicine and board of nursing. Write the address and phone number for each.

Prescriptions and Labels

*P*rescription drugs require the control of a prescriber to ensure that the patient does not take dangerous or inappropriate medication. The physician or other prescriber must first evaluate the patient to diagnose the illness or condition requiring medication. For example, although patients may be able to choose an over-the-counter (OTC) medication to treat mild headaches, they need health-care providers with medical training to evaluate the cause of severe or debilitating headaches and to identify an appropriate medicine. The more serious the illness requiring medication is, the more likely it will be that the medication is available by prescription only.

A key element in keeping the patient safe is ensuring the accuracy of prescriptions for medications. Drugs have a variety of names, are developed from several sources, are administered by different routes, and act in various ways. Therefore, the prescriber must give specific information to avoid mistakes when prescriptions are filled or medications are administered. As a health-care professional, you must ensure the safe transfer of information from the prescriber through the patient to the pharmacist. To do so, you must memorize abbreviations and understand the parts of the prescription. You also need to be able to read labels and prescriptions to educate patients about taking their medication safely. This chapter discusses the types of prescriber orders, the parts of prescriptions, and medication labels.

LEARNING OUTCOMES

At the end of this chapter, you should be able to:

5.1 Define all key terms.
5.2 Discuss precautions to ensure patient safety.
5.3 Identify the parts of a legal prescription.

5.4 Differentiate among three different types of medication orders.

5.5 List which health-care providers are able to write prescriptions.

5.6 Define abbreviations used in prescriptions.

5.7 Interpret labels safely.

5.8 Discuss the impact of e-prescribing on health-care consumers.

KEY TERMS

Automatic stop orders	Medication orders	Standing orders	Superscription
Electronic prescription	Rx	STAT orders	Verbal orders
Inscription	Signature	Subscription	

■ MEDICATION ORDERS

Medication orders are the prescriptions provided by a physician for a patient for a specific medication. Medication orders include written orders, verbal or standing orders, and stop orders. Prescriptions are dispensed only by health-care professionals who are licensed to do so. Pharmacists are licensed in all 50 states to dispense medications, and therefore must understand all of the different types of medication orders and the prescription itself. The prescription order itself contains some basic information, such as the preprinted prescriber's name and contact information. Knowing the basic parts of a medication order aids in ensuring the patient's safety because of the many different medications, routes of administration, and times for taking them. This knowledge also helps to prevent errors and to teach patients important facts about their medications. Review the abbreviations presented in Chapter 3 (Tables 3-2 and 3-3); in addition, Table 5-1 lists common abbreviations used. Abbreviations can vary from one setting to the next, so be sure to check which are—and are not—accepted at your workplace. The most accepted abbreviations along with the commonly misinterpreted abbreviations can be found on the Institute for Safe Medication Practices website (www.ismp.org).

Written Orders

Obtain a written order for a prescription whenever possible, to decrease the chance of misinterpretation of information written on the order and subsequent errors. Legally, every drug that is ordered, administered, or dispensed must also have written documentation by the prescriber. Having this information in writing protects the health-care professional who administers or dispenses the drug from possible later discrepancies between what the prescriber meant to order and what was actually given or administered. The prescriber should write or type the prescription accurately. A health-care facility is a busy workplace, and errors result from haste or sloppy penmanship. As a health-care professional, you help ensure the patient's safety by proofreading a prescription before the patient takes it to the pharmacy. If a prescriber has poor handwriting, offer to write or type the prescription, and then have the prescriber

---

TABLE 5.1 Abbreviations Related to Medication Administration

Abbreviation	Meaning	Abbreviation	Meaning
cap	capsule	mL	milliliter
elix	elixir	Mg	milligram
G	gram	Oz	ounce
Gr	grain	Tab	tablet
Gtt	drops	T, Tb	tablespoon
mcg	microgram	t, tsp	teaspoon
mEq	milliequivalent		

read and sign it. The exception is a prescription for a Schedule II drug, which must be written by the prescriber.

Verbal Orders

When a prescriber has the health-care professional write the prescription, these instructions are **verbal orders.** For example, a physician may not be present, so the order is given over the telephone. Check with your supervisor to see whether you are allowed to take a verbal order. If so, write words and numbers carefully, and be sure to read what you have written back to the prescriber to ensure that the information is correct. Some offices require that the prescriber also repeat the information back to you. In rare instances, a physician may give a verbal order during an emergency situation. This is known as a **STAT** order, meaning to give immediately. This should be the only instance in which you give a patient a medication without a written order when the prescriber is present. If the situation is not an emergency, you should write the order, and have the prescriber sign it before the medication is administered or dispensed. In all instances, the prescriber must sign the order as soon as possible. Again, this procedure legally protects the health-care worker from discrepancies between what the prescriber intended and what was administered. Verbal orders are not permitted for Schedule II drugs unless it is an emergency and meets specific criteria. Those criteria include the following:

- The quantity prescribed and dispensed is limited to the amount required for the emergency period.
- The pharmacist will immediately write the prescription, which will contain all information required except for the signature of the prescribing individual.
- The pharmacist will make a reasonable effort to determine that the oral authorization legitimately came from the prescribing individual.
- Within 7 days of authorizing an emergency oral prescription, the prescribing individual will have a written prescription for the emergency quantity prescribed and delivered to the dispensing pharmacist including "Authorization for Emergency Dispensing" and the date of the oral order listed on the prescription.

Electronic Prescription Orders

A newer type of medication order is the **electronic prescription** (e-prescription). The prescriber creates the prescription electronically and sends it directly to the patient's pharmacy. In many instances, the electronic prescribing network used by the medical insurance companies and pharmacies can immediately verify insurance coverage for medications. Some electronic prescribing network programs manage the patient's medication history, to identify any medication interactions or other problems before the patient receives the ordered medication. E-prescriptions bypass the typical problems of written prescriptions, such as illegible writing, loss of the written document, and missing information on the prescription.

A CLOSER LOOK 5.1: Internet Pharmacies

With the soaring cost of prescription medication in the United States and the high numbers of Americans without medical insurance, many people are turning to Internet pharmacies. Many legitimate Canadian companies take a written prescription and fill it with lower-cost Canadian medications.

Standing Orders

A prescriber may leave a list of **standing orders** to be used in specific routine circumstances. For example, before a diagnostic test, a prescriber may require the patient to have nothing by mouth (NPO) after midnight, have an enema, follow with a clear liquid diet, and take an antibiotic. It is important to verify standing orders with the prescriber. These standing orders need to be reviewed and updated regularly, usually on an annual basis. Like all other orders, standing orders are not exempt from a timely signature and must be signed by the prescriber as soon as possible.

Stop Orders

Automatic stop orders are given for a limited time only. A common example is an order for Schedule II and III drugs after an injury or surgical procedure. Most likely, the patient will experience some level of pain for a short time following the injury or surgery, and the physician therefore orders a Schedule II narcotic analgesic to be taken every 4 hours as needed. Because this prescription cannot be refilled unless the prescriber renews it, the patient is less likely to become addicted to the medication. Another example is an antibiotic to be taken twice a day for 10 days. The order stops after 10 days and is not refilled unless the prescriber renews it. To "d/c" an order is to discontinue it.

Regardless of the order, the prescription must be clear. Patients can suffer serious consequences or possibly die if a pharmacist misinterprets a prescription and gives the wrong medication or the wrong dose. Your role is to be the safety check before the prescription is sent to the pharmacist, to make sure the information is accurate and legible.

 CRITICAL THINKING

You review a prescription and find that you cannot determine whether the medication is Trileptal (an antiseizure medication) or Tylenol 3 (a narcotic pain reliever). What would the difference mean to the patient if the wrong drug were given? What should you do in this situation?

■ PARTS OF A PRESCRIPTION

The prescription is a written record of the prescriber's order. In addition to physicians, nurse practitioners and physician assistants are allowed to prescribe medications. Prescription privileges differ from state to state. Research and learn who can prescribe medications in your state. Be sure the person ordering the medication is lawfully allowed to do so. On every prescription pad, the prescriber is identified by name and, if he or she is licensed to prescribe scheduled drugs, the prescriber's Drug Enforcement Administration (DEA) number. Only the patient whose name is on the prescription should take the medication.

Drugs are ordered in facilities such as hospitals, outpatient surgery centers, and prescribers' offices. Because you will probably have the most contact with prescriptions in a prescriber's office, that setting is the main focus of this discussion.

Every prescription must include two types of information, administrative information and specific information relating to the dispensing of the medication. The administrative information for controlled dangerous substances (CDS) must include the name, address, telephone number, and DEA number of the prescriber; the name and address of the patient; and the date of the order. For non-CDS prescriptions, it is not required by law to obtain either the patient's or the prescriber's address. The following list provides details for some of these parts:

■ Date. Including the date of the order is important for filing insurance claims and for linking the drug therapy with the office visit. The date of the order should match the date of the office visit, even though patients may not fill the prescription for up to 1 month after the visit because they may receive free samples at the office or emergency department. Prescriptions should never be postdated.

■ Physician's name, contact information, and DEA number. Large medical groups may use one prescription form with all the legal prescribers listed, or they may have separate prescription forms for each prescriber. All prescribers licensed to prescribe scheduled drugs must have their DEA numbers preprinted on the prescription form.

> ### A CLOSER LOOK 5.2: **Drug Enforcement Administration Numbers**
>
> Pharmacists can verify the legitimacy of the DEA number found on a prescription by the following method: Each number has two letters followed by seven digits. The first letter is always A or B, based on when the number was issued (A is earlier than B). The second letter is the first letter of the prescriber's name. The seven digits have a mathematical relationship that is always followed. Try the formula to see whether BW1342586 is a valid DEA number:
>
> Add the first, third, and fifth numbers. In this case, 1 + 4 + 5 = 10
>
> Now add the second, fourth, and sixth numbers: 3 + 2 + 8 = 13
>
> Double the sum just calculated: 13 × 2 = 26
>
> Add this to the first sum: 26 + 10 = 36
>
> Take the last digit in that sum (36, the first digit is 3, the last digit is 6).
>
> The final digit in this DEA number must be 6.
>
> If the final digit in this number were anything but a 6, the DEA number would be fraudulent.

■ **Patient's name, address, and date of birth.** Be sure that the current address of the patient appears on the prescription form; write it on the form if it is not there already, and check with the patient to be sure it is correct. Including the patient's birth date on the prescription helps the pharmacist ensure that the drug and dosage prescribed are appropriate for the age group of this patient.

The second type of information on the prescription that relates to the dispensing of the medication includes **Rx** or the **superscription,** which means "take thou" and is an abbreviation for prescription or treatment; **inscription** (name of drug, dosage, and quantity to be dispensed); directions for taking the drug **(signature);** refill numbers **(subscription);** a notation about whether a generic drug can be used; and the signature of the prescriber (Fig. 5-1).

■ **Inscription (name of drug, dosage, and quantity to be dispensed).** The drug name must be clearly identified. The prescriber may write the generic or brand name on the order. The prescriber also notes whether a generic drug can be substituted for a brand name drug. This information may be indicated with a checked box, or it may be written out as "do not substitute" or "dispense as written" if the prescriber prefers the brand name drug. As noted in Chapter 4, insurance companies and health maintenance organizations (HMOs) usually prefer paying for the less-expensive drug. However, some patients are allergic to dyes or fillers found in certain generic drugs. For these patients, the brand name drug is the best choice.

The dosage is a crucial piece of information. Make sure that the strength of the drug is clearly indicated. Missing a decimal point or a zero (e.g., 25 mg instead of 2.5 mg or 0.25 mg instead of 25 mg) can harm a patient. Again, the Institute for Safe Medication Practices covers the appropriate and inappropriate use of decimals (www.ismp.org). If a dose seems inappropriate, check your drug resources before giving the patient the prescription, and if the dose still does not seem right, check it with the prescriber.

The quantity to be dispensed is indicated by a number after a pound sign (#). In addition, this number should be written out. Adding a zero at the end or a 1 in front of a number is simple, but a number that is also written out is not so easily changed. For an acute problem, the drug may be given for only a short time. Thus, perhaps only a 1-week or 1-month supply is given. A patient with a chronic condition may require a 90-day supply and three refills to continue the drug treatment for 1 year.

■ **Signature.** The signature is from *signetur,* a Latin word for "write on the label." It instructs the patient when and how to take the drug. Prescribers use standardized abbreviations when

```
              Ⓐ CARL NEWELL, M.D.          DEA# _____
                   125 Main Street
                 Hometown, VA 22958
                  (703) 555-0106


Ⓑ  Connie Martin                    Ⓒ  Date: __11/14/20xx__
   789 Beach Tree Drive
   Hometown, VA 22958
   D.O.B. 6/2/78

        Ⓓ  Rx

         Ⓔ  Colace 100 mg
             Tablets #30
         Ⓕ  1 tab PO qhs
Ⓖ  Refills:    None   1   2  ③  4

   May substitute generic          ☐
Ⓗ
   May not substitute generic      ☐   Ⓘ  _____
                                              Signature
```

FIGURE 5-1: Sample prescription. A prescription has several parts: (A) name, address, telephone number, and Drug Enforcement Administration (DEA) number of the prescriber; (B) patient's name, address, and date of birth; (C) date; (D) Rx (abbreviation for prescription or treatment); (E) inscription (name of drug, dosage, and quantity to be dispensed); (F) signature (directions to the patient); (G) number of refills; (H) whether a generic drug can be used; and (I) prescriber's signature.

writing prescriptions. For example, a prescriber may write "1 tab q4h prn." This Latin is not understood by most patients, so the pharmacist writes the following on the medication label: "Take one tablet by mouth every 4 hours as needed."

■ **Subscription (refill).** The prescriber may specify how many refills are allowed before the patient must return to the office. Patients with chronic conditions may not return to the office for some time. For these patients, refill orders facilitate the continuity of care.

■ **Physician's signature.** Prescriptions are not valid unless they are signed by the physician. Although the prescription may be completely written by the health-care professional (except for Schedule II drug prescriptions), the prescriber must sign the prescription.

CRITICAL THINKING

If most patients do not understand Latin, why do you think physicians write the signature in Latin?

If a patient calls for a refill, the prescriber may refill the prescription without asking to see the patient again, especially if the patient has a chronic condition or is taking birth control pills. After the refill has been approved, the health-care professional must document in the patient's medical record that the prescription was telephoned to the pharmacy.

CRITICAL THINKING

You work in a busy gynecologist's office. Many women run out of birth control pills before you can schedule them to come to the office. Create a protocol for refilling oral contraceptives without seeing the patient.

◼ DRUG LABELS

Drug labeling is all the printed information that is provided with a drug. This labeling is regulated by the Food and Drug Administration (FDA), which specifies exactly what must appear on the label.

Manufacturer Labels

The manufacturers place their information on the medication bottle or package they provide to the health-care facilities and pharmacies. The manufacturers also include information on the package insert they include with the medication. The label contains the strength of the medication, the form it comes in, the quantity of medication in the container, the lot and NDC numbers, the manufacturer name, storage information, and expiration dates. Prescription medications will have "RX ONLY" on the label. A controlled dangerous substance (CDS) will have the schedule number on the label and a large C with the Roman numeral inside, e.g., ℂ. The package insert provides more detailed information for the health-care provider in regard to this medication, including, but not limited to, forms and strengths of the drug available, mixing of and stability of the medication, adverse reactions, patient counseling information, and full prescribing information.

Medication Labels

The medication label placed on the container by the dispensing pharmacist contains important information (Fig. 5-2). It includes the pharmacy's name, address, and telephone number, which are useful in case the patient needs to contact the pharmacy with problems or questions. The dispensing date is also on the label. This date may differ from the date when the prescriber wrote the prescription. The pharmacist originates an Rx number that identifies this unique prescription in the computer system and on the label. The patient can refill the prescription by using this number. The patient's full name and address is included, as are the name of the medication. In addition, the following must be included on the label:

◼ **Strength of drug dispensed:** It is important to know the concentration of the medication, meaning how weak or strong it is.

◼ **The dosage form:** It is the ordered medication being dispensed in the form of a tablet, liquid, or aerosol, for example.

◼ **Amount of drug dispensed.** The amount of medication contained in the prescription bottle must be listed. This information is listed as a number and, if the medication is in liquid form,

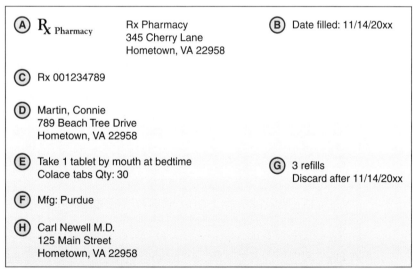

FIGURE 5-2: Sample medication label. A drug label has several parts: (A) name, address, and telephone number of the pharmacy; (B) date when the prescription was filled; (C) Rx (prescription) number; (D) name and address of the patient; (E) directions to the patient (Latin abbreviations translated into English for the patient), and name and quantity of medication; (F) the manufacturer; (G) number of refills and expiration date; and (H) name of the prescriber.

the unit of measure, such as 120 mL or 8 ounces. Labels for liquid medications also give the concentration of the liquid (e.g., 100 mg per 5 mL). Labels for pills, tablets, and capsules usually state simple quantity (e.g., Qty: 60).

- **Warning labels.** The pharmacist places appropriate warning labels on the prescription container to make sure that patients understand the best way to take the medication and become aware of possible situations to avoid. These warning labels are usually a bright color, to make sure they are not overlooked (Fast Tip 5.1).

- **The manufacturer:** If the drug is generic, it is important to know which manufacturer made this particular medication as each one has slightly different ingredients and may affect the patient in a different way.

- **Refill information:** It is important for the patient to know how many refills, if any, they are allowed to have on this medication.

- **The prescriber name:** The label contains the name of the prescribing professional. For accuracy, the prescriber's name and perhaps license classification (e.g., MD or FNP) are included.

- **Expiration date:** The pharmacist also adds the date when the medication will expire or lose its potency and should be discarded.

The pharmacist translates the Latin abbreviations into English for the patient (compare Fig. 5-1 with Fig. 5-2). It is important for the patient to understand the order, but the patient may be hesitant to ask a pharmacist about it. Therefore, before the patient leaves the medical office, be sure he or she knows how to take the drug. Also, instruct the patient to read the label on the medication bottle carefully.

CHECK UP 5.1: ABBREVIATIONS

Before completing the rest of the chapter, test yourself on the following abbreviations. If you do not know some of them, make flash cards to help you memorize them.

$\bar{a}$ _____	gtt _____	o.u. _____
a.c. _____	hs _____	oz _____
a.d. _____	ID _____	$\bar{p}$ _____
a.s. _____	IM _____	p.c. _____
a.u. _____	IV _____	prn _____
bid _____	mcg _____	$\bar{s}$ _____
$\bar{c}$ _____	mEq _____	SC _____
cap _____	mg _____	STAT _____
d/c _____	mL _____	Tb _____
elix _____	NPO _____	tid _____
g _____	o.d. _____	tsp _____
gr _____	o.s. _____	

Fast Tip 5.1 Warning Labels

Remind patients to check for any warning and instruction labels the pharmacist added to the container. Examples of warnings and instructions include:

- Shake well.
- Keep refrigerated.
- For the ear.
- Take medication on an empty stomach.
- Do not drink alcoholic beverages when taking this medication.
- Do not take dairy products, antacids, or iron preparations within 1 hour of taking this medication.
- Avoid prolonged or excessive exposure to direct or artificial sunlight while taking this medication.

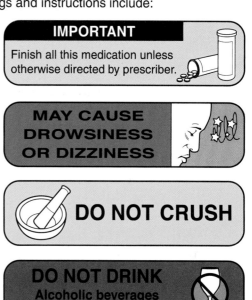

Manufacturer Information

Stock medications stored in the office must be labeled with the necessary information to ensure safe administration. This information should include the brand (trade) name, generic name, drug strength and drug form, route of administration, total amount of medication in the container, directions for reconstitution if necessary, National Drug Code (NDC), expiration date, and lot number (Fig. 5-3).

- **Trade name.** This is the brand name given to the drug by the manufacturer with the patent rights to this drug. The trade name is always capitalized to differentiate it from the generic name.

- **Generic name.** This is the official name given to the drug by the U.S. Pharmacopeia. The generic name is almost always lowercase except when it is capitalized to begin a sentence.

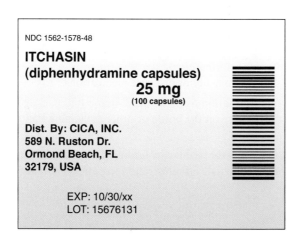

FIGURE 5-3: Sample manufacturer label. The manufacturer's label should include the brand (trade) name, generic name, drug strength and drug form, route of administration if other than oral, total amount of medication in the container, directions for reconstitution if necessary, manufacturer, National Drug Code (NDC), expiration date, and lot number.

■ **Drug strength and form.** The amount of active drug (e.g., milligrams, micrograms, grains) is listed on the label, as is the form or unit of measure in which the active drug is contained (e.g., tablets, capsules, teaspoons, milliliters).

■ **Route of administration.** This instruction explains how the patient is to take the medication. Most medication labels on drugs for parenteral use list the acceptable administration routes. For oral drugs, the common assumption is that a tablet will be given by mouth, and the oral route therefore is not listed.

■ **Total quantity.** The quantity indicates the total amount of medication in the container in tablets, capsules, caplets, or milliliters. If the drug is in powder form, the quantity designation will identify the total medication weight in the package, as well as the total concentration and total number of milliliters in the package if reconstituted according to label instructions.

■ **NDC number and lot number.** The NDC number assigned to each medication identifies the manufacturer, product, and size of the container. This information is listed on the label as NDC followed by a 10-digit number. The lot number links this package to a specific batch of drugs manufactured in a particular place over a given period of time. This information is important when a problem is found with a drug, such as contamination by a pesticide or other substance. The FDA can usually pinpoint the problem to a specific lot and can issue a recall for that lot number alone.

More contact information is available on the package insert in regard to the manufacturer as well as more detailed drug information than that included on the label or packaging.

Prescription drugs are not the only medications that include medication labels. OTC drugs, purchased without a prescription, also contain labels or instructions on drug use based on age and weight. The FDA has determined that, if the consumer takes an OTC medication as directed on the label, the drug is safe for the general population, although the medication may cause side effects, which are also listed on the label. As with prescription drugs, it is important for patients taking OTC drugs to read the label, including the dosage and any possible side effects. OTC drugs can interact negatively with prescription drugs. For example, some cold medicines increase the action of sedatives, so a person taking both medications would be sleepier than expected.

●●● SUMMARY

■ Medication orders take a variety of forms including handwritten or typed, verbal, or electronic directly to the pharmacy.

■ Standing medication orders are used in specific routine circumstances such as diagnostic tests.

■ Stop medication orders are given for a limited time. Stop orders cannot be refilled unless the prescriber renews it.

■ Prescriptions must contain a set amount of information allowing the pharmacist to safely dispense medications to the patient. There are two types of information required. The administrative information includes the doctor's and patient's contact information as well as the physician's credentials and the patient's date of birth. The second type of information give specifics such as which drug is to be dispensed and in what quantity, strength, and form.

■ Drug labels are required to provide information to allow patients to safely receive medications.

   ■ The manufacturer must provide information on the label and on a package insert to allow health-care providers to safely administer or dispense medications.

   ■ Pharmacists must translate information from the prescription and package labeling onto the medication label that they place on the bottle or other packaging they provide to the patient.

   ■ Medications that are kept as stock in the health-care facility must also have the manufacturer-provided information label to allow safe administration to patients in that facility.

Activities

To make sure that you have learned the key points covered in this chapter, complete the following activities.

True or False

Write true if the statement is true. Beside the false statements, write false and correct the statement to make it true.

1. Physicians are the only health-care professionals allowed to write prescriptions. _____

2. The DEA issues a specific number to those prescribers who write prescriptions for scheduled drugs. _____

3. There is only one type of medication order. _____

4. The abbreviation gtt stands for drops. _____

5. NDC code stands for National Drug Code. _____

6. OTC medications are never dangerous. _____

7. A pharmacist can decide whether a generic drug can be used for a brand name drug.

8. A STAT order is a standing order. _____

9. An automatic stop order means to discontinue the medication after a specified period of time. _____

10. Rx is the abbreviation for prescription or treatment. _____

Choose the best answer for each question.

1. Which of the following explains how to take a medication?

A. Inscription

B. Superscription

C. Subscription

D. Signature

2. The abbreviation for three times per day is:

A. bid

B. o.d.

C. hs

D. tid

3. Which abbreviation means without?

A. $\bar{p}$

B. x

C. $\bar{s}$

D. $\bar{c}$

E. w

4. Which abbreviation means drops?

A. g

B. gr

C. gtt

D. mg

5. Which abbreviation means to give the drug immediately?

A. prn

B. STAT

C. NPO

D. d/c

6. The abbreviation for two times per day is:

A. bid

B. o.d.

C. hs

D. tid

7. Which abbreviation means with?

A. w

B. x

C. $\bar{c}$

D. $\bar{s}$

8. Which abbreviation means to take as needed?

    A. STAT

    B. prn

    C. NPO

    D. tid

9. Which abbreviation means that the patient should take nothing by mouth?

    A. prn

    B. STAT

    C. NPO

    D. d/c

10. Which of the following are examples of warning labels?

    A. Shake well.

    B. Keep refrigerated.

    C. Do not take with dairy products.

    D. Avoid prolonged exposure to the sun.

    E. All of the above.

Application Exercises

Respond to the following situations.

1. What standing orders may be necessary for Henry to have a barium enema diagnostic

    test? _____

    _____

    _____

2. Write a prescription for Brittany for the following: Feldene 20-mg capsules. Quantity of 30.

    Take one every day before breakfast. _____

    _____

    _____

3. The physician frequently misplaces prescription pads. How should these pads be stored to

    ensure that they are not misused? _____

    _____

    _____

4. Prednisone is ordered: four pills today, three tomorrow, two the day after tomorrow, one

    the day after that, and then stop. How many pills are dispensed? _____

    _____

    _____

5. How does the label read for the following prescription? Warren Short. Nitroglycerin tablets. 0.4 mg sublingually every 5 minutes, up to three tablets for chest pain. Dr. Clark Castillo wants him to have 60 tablets. The prescription may be refilled as needed, but once the bottle is opened, the tablets should be used for only 6 months. _____

_____

_____

6. Donna is prescribed doxycycline 100-mg tablets. This prescription is for 20 tablets, with two taken as an initial dose, then one tablet every 12 hours until the supply is exhausted. How would you document this prescription in Donna's chart? _____

_____

_____

7. Create a prescription for the following: Dr. Campbell wants Peter to have Tylenol 3 (a controlled substance) for pain: one to two tablets every 4 to 6 hours as he needs the medication. Dr. Campbell wants the patient to have 30 tablets. No refills. _____

_____

_____

8. Theresa, a nurse practitioner, wants Sharon to take potassium tablets daily. Write the prescription for K-Dur, 20 mEq once daily in the morning for 90 days. The prescription can be refilled three times. _____

_____

_____

Internet Research
Visit http://bemedwise.org, and:

■ Click on the "Be MedWise" pulldown menu. Select "Use Your Prescription Medicines Safely," and then "How to Read Prescription Drug Labels." Identify the two warnings listed on the "Prescription Label."

■ Search for "College Resource Kit." Select one of the PDFs and create a plan for implementing the plan on your campus.

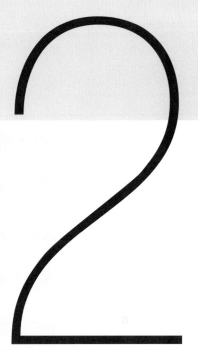

Calculations

Review of Mathematics

In your career as a health-care professional, you may be required to use calculations to care competently for the patients you serve. The next three chapters cover dosage calculations. This chapter includes a review of fractions, decimals and percents, ratios and proportions, and solving for unknowns. If you fear mathematics and do not master the problems included in the chapters, you will continue to struggle with mathematical concepts. The more you read these chapters and the more problems you solve, the easier it will be to understand how to calculate dosages safely. If you are still uncomfortable with any of these problems, review the exercises in this chapter, and ask your instructor for further guidance. See Appendix H for a basic review of whole numbers calculation (addition, subtraction, multiplication, and division).

You should also use the Calculating Drug Dosages tutorial (available online at www.davisplus.com). This interactive tutorial contains many dosage calculation problems and takes you step-by-step through solving them. It is a great tool for learning dosage calculations, and you should use it frequently to become comfortable with this important aspect of health care.

LEARNING OUTCOMES

At the end of this chapter, you should be able to:

6.1 Define all key terms.
6.2 Discuss numerical relationships.
6.3 Perform calculations involving whole numbers.
6.4 Calculate problems using fractions.
6.5 Find the least common denominator.
6.6 Perform calculations involving decimals.
6.7 Calculate percents, ratios, and proportions.
6.8 Solve problems for an unknown quantity.

KEY TERMS		
Decimal	Improper fraction	Percents
Denominator	Invert	Proper fraction
Dividend	Least common	Proportion
Divisor	denominator	Ratios
Extremes	Means	Scored
Factors	Mixed number	Whole numbers
Fraction	Numerator	

■ WORKING WITH FRACTIONS

A **fraction** is simply a part of a whole. Understanding fractions is important because often a dose that must be administered is not a **whole number.** If we do not understand how fractions function, patients will be in danger of receiving the incorrect dosage.

Suppose you have a whole pizza and want to give some to your friends. You can divide the pizza into slices of varying sizes (Fig. 6-1). For example, you can divide the pizza into three pieces or four pieces; a slice of pizza from the three-piece division is larger than a slice of pizza from the four-piece division. In other words:

1/3 is greater than 1/4
1/4 is less than 1/3

The number on the top is called the **numerator.** It is part of the whole being divided. The **denominator** is the number on the bottom. It represents the total number of equal parts in the problem.

If the numerator is smaller than the denominator, the fraction is called a **proper fraction** (Fig. 6-2). In the pizza example, if you have three friends and divide the pizza into four pieces, each of your three friends will have a piece, and that leaves one piece (1/4) for you.

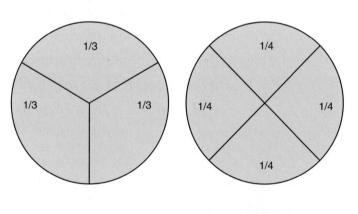

FIGURE 6-1: Fractions. Slices of a pie (represented as this circle) divided into three sections are larger than slices of a pie divided into four sections: 1/3 is larger than 1/4.

FIGURE 6-2: Proper fraction. This figure shows the proper fraction 2/5. It is a proper fraction because the numerator (top number) is smaller than the denominator (bottom number).

CRITICAL THINKING

What happens to the pizza slices when a numerator becomes larger? A denominator becomes larger? If you have trouble remembering this concept, ask yourself what would happen if you and your siblings were inheriting money? The more brothers and sisters you have, the smaller your share would be.

An **improper fraction** means that the numerator is larger than the denominator. It is top-heavy. For example, you divide a pizza into four pieces but have five friends (5/4). You will need to find another pizza or cut smaller pieces (Fig. 6-3 and Check Up 6.1 to 6.3).

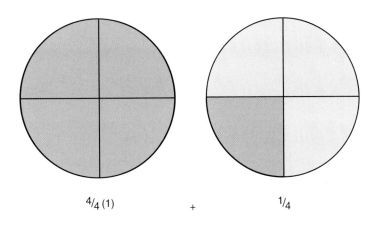

4/4 (1)   +   1/4

= 5/4 or 1 1/4

FIGURE 6-3: Improper fraction. If you divide a pie into four pieces but have five friends, you need to find another pie, be "improper," or cut smaller pieces. This illustration shows the improper fraction of 5/4. You can also write 1 1/4 because 5/4 = 4/4 (or 1) + 1/4.

 CHECK UP 6.1: FRACTION SIZES

Circle the fraction with the largest value in each listing. Then, using the same numbers, underline the lowest value in each listing.

4/25, 5/25, 10/25   1/75, 1/100, 1/125

1/300, 1/200, 1/100   4/8, 1/8, 2/8

5/3, 2/3, 4/3

Circle the fraction with the lowest value, and underline the highest.

1/10, 1/8, 1/6   2/16, 1/16, 4/16

3/6, 2/6, 5/6   2/12, 1/12, 6/12

1/25, 1/75, 1/50

CHECK UP 6.2: SHADE THE PIZZAS

In each of the circles, divide the pizza into the denominator, and shade the numerator.

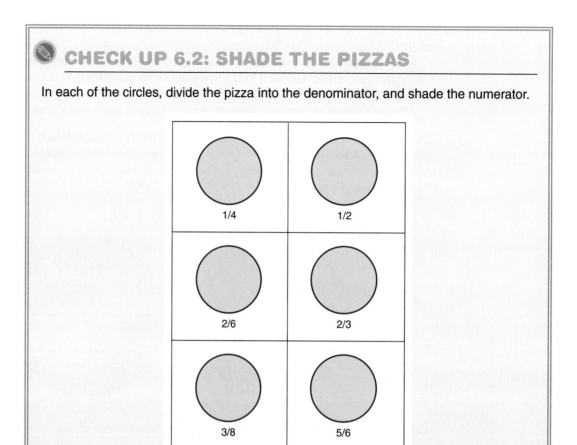

CHECK UP 6.3: IMPROPER FRACTIONS

1. Shade the circles to represent the improper fraction 16/5.
2. Draw each fraction on a separate sheet, and use shading to represent the fraction.

| 8/4 | 13/5 | 5/3 | 3/2 | 15/6 |

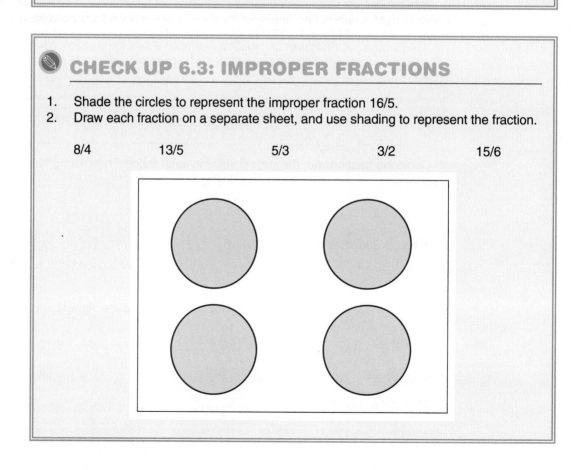

Least Common Denominators

A common denominator is a number that is a common multiple of two (or more) denominators. Finding the lowest number into which both denominators can be divided to keep the fraction small makes it easier to work with and is called the **least common denominator (LCD).** To find the LCD of two or more fractions:

■ List the multiples of each denominator.

■ Compare the lists. Any numbers that appear on all lists are common denominators.

■ The lowest number that appears on all lists is the LCD.

Example: 1/9 + 1/6
Write the multiples of each denominator:
9 » 9...**18**...27...36
6 » 6...12...**18**...24...36

As you can see, both 18 and 36 are common denominators of 9 and 6. However, 18 is the LCD. Once you have the LCD, it becomes the denominator of each fraction. Using this example, determine what number, when multiplied, would give you the LCD. In this case, if you multiplied 9 by 2, you would have 18, which would become the denominator.

$$9 \times 2 = 18$$

Next, multiply 2 by the numerator, which is 1. Your fraction would then be 2/18. For the fraction of 1/6, the denominator is 6. You would multiply 6 by 3 to make 18, and then multiply the 1 by 3 and place it over 18. Thus:

$$1/9 + 1/6 = 2/18 + 3/18 = 5/18$$

In Check Up 6.4 and 6.5, test your knowledge of working with fractions.

Mixed Numbers and Improper Fractions

A **mixed number** is a whole number plus a fraction (for example: 5 1/2). You will need to know how to convert mixed numbers into improper fractions as you work with various medication orders and dosages. To do this:

Multiply the denominator by the whole number.

$$2 \text{ (denominator)} \times 5 \text{ (whole number)} = 10$$

■ Add the result from the first step to the numerator.

$$10 + 1 \text{ (numerator)} = 11$$

■ Keep the denominator.

11/2

 CHECK UP 6.4: LEAST COMMON DENOMINATORS

Find the least common denominator, and then work out the problem on a separate sheet.

1/15 + 1/45 = _____   3/8 + 1/6 = _____   3/25 + 4/75 = _____

1/3 + 3/8 = _____   4/5 + 5/12 = _____   1/4 + 3/16 = _____

5/12 + 1/10 = _____   5/6 + 3/5 = _____

1/4 + 1/5 = _____   1/2 + 1/19 = _____

CHECK UP 6.5: TAKING FRACTIONS APART

Examine the fraction 3/4.

1. What are the total equal parts in one whole? _____

2. What is the size of each part? _____

3. How many parts are being talked about? _____

4. The numerator is _____.

5. The denominator is _____.

The reverse is also necessary—learning how to convert improper fractions to mixed numbers. The process for this is as follows:

■ Divide the numerator by the denominator.

29 (numerator) ÷ 5 = 5 (remainder of 4)

■ The remainder becomes the numerator.

5 4/5

■ The denominator stays the same.

29/5 = 5 4/5

In Check Up 6.6 and 6.7, convert the mixed numbers to improper fractions and vice versa.

 ## CHECK UP 6.6: CONVERTING

Convert these mixed numbers to improper fractions.

3 1/3 = _____   6 1/4 = _____   1 1/6 = _____

9 1/2 = _____   10 2/5 = _____

 ## CHECK UP 6.7: CONVERTING

Convert these improper fractions to mixed numbers.

28/5 = _____   30/7 = _____   7/6 = _____

42/5 = _____   52/10 = _____

Reducing to Lowest Terms

Because large numbers can be more difficult to work with, learning how to reduce a number to its lowest term is important. **Factors** (numbers multiplied together to make another number) are used to determine the largest common divisor (the biggest whole number that reduces multiple whole numbers) to divide the **dividend** (the number you want to reduce). In this case, both the numerator and denominator are divided.

To reduce a larger fraction, such as 6/10, to its lowest term, follow these steps:

■ Determine the largest common divisor.

Determine the factors of each number:

$$6$$
$$1 \times 6 = 6$$
$$2 \times 3 = 6$$
Factors of 6 are therefore 1, **2**, 3, and 6.
$$10$$
$$1 \times 10 = 10$$
$$2 \times 5 = 10$$
Factors of 10 are therefore 1, **2**, 5, and 10.

Compare the two lists of factors, and determine the highest number common to both lists. In this instance, 2 is the highest number on both lists; thus, both 6 and 10 are divisible by 2.

■ Divide the numerator and denominator by this number to reduce it to its lowest terms (Check Up 6.8).

$$6 \div 2 = 3$$
$$10 \div 2 = 5$$

Adding Fractions

At times, a patient is required to take partial tablets. When computing a month's supply of medication, you must be able to calculate how many tablets the patient takes per day because pharmacies do not dispense partial tablets. Adding fractions is easy when they have the same denominator.

■ Add the numerators.

Example: 1/4 +1/4
$$1 + 1 = 2$$

■ Place the sum (what you find when you add) over the denominator.

2/4

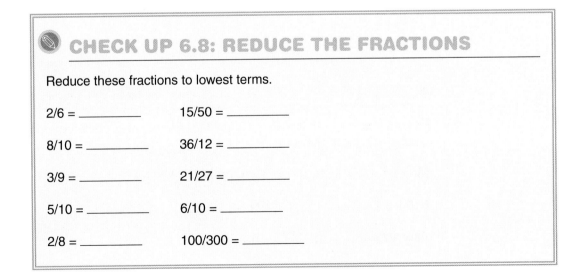

✎ CHECK UP 6.8: REDUCE THE FRACTIONS

Reduce these fractions to lowest terms.

2/6 = _____   15/50 = _____

8/10 = _____   36/12 = _____

3/9 = _____   21/27 = _____

5/10 = _____   6/10 = _____

2/8 = _____   100/300 = _____

■ Reduce to the lowest terms.

$$2 \div 2 = 1$$
$$4 \div 2 = 2$$

Adding fractions with different denominators:

■ Change fractions to an equal fraction with the LCD.

Example: 1/3 + 1/4 = LCD for both 3 and 4 is 12. Multiply this number by the numerator.

$$3 \times 4 = 12; \text{ so, } 4 \times 1 = 4/12$$
$$4 \times 3 = 12; \text{ so, } 3 \times 1 = 3/12$$

■ Add the numerators.

$$4 + 3 = 7$$

■ Place the sum over the denominator.

7/12

■ Reduce to the lowest terms.

The largest common divisor for 7 and 12 is 1; therefore, 7/12 constitutes the lowest terms (Check Up 6.9).

Subtracting Fractions

Subtracting fractions with the same denominator follows the same process as adding fractions.

■ Subtract the numerator.
■ Preserve the same denominator.
■ Reduce if necessary.

Example: 5/6 – 1/6 = 4/6 = 2/3

If the denominators are different, you must:

■ Find the LCD.

Example: 12/5 – 1/2
5 **10** 15 20 25 30
2 4 6 8 **10** 12 14 16

■ Change to equivalent fractions.

$$5 \times 2 = 10; \text{ thus, multiply } 12 \times 2 = 24, \text{ which results in } 24/10$$
$$2 \times 5 = 10; \text{ thus, multiply } 1 \times 5 = 5, \text{ which results in } 5/10$$

 CHECK UP 6.9: ADD THE FRACTIONS

Add the fractions with both a common denominator and a different denominator based on what you have reviewed.

1/2 + 1/3 = _____   1/4 + 1/6 = _____

1/10 + 2/5 = _____   1/9 + 2/3 = _____

5/8 + 3/7 = _____

■ Subtract the numerators.

$$24 - 5 = 19$$

■ Place the remainder over the common denominator.

$$19/10$$

■ Reduce if necessary (Check Up 6.10).

$$1\ 9/10$$

Multiplying Fractions

Multiplying fractions is also fairly straightforward. You do not have to worry about common denominators.

■ Multiply the numerators.

■ Multiply the denominators.

■ Reduce if necessary.

Example: $\dfrac{2}{5} \times \dfrac{3}{4} = \dfrac{2 \times 3}{5 \times 4} = \dfrac{6}{20} = \dfrac{3}{10}$

In Check Up 6.11, multiply the fractions.

 CRITICAL THINKING

Your patient is getting 1/3 tablespoon of a medication four times daily. How would you help your patient plan ahead to make sure he or she has enough medication for a week away at camp?

 CHECK UP 6.10: SUBTRACT THE FRACTIONS

Subtract these fractions.

2/3 – 1/3 = _____   10/6 – 2/3 = _____

5/6 – 5/12 = _____   15 – 7 1/2 = _____

250/500 – 50/500 = _____

 CHECK UP 6.11: MULTIPLY THE FRACTIONS

Multiply these fractions.

1/3 × 4/6 = _____   5/6 × 1/6 = _____

1/8 × 5/10 = _____   5/25 × 5/3 = _____

2/3 × 8/9 = _____

Dividing Fractions

Division is multiplication in reverse. When you multiply 1/5 × 2/3, you have 2/15. Suppose you divide 2/15 by 1/3. You should have 2/3.

To reverse multiplication, **invert** the fraction you are dividing by (flip the numerator and denominator over), and change the process to multiplication instead of division.

$$\text{Example: } \frac{2}{15} \div \frac{1}{5} \rightarrow \frac{2}{15} \times \frac{5}{1} = \frac{10}{15} = \frac{2}{3}$$

Therefore, the steps for dividing fractions are as follows:

■ Invert the second fraction.

■ Multiply the two fractions.

■ Reduce if needed.

In Check Up 6.12, try dividing the fractions.

CRITICAL THINKING

Sometimes patients don't take a whole pill, but part or multiples of a pill, and we may have to help them with this concept. For example, if Colleen E. takes 1 1/2 pills per dose, how will she plan to take enough medication with her for a 14-day vacation?

■ DECIMALS

A **decimal** is similar to a fraction, but with 10, 100, 1,000, and so on in the denominator. However, rather than writing it as a fraction, you can use a decimal point. Because drug doses often contain decimal points, it is important to understand decimals and how they work. Figure 6-4 illustrates how to identify units in numbers that have a decimal.

Rounding Decimals

Tablets are not usually dispensed in parts unless they are specifically **scored** (easily divisible into accurate doses) to do so. Capsules cannot be broken apart and separated evenly. Thus, you would usually round up or down if a dosage calculation does not produce a whole number. With fluids, you can give an exact decimal (e.g., 1.3 mL), but you may need to round up or down between 1.3 and 1.4 if the decimal is between those marks on the syringe or a measuring cup.

If a tablet is not scored, and you must round the amount:

For 0.5 to 1.49 → give one tablet
For 1.50 to 1.99 → give two tablets

 CHECK UP 6.12: DIVIDE THE FRACTIONS

Divide these fractions.

1/6 ÷ 1/2 = _____   6/2 ÷ 3/4 = _____

15/30 ÷ 5 = _____   2/3 ÷ 6/8 = _____

2/3 ÷ 3/2 = _____

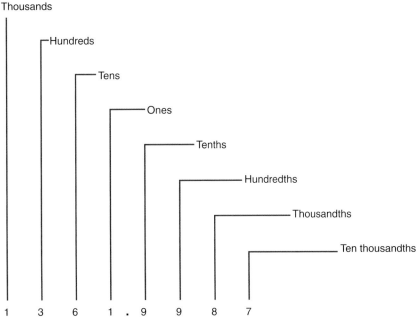

FIGURE 6-4: Decimal system. The decimal system is based on units of 10. Each numerical place in the number 1,361.9987 has a specific unit name. The first number in front of a decimal point is a whole number, in this case 1. The next numbers are based on units of 10 (tens, hundreds, thousands). The numbers behind the decimal point are also based on 10, but because they are less than a whole number, the unit names are tenths, hundredths, thousandths, ten thousandths, and so on.

For dosage calculations, it is rarely necessary to go past the hundredths place. When you are making a dosage calculation requiring more than one step, it is important to wait to round until the final calculation is completed. Rounding after each step could potentially change the final amount of medication you are giving.

Identifying Decimal Values

Determining whether you are giving a correct dosage requires a basic understanding of how decimals change the value of a number. Moving the decimal by one place increases or decreases the value of the number by 10; moving it two places changes the value by 100, and so forth. Those differences are significant in the amount of medication given to a patient. Thus, it is important to know how to compare numbers with decimals.

When decimal numbers contain whole numbers, the whole numbers must be compared to determine which is larger. For example, 5.8 is larger than 2.9, and 7.37 is larger than 6.39. When the whole numbers are the same or zero and the numbers in the tenths place are the same, the decimal with the higher number in the hundredths place is larger. For example, 0.66 is larger than 0.64, and 2.17 is larger than 2.15.

In Check Up 6.13, solve the problems regarding scored and unscored tablets.

The addition of zeros to the right of the end of a decimal does not alter its value, so these zeros are usually deleted. For example, if the number is 3.0, we would write 3 instead of 3.0. In addition, if the decimal is somehow missed (read as 30 instead of 3.0), an error would occur, resulting in a dosage 10 times too high. The zero to the left of the decimal point, however, is very important; it shows that the dosage is very small; 0.35 would be written instead of .35. Again, if the decimal point were missed (read as 35 instead of .35), this particular error would cause the patient to receive 100 times too much medication. Therefore, use of the decimal point in relation to zeros is a safety issue.

In Check Up 6.14, circle the larger number.

CHECK UP 6.13: SCORE THE TABLETS

If you had a scored tablet, what would you give for each of the following doses?

1.1 = _____   2.1 = _____

1.5 = _____   2.49 = _____

1.0 = _____

If you had an unscored tablet, what would you give?

1.1 = _____   2.1 = _____

1.5 = _____   2.59 = _____

1.9 = _____

 CHECK UP 6.14: DECIMAL SIZES

Circle the larger number, if there is one.

0.25 or 0.52   0.5 or 0.05

0.24 or 0.355   4.4 or 4.40

0.322 or 0.321

Adding Decimals

To add decimals, line up the decimal points and add each column; carry over a number as necessary.

$$\text{Example:} \quad \begin{array}{r} 1.25 \\ + \ 2.56 \\ \hline 3.81 \end{array}$$

In Check Up 6.15, add the decimals.

Subtracting Decimals

To subtract decimals, line up the decimal points and subtract.

$$\text{Example:} \quad \begin{array}{r} 4.3000 \\ - \ 1.7942 \\ \hline 2.5058 \end{array}$$

In Check Up 6.16, subtract each of the decimal values.

CHECK UP 6.15: ADD THE DECIMALS

Add the following. You may want to rewrite them on top of each other.

0.3 + 0.07 = _____   5.44 + 60.66 = _____

219.8 + 14.02 = _____   8.774 + 0.26 = _____

9.07 + 19.1 = _____

 CHECK UP 6.16: SUBTRACT THE DECIMALS

Subtract these decimals. You may want to rewrite them so that the first value is on top of the second value.

13.2 – 6.82 = _____   64.1 – 1.999 = _____

3.005 – 1.882 = _____   25.4 – 3.9 = _____

29 – 10.03 = _____

Multiplying Decimals

To multiply decimals, multiply as for whole numbers and insert the decimal point into the product so that the number of places to the right is equal to the sum of the decimal places in the factors.

Example:

$$21.4 \times 0.36 = 7.704$$

Multiply as a whole number:

$$
\begin{array}{r}
214 \\
\times\ 36 \\
\hline
1284 \text{ (the result of } 6 \times 214) \\
642 \text{ (the result of } 3 \times 214) \\
\hline
=\ 7704
\end{array}
$$

Add the number of decimal places:

$$
\begin{array}{r}
21.4 \rightarrow \text{one place to the right of the decimal point} \\
\times\, 0.36 \rightarrow \text{two places to the right of the decimal point} \\
\hline
=\ 7.704 \rightarrow \text{three places to the right of the decimal point}
\end{array}
$$

To multiply a decimal by a power of 10 (10, 100, 1,000 ....), move the decimal point to the right the same number of places as there are zeros in the power of 10. This is important in case a prescriber orders a medication in a unit of measure different from what is on the label (Fast Tip 6.1). Chapter 8 discusses this issue in more detail.

In Check Up 6.17, multiply the decimal values.

Fast Tip 6.1 Power of 10

As a zero is added to the number 1 (i.e., 10, 100, 1,000), the decimal point moves to the right the same number of places as the number of zeros. When two zeros are added, you have 100, and when three zeros are added, you have 1,000. Add the number of zeros that correspond to the power of 10. For example, 100 is 10 to the power of two; thus, it has two zeros. The number 1,000 is 10 to the power of three and has three zeros.

$$\overset{1}{3.9825 \times 10} \quad = \quad \overset{1}{39.825}$$
$$\overset{2}{3.9825 \times 100} \quad = \quad \overset{2}{398.25}$$
$$\overset{3}{3.9825 \times 1,000} = \quad \overset{3}{3,982.5}$$

 CHECK UP 6.17: MULTIPLY THE DECIMALS

Multiply these decimals.

9.68 × 10 = _____   9.86 × 2.2 = _____

10.02 × 100 = _____   42.47 × 4.01 = _____

100.2 × 10 = _____

Dividing Decimals

To divide decimals, follow these steps.

Move the decimal in the **divisor** (number doing the dividing) to the right of the decimal place to make the divisor a whole number. If you are dividing 100 by 0.5, 0.5 would become 5.0.

■ Move the decimal the same number of places in the dividend (number being divided). In this example, 100 would become 1,000.

■ Then do the long division. In this case, 1,000 ÷ 5 = 200.

In Check Up 6.18, divide the decimal values.

 CHECK UP 6.18: DIVIDE THE DECIMALS

Divide these decimals.

70 ÷ 4.4 = _____   200 ÷ 0.25 = _____

1,000 ÷ 3.5 = _____   400 ÷ 1.6 = _____

200 ÷ 2.5 = _____

Decimal and Fractional Forms

Have you noticed that decimals are really fractions? For example, 0.3 is simply 3/10, and 0.95 is 95/100.

To convert a decimal to a fraction, place the decimal over the number of the places it signifies. For example:

0.4　 = 4/10 (four tenths)

0.04　 = 4/100 (four hundredths)

0.004 = 4/1,000 (four thousandths)

Another way to do this is to count the number of places to the right of the decimal point, add that number of zeros to "1," and use it as the denominator. For example:

0.3　 = 3/10 (Use zero because there is one place after the decimal point.)

0.95　 = 95/100 (Use 2 zeros because there are two places after the decimal point.)

0.002 = 2/1,000 (Use 3 zeros because there are three places after the decimal point.)

To convert a fraction to a decimal, simply put the decimal point one place to the left of the decimal for each 0 in the denominator. For example:

3/10 = 0.3 (The decimal point is one to the left of the number because there is one zero in the denominator.)

95/100 = 0.95 (The decimal point is two places to the left of the number because there are two zeros in the denominator.)

2/1,000 = 0.002 (The decimal point is three places to the left of the number because there are three zeros in the denominator.)

Of course, if the fraction is not over a number divisible by 10, you must perform long division. In Check Up 6.19, convert each fraction to a decimal.

Percentages

Percents, quite simply, are numbers "over the denominator" 100.

A quarter = 25 cents = 0.25 = 25/100, or 25%

A penny = 1 cent = 0.01 or 1/100, or 1%

If you are asked to leave a 15% tip on a $15.00 dinner:

Convert the percentage to a decimal
15% = 0.15

 CHECK UP 6.19: FRACTIONS TO DECIMALS

Convert each of these fractions to a decimal. Use a separate sheet.

4/10 = _____   3/10 = _____

6/100 = _____   43/100 = _____

71/100 = _____   5/1,000 = _____

192/1,000 = _____   5/12 = _____

20/1,000 = _____   55/1,000 = _____

Multiply as a whole number:

$$
\begin{array}{r}
1500 \\
\times\,15 \\
\hline
7500 \text{ (the result of } 5 \times 1500) \\
1500 \text{ (the result of } 1 \times 1500) \\
\hline
= 22500
\end{array}
$$

Add the number of decimal places:

$$
\begin{array}{r}
\$15.00 \text{ (2 decimal places)} \\
\times\,0.15 \text{ (2 decimal places)} \\
\hline
\$2.2500 \text{ (the decimal point is inserted four places to the right of the decimal point)}
\end{array}
$$

The tip would be $2.25. In this case, you have converted percentage to a decimal.
In Check Up 6.20, convert each number to a percentage.

■ RATIOS AND PROPORTIONS

Ratios and proportions are ways to compare items. A **proportion** is a statement to say that two **ratios** (mathematical relationships) are equal. In the following example, both sides of the equation (ratios) are equal.

100 syringes is to	=	200 syringes is to
one box	as	two boxes

This could also be written using colons as follows:

100 syringes : one box = 200 syringes : two boxes

Both sides of the equal sign must relate to each other in the same way. For example:

$$1/1 = 2/2 = 3/3 = 4/4 = 5/5 = 6/6 = 7/7$$

All these relate to each other in the same way because they all are equal to 1. They could instead be equal to 1/2.

$$1/2 = 2/4 = 3/6 = 4/8 = 5/10 = 6/12 = 7/14$$

To go from 1/2 to 2/4, you multiply the numerator and denominator by 2. They are still equal. To go from 1/2 to 3/6, you multiply the numerator and denominator by 3.

As you multiply the numerator and denominator by the same number, you are simply multiplying by 1 and thus are not changing the relationship of the numbers.

Ratios and proportions are also expressed as fractions. If you are asked to make a 1:10 bleach solution, it is a 10% or 10/100 bleach solution.

$$1:10 \rightarrow 1/10 = \text{one tenth bleach and nine tenths water}$$

 CHECK UP 6.20: NUMBERS TO PERCENTAGES

Convert each of these numbers to a percentage.

20/100 = _____   0.20 = _____

2/100 = _____   0.02 = _____

0.2 = _____

Or if you are going to perform a dressing change requiring a 40% Betadine solution and the policy manual states that Betadine will be mixed with sterile saline solution, you know that the two solutions must be mixed together. The formula would be a 4:10 or 40/100 Betadine solution.

$$4:10 \rightarrow 4/10 = \text{four tenths Betadine and six tenths sterile saline}$$

Ratios as Decimals

Ratios also relate to decimals. Most medications are administered using the metric system, which has decimals. To convert a ratio to a decimal, write it as a fraction over a number divisible by 10, and convert it to a decimal.

$$1:10 = 1/10 = 0.1$$

In Check Up 6.21 and 6.22, determine what number makes each ratio correct, and then write each ratio as a decimal.

If a number is not divisible by 10, you will need to perform long division. For example:

$$1:9 = 1/9 = 1 \div 9 = 0.11$$

Converting Decimals to Ratios

To convert a decimal to a ratio, write the decimal as a fraction in lowest terms. Restate the fraction as a ratio, as in the following example:

Write 0.14 as a ratio.

■ Place 14 as the numerator and 100 as the denominator because the hundredths place is occupied.

$$14/100$$

✎ CHECK UP 6.21: RATIOS

What number makes each ratio correct?

1:10::4: _____   10:100::1: _____

3:6::5: _____   250:500:: _____:2

6:3:: _____:4

✎ CHECK UP 6.22: RATIOS TO DECIMALS

Write each ratio as a decimal.

1:8 = _____   1:100 = _____

1:5 = _____   1:1,000 = _____

1:10 = _____

■ Reduce if necessary.

$$\frac{14 \div 2}{100 \div 2} = \frac{7}{50}$$

■ Change 7/50 to a ratio.

$$7{:}50$$

In the Check Up 6.23, convert the decimals to ratios.

Converting Ratios to Percents

To convert a ratio to a percentage, change it to a decimal first, and then multiply the decimal by 100 and add the % sign.

$$1{:}50 = 1/50 = 0.02$$
$$0.02 \times 100 = 2\%$$
$$1{:}50 = 1/50 = 0.02 = 2\%$$

In Check Up 6.24, convert each ratio to a percentage.

Converting Percents to Ratios

To convert a percentage to a ratio, write it as a fraction in lowest terms. Write the faction as a ratio.

$$25\% = 25/100 = 1/4 = 1{:}4$$

In Check Up 6.25, convert each percentage to a ratio.

 CHECK UP 6.23: DECIMALS TO RATIOS

Convert these decimals to ratios.

0.125 = _____   0.2 = _____

0.12 = _____   0.22 = _____

0.1 = _____

 CHECK UP 6.24: RATIOS TO PERCENTAGES

Convert each ratio to a percentage.

2:3 = _____   1:10 = _____

1:2 = _____   1:3 = _____

100:200 = _____

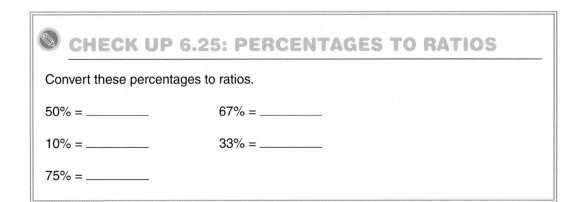

CHECK UP 6.25: PERCENTAGES TO RATIOS

Convert these percentages to ratios.

50% = _____   67% = _____

10% = _____   33% = _____

75% = _____

Checking Ratio and Proportions

If you are not sure whether you calculated a ratio correctly, there is an easy way to check yourself.

Consider: 1:3::100:?

Suppose you thought the correct answer was 300. To check yourself, you could multiply the **means** (middle numbers) by the **extremes** (outer numbers). If you have calculated correctly, the means and extremes should be equal (Fig. 6-5).

Here are two examples to illustrate this point.

■ Problem: 1:2::3:?

Proposed answer: 1:2::3:6

Means: $2 \times 3 = 6$

Extremes: $1 \times 6 = 6$

6 = 6, so the answer is correct

■ Problem: 2:3::4:?

Proposed answer: 2:3::4:7

Means: $3 \times 4 = 12$

Extremes: $2 \times 7 + 14$

12 does not equal 14, so the answer is incorrect

You can also use the means and extremes method to check your work when you have an answer. In Check Up 6.26 and 6.27, test your knowledge of ratios and proportions.

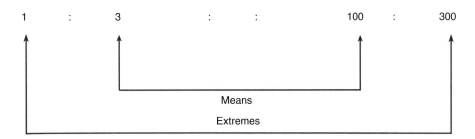

Means
3 X 100 = 300

Extremes
1 X 300 = 300
300 = 300 correct

FIGURE 6-5: Means and extremes. Means and extremes check for proportions. To verify that your answer for a proportion is correct, multiply the means and the extremes. The two results should be equal.

CHECK UP 6.26: PROPORTIONAL RATIOS

Check whether these ratios are proportional. Write true or false.

1:4::100:200 _____   1:5::20:100 _____

1:2::50:100 _____   1:6::2:7 _____

1:3::3:6 _____

 CHECK UP 6.27: EQUAL RATIOS

Check whether these ratios are equal. Write true or false.

1:2::2:5 _____   200:150::1:2 _____

2:3::4:6 _____   250:200::5:4 _____

10:100::2:20 _____

■ SOLVING FOR AN UNKNOWN

A prescriber writes orders for a dose of medication. When you go to the medication cupboard, you find a vial of the correct medication, but not in the dosage you need. Because you must solve for the unknown amount of medication you need to administer, you must know how to solve for an unknown.

If you are given a ratio or fraction, you need to find an unknown. For example:

$$\frac{100}{200} = \frac{1}{?}$$

This could also be written 100:200::1:?

There are several ways to solve for the unknown value (indicated by the question mark). One way is to use words.

100 relates to 200 as 1 relates to an unknown number.

100 is 100 times greater than 1.

Therefore, 200 is 100 greater than the unknown number, which is 2.

Another way is to use means and extremes.

$$100:200::1:?$$
$$200 \times 1 \text{ (means)} = 200$$
$$100 \times ? \text{ (extremes)} =$$
$$? = 200/100$$
$$? = 2$$

You can also use fractions and cross-multiply.

$$\frac{100}{200} = \frac{1}{?}$$
$$100 \times ? = 1 \times 200$$
$$100? = 200$$
$$100?/100 = 200/100$$
$$? = 2$$

CHECK UP 6.28: SOLVING FOR UNKNOWNS

Solve for the ? (unknown) value.

100:200::?:2 _____   50:150::?:3 _____

2:1::400:? _____   250:1::500:? _____

300:?::100:1 _____

CRITICAL THINKING

Did you notice how similar the last two methods are? Why does cross-multiplying work?

In Check Up 6.28, try solving for the unknown value. Try using each of the different methods mentioned earlier, and then use the one you find easiest to determine the value.

CRITICAL THINKING

Sometimes it is easier to leave a calculation in a fractional form, and sometimes it is better to work with a decimal. When would you use a decimal rather than a faction? When would it be easier to write a numerical equation as a fraction, and when would it be easier as a ratio?

●●● SUMMARY

■ Understanding basic math concepts is essential for calculating dosages safely.

■ A fraction is a part of a whole. The numerator is number on the top. The denominator is the number on the bottom. The fraction is called a proper fraction if the numerator is smaller than the denominator. An improper fraction means that the numerator is larger than the denominator

■ A common denominator is a number that is a common multiple of two (or more) denominators. The lowest number into which both denominators can be divided (keeping the fraction small makes it easier to work with) is called the least common denominator (LCD).

■ A mixed number is a whole number plus a fraction.

■ Factors are used to determine the largest common divisor to divide the dividend.

■ A decimal is similar to a fraction, but with 10, 100, 1,000, and so on in the denominator. Moving the decimal by one place increases or decreases the value of the number by 10, moving it two places changes the value by 100, and so forth. The zero to the left of the decimal point is very important; it shows that the dosage is very small.

■ Ratios and proportions are ways to compare items. A proportion is a statement to say that two ratios (mathematical relationships) are equal.

Activities

To make sure that you have learned the key points covered in this chapter, complete the following activities.

Calculations

Find the least common denominator.

1. 1/3 and 1/4 _____

2. 1/8 and 1/6 _____

3. 1/2 and 1/3 _____

4. 1/5 and 1/15 _____

5. 1/15 and 1/90 _____

6. 1/7 and 1/9 _____

7. 1/4 and 1/9 _____

8. 1/10 and 1/4 _____

9. 1/100 and 1/25 _____

10. 1/2 and 1/10 _____

Add the following.

1. 3/4 + 1/4 = _____

2. 1/5 + 2/5 = _____

3. 1/6 + 2/3 = _____

4. 1 1/3 + 1/3 = _____

5. 1 1/3 + 2/3 = _____

6. 8/17 + 6/17 + 2/17 = _____

7. 2/3 + 3/8 = _____

8. 2/5 + 1/3 = _____

9. 1/4 + 1/6 = _____

10. 1 1/3 + 1/2 = _____

Subtract the following.

1. 1 1/2 – 1/2 = _____

2. 15/7 – 8/7 = _____

3. 150/50 – 75/50 = _____

4. 21/1 – 3/1 = _____

5. 5/6 – 3/6 = _____

6. 3/4 – 2/4 = _____

7. 6/3 – 1 1/2 = _____

8. 3/4 – 1/4 = _____

9. 7/18 – 3/24 = _____

10. 4/6 – 1/6 = _____

Multiply the following.

1. 1/3 × 1/4 = _____

2. 250/1 × 1/500 = _____

3. 200/400 × 1/2 = _____

4. 5/1 × 1/4 = _____

5. 3/1 × 10/1 = _____

6. 1/2 × 90 = _____

7. 4/1 × 2 1/2 = _____

8. 3/7 × 3/9 = _____

9. 300/600 × 1 = _____

10. 150/450 × 2 = _____

Divide the following.

1. 4/4 ÷ 5/9 = _____

2. 5/10 ÷ 2/4 = _____

3. 1/6 ÷ 1/6 = _____

4. 9/10 ÷ 3/5 = _____

5. 6/9 ÷ 9/10 = _____

6. 6 ÷ 1/6 = _____

7. 1 2/3 ÷ 2/4 = _____

8. 3/5 ÷ 5/9 = _____

9. 100 ÷ 4 = _____

10. 6 ÷ 6/8 = _____

Reduce the following fractions.

1. 500/250 = _____

2. 600/3 = _____

3. 1,000/10 = _____

4. 100/4 = _____

5. 75/150 = _____

6. 240/3 = _____

7. 250/25 = _____

8. 50/500 = _____

9. 100/150 = _____

10. 15/150 = _____

Calculate these decimal problems.

1. $0.04 \div 0.2$ = _____

2. $10.87 - 0.345$ = _____

3. 100×9.8 = _____

4. Arrange from smallest to largest: 0.135, 0.13, 0.003 _____

5. Write 52 thousandths as a decimal. _____

6. Divide 17.25 by 0.85. Round to the nearest tenth. _____

7. Round to the nearest tenth: 18.75 _____

8. Convert to a decimal: 6 1/4 _____

9. Write as a decimal: 7 1/5 _____

10. $1.054 + 3.15$ = _____

11. $0.05 + 0.005$ = _____

12. $250.98 - 5.55$ = _____

13. 250×0.2 = _____

14. $250 \div 500$ = _____

15. $250 \div 0.5$ = _____

Which is greater?

1. 0.12 or 0.012 _____

2. 4.4 or 0.44 _____

3. 0.15 or 0.16 _____

4. 1.6 or 0.16 _____

5. 0.05 or 0.50 _____

Answer the following questions.

1. What is 10% as a fraction?

2. What is 5/100 as a percentage?

3. What is 50% of 60?

4. What is 0.25 as a percentage?

5. What is 75% as a decimal?

Convert these decimals to ratios.

1. 0.33 _____

2. 0.50 _____

3. 0.67 _____

4. 0.75 _____

5. 0.90 _____

Convert these ratios to percentages.

1. 1:2 _____

2. 2:3 _____

3. 1:4 _____

4. 2:5 _____

5. 4:6 _____

Convert these percentages to ratios.

1. 50% _____

2. 67% _____

3. 80% _____

4. 99% _____

5. 60% _____

Check whether the following ratios are correct. Write true or false.

1. 1:10::4:50 _____

2. 250:500::1:2 _____

3. 100:400::3:5 _____

4. 1:2::200:400 _____

5. 50:150::1:2 _____

Solve for the ? (unknown).

1. 1:10::3:? _____

2. 100:1::400:? _____

3. 200:400::2:? _____

4. 2:3::4:? _____

5. 1:2::?:8 _____

6. 100:300::?:3 _____

7. 100:300::?:6 _____

8. 100:200::?:4 _____

9. 200:1::400:? _____

10. 1:200::?:400 _____

11. 100:1::200:? _____

12. 1:3::2:? _____

13. 0.5:1::?:2 _____

14. 0.25:1::25:? _____

15. 75:150::1:? _____

Application Exercises

Solve the following word problems:

1. One slice of bread contains 100 calories. How many calories do you reduce if you omit 1/4 of a slice of bread per day for 30 days? _____

2. One serving of crisp bread is 60 calories. If you ate 3/4 of a serving, how many calories did you eat? _____

3. A banana split has 550 calories. If you burned 2/3 of those calories, how many calories do you still have to burn to work off the banana split calories? _____

4. Jamie received 21 sample pills from her physician. If she must take half of a pill 3 times per day, how many days will the pills last before she needs to fill the written prescription her physician gave her? _____

5. Jane weighed 102 lb at the end of January. She gained 2% in February. How much does she weigh now? _____

6. Joyce gives her daughter 1/2 T at each of three meals each day. How much does she give in 1 day? _____

7. Diana drank 2 1/2 cups of water, 1 1/4 cups of milk, and 1 cup of orange juice. How many cups did she drink? _____

8. At the beginning of the day, you have a 30-oz bottle of medication. If each dose is 1/2 oz, how many doses in total do you have? _____

9. Jasmine weighed 100 lb at the last visit. She has lost 4 1/2 lb this month. How much does she now weigh? _____

10. Annabelle is receiving 500 mL of fluid IV. A total of 100 mL has been used in 1 hour. What percent of the fluid is left? _____

11. Peter makes $12.00 per hour. If he works for 32 hours, how much does he make? _____

12. Colleen is feeling very drowsy on 50 mg of Zoloft. The nurse practitioner says to cut the prescription by 50%. How much should Colleen take? _____

13. Donnie made sales totaling the following this hour: $15.28, $77.42, $35.00, $10.00, $35.00, $98.99, and $17.44. How much in total did he make this hour? _____

14. Kelly owes a medical office $498.43 and pays $35.00. How much does she now owe? _____

15. Gary sees the physician four times this month. Each time he pays $35.50. How much does he pay in total? _____

16. Dr. Binderwald has allotted $240.60 in bonuses to be split equally among his six staff members. How much should each person receive? _____

17. In this medical office, the ratio of allied health professionals to patients is 1:3. If there are 60 patients, how many allied health professionals are needed at this time? _____

18. If there are 50 vials of flu vaccine in a box and that is 25% of your requirements, how many boxes do you need? _____

19. If 3 grams of a drug are contained in 50 mL of solution, write the ratio. _____

20. Describe a 10% bleach solution as a ratio. _____

21. How much bleach is in the solution mentioned in question 20? How much water? _____

22. David weighs 50 lb. He is about one third of an adult's weight. How much of an adult dose should he receive? _____

23. Ian weighs 300 lb. If an adult dose is based on 150 lb and he is twice that size, how much of an adult dose should he receive of a medication with a dosage based on weight? _____

24. Judith is slicing a pie. She sliced six pieces for her three children. If the children are given equal shares, how many slices does each child receive? _____

25. Sheri is adding up her paychecks for this month. She received $355.60, $320.00, $440.00, and $350.40. How much did she make this month? _____

7

Measurement Systems

*U*nderstanding units of measure and knowing how to convert them from one unit to another are critical when calculating dosages. Now that you have reviewed the basic mathematics necessary to determine dosage calculations, the next steps are to examine and review the four systems of measurement used for drug dispensing: avoirdupois, apothecary, household, and metric.

The large amount of information presented in this chapter is critical to safe administration of medication to patients. Continue to work on learning this material; make flash cards, or use the resources available with this book online at www.davisplus.com to practice further. As a future health professional, do not think you can learn this material, take a test, and then forget it. You will use most of this information on a daily basis and must become confident and competent in your practice.

LEARNING OUTCOMES

At the end of this chapter, you will be able to:

7.1 Define all key terms.
7.2 Compare the four systems of measurement used for drug dispensing.
7.3 State the basic units of measurement in the metric system.
7.4 Use conversion methods for each system of measurement correctly and accurately.

KEY TERMS

Apothecary system	Avoirdupois system	Compound

■ MEASUREMENT SYSTEMS

Before the metric system was developed, pharmacists used to **compound,** or mix, and dispense drugs. Patients and their families often measured drugs with whatever utensils were handy, such as teaspoons, tablespoons, and cups of various sizes. Today, medications are ordered using the metric system. The four measurement systems discussed here are the avoirdupois, apothecary, metric, and household systems.

Avoirdupois System

The units in the **avoirdupois system** are the familiar pounds and ounces. This system is used for measuring medications, as well as for general purposes. Most scales used to weigh patients measure weight in pounds and ounces. As a health-care professional, you need to learn how to convert pounds to kilograms to calculate drug dosages. Dosages of some medications are strictly based on a patient's weight, and others must be adjusted if the patient is either obese or very small. The two accepted conversion methods have results that differ slightly, as shown in the examples given here. The conversion of kilograms to pounds and pounds to kilograms is as follows:

$$1 \text{ kg} = 2.2 \text{ lb}$$
$$1 \text{ lb} = 0.45 \text{ kg}$$

Therefore, if a patient weighs 95 lb and you need to convert this weight to kilograms, you would multiply by 0.45:

$$95 \times 0.45 = 42.75 \text{ kg, rounded to } 43 \text{ kg}$$

An alternative would be to divide by 2.2:

$$95 \div 2.2 = 43.18 \text{ kg, rounded to } 43 \text{ kg}$$

CRITICAL THINKING

Harold F. is seen in the office. He has a history of congestive heart failure and is concerned that he is gaining a lot of weight. You determine that he weighs 185 lb. When he asks you how much weight he has gained since his last checkup the previous month, you check the chart and find that he weighed 79 kg. What will you tell him?

The foregoing conversions work well with whole numbers. However, suppose a pediatric patient weighs 9 lb 8 oz. In this case, to calculate accurately, you must know how many ounces are in 1 lb. Ounces are most commonly used when weighing infants and children, whose weight is typically much less than an adult's and in whom every ounce counts. In addition, as discussed in Chapter 8, because infants' body systems are not fully developed, infants are extremely susceptible to inappropriately high drug doses. The nervous system, kidneys, and liver of these small patients are not mature enough to process the medications as a healthy adult does. Therefore, we must be extremely precise when weighing infants and small children and again when converting their weights between systems, to ensure appropriate medication doses.

$$1 \text{ pound (lb)} = 16 \text{ ounces (oz)}$$

Example: The foregoing patient weighs 9 lb 8 oz; therefore:

$$\text{Divide 8 by 16} = 0.5$$
$$9.5 \text{ lb} \times 0.45 = 4.28 \text{ kg or } 4.3 \text{ kg (rounded)}$$

Or

$$9.5 \text{ lb} \div 2.2 = 4.31 \text{ kg or } 4.3 \text{ kg (rounded)}$$

CRITICAL THINKING

Sally S. brings her 3-month-old baby to the clinic because of a fever and possible ear infection. You find that the infant weighs 13 lb, 4 oz. The physician writes an order for you to give a dose of antibiotics based on the infant's weight in kilograms. Before you give the medication, you must convert the child's weight to kilograms. How will you do this, and what is her weight in kilograms?

Conversely, the scale used may be calibrated in the metric system, and you may need to convert kilograms to pounds and ounces for the patient or the patient's family. For example, if a patient is told that he lost 5 kg, this value may not mean as much to him as if you told him that he lost 11 lb. It is also more likely that a home scale will measure in pounds and not in kilograms. Parents of infants may also want to know their infant's weight in pounds rather than kilograms.

Example 1: The patient weighs 14 kg.

$$14 \times 2.2 = 30.8, \text{ or 31 lb (rounded)}$$

Or

$$14 \div 0.45 = 31.1, \text{ or 31 lb (rounded)}$$

Example 2: The patient weighs 4.3 kg.

$$4.3 \times 2.2 = 9.5 \text{ lb and}$$
$$9.5 \text{ lb} = 9 + (0.5 \times 16) = 9 \text{ lb 8 oz}$$

Or

$$4.3 \div 0.45 = 9.5 \text{ lb and}$$
$$9.5 \text{ lb} = 9 + (0.5 \times 16) = 9 \text{ lb 8 oz}$$

In Check Up 7.1, practice converting weights from pounds to kilograms.

 CRITICAL THINKING

Would you rather be weighed in kilograms or pounds? Why?

 ## CHECK UP 7.1: POUNDS TO KILOGRAMS

Convert these weights from pounds (lb) to kilograms (kg).

195 lb = _____ kg   300 lb = _____ kg

55 lb = _____ kg   125 lb = _____ kg

40 lb = _____ kg

Convert these weights from pounds (lb) to kilograms (kg).

2 lb 4 oz = _____ kg   6 lb 12 oz = _____ kg

7 lb 3 oz = _____ kg   12 lb 6 oz = _____ kg

4 lb 8 oz = _____ kg

Convert these weights from kilograms (kg) to pounds (lb).

85 kg = _____ lb   200 kg = _____ lb

10 kg = _____ lb   21 kg = _____ lb

120 kg = _____ lb

Apothecary System

The **apothecary system,** which uses fractions instead of decimals, is one of the oldest systems of measurement. In addition, Roman numerals are common in this system, as opposed to Arabic numerals used in all other systems. Pharmacists, or apothecaries as they were known, used this system for compounding drugs. The apothecary system is rarely used today, as it is complicated and less accurate. There is not a specific conversion for each unit, but a range of possible numbers. For example, 1 grain is equivalent to anywhere from 60 to 65 mg. However, some prescribers continue to use it, just as some patients continue to use nonmetric measuring utensils, so you must be familiar with it. Common drugs that follow the apothecary system of measurement are Tylenol (Tylenol gr V) and morphine (morphine gr 1/4), which may be ordered or available in grains. Therefore, if you are using these medications, it is important to remember that there is not one correct dosage, but a range of correct dosages. For the purposes of medication administration in this textbook, we will use a specific number instead of a range of numbers, but remember that the apothecary system is not a precise system. Chapter 8 discusses how to convert grains into metric measurements.

A CLOSER LOOK: Apothecary Symbols and Abbreviations

Although symbols and abbreviations for some apothecary measurements are not recommended, some prescribers still use them, so you should be familiar with them.

Unit	Abbreviation	Symbol
Grain	gr	None used
Minim	—	ℳ
Dram	dr	ʒ
Ounce	oz	

Household System

At home, a patient may use available teaspoons, tablespoons, cups, glasses, teacups, or other utensils to measure medication. However, this practice is unsafe because household utensil sizes are not standardized. Encourage your patients to use the metric system or standardized measuring tools. Box 7-1 provides common household measures.

In Check Up 7.2, convert the measurements based on the content in Box 7-1.

Equivalents Between Apothecary and Household Systems

Before discussing the metric system, it is important to understand the equivalents between the apothecary and household measuring systems. If a doctor writes an order in the apothecary system, you must convert it to the household system so that patients understand how much medication to take. You may be able to come up with some shortcuts to help you remember a conversion. For example, think about the number of minutes your favorite television drama lasts. Most likely, it is 60 minutes; therefore, one drama equals 60 minutes. This association may help you remember that 1 dram (a measurement used for fluids) equals 60 minims.

Larger fluid measurements are pints, quarts, and gallons. Some equivalents are minute. In fact, these equivalents are so small that the number of tiny amounts in a larger amount can vary greatly, similar to grains of sand in a cup.

One drop (gt) is so small that 360 to 480 drops (gtt) = 1 oz.
There are 360 to 480 grains or minims in an ounce.
One drop (gt) = 1 grain = 1 minim because they are all about the same size.

In Check Up 7.3, write the equivalents based on the foregoing relationships.

How did you do? Be sure to familiarize yourself with these equivalents. Fast Tip 7.1 offers a quicker way to learn different measurements, with less to memorize.

BOX 7.1 Household Measurements

Measurement	Equivalent
3 teaspoons (t or tsp)	1 tablespoon (T or Tbs)
2 T	1 fluid ounce (oz)
8 oz	1 cup (c)
2 cups	1 pint (pt)
2 pints	1 quart (qt)
4 quarts	1 gallon (gal)
1 juice glass	4 oz
1 teacup	6 oz
1 glass	8 oz

CHECK UP 7.2: HOUSEHOLD EQUIVALENTS

Write the equivalent household measurement.

1 juice glass = _____ oz   1 cup = _____ oz

1 teacup = _____ oz   1 pint = _____ cups

1 glass = _____ oz   1 quart = _____ pints

1 T = _____ oz   1 gallon = _____ quarts

1 oz = _____ t   1 cup = _____ pint

CHECK UP 7.3: MORE EQUIVALENTS

1 oz = _____ dr   4 pints = _____ quarts

16 dr = _____ oz   8 fluid ounces = _____ pint

1 dr = _____ minims   1 gallon = _____ quarts

120 minims = _____ dr   360 gtt = _____ oz

80 dr = _____ oz   1 oz = _____ grain

1 quart = _____ gallon   1 gt = _____ oz

1 pint = _____ fluid ounces

Fast Tip 7.1   One-Ounce Conversions

The following may be an easier way to learn how different measurements relate to each other and how they relate to an ounce.

$$
\begin{aligned}
1 \text{ oz} &= 2 \text{ T} \\
&= 6 \text{ t} \\
&= 8 \text{ dr} \\
&= 360 \text{ to } 480 \text{ gtt, grains, minims} \\
&= 30 \text{ mL}
\end{aligned}
$$

If you memorize these relations, you can always move through the ounce for conversions.

CRITICAL THINKING

Does it bother you that 1 oz is equivalent to something between 360 and 480 gtt, minims, or grains? What does this say about the accuracy of these systems?

Sometimes Roman numerals are used when ordering grains. The most common examples are Tylenol and morphine, as discussed earlier. Roman numerals can be written one of three ways. If you are unsure about the order written, always check with the prescriber. For example, grains (gr) V = 5 grains. Table 7-1 provides a list of the two most common ways Roman numerals are written.

The Metric System

The metric system is based on the decimal system of places of 10 (10, 100, and 1,000). This system is used by many countries and most researchers. It has become the standard for calculating drugs because it is the most accurate. The base units of measure are as follows:

Mass or weight = gram
Length = meter
Volume or fluids = liter

TABLE 7.1 Values of Roman Numerals

Value	Roman Numeral	Options
1	i	I
2	ii	II
3	iii	III
4	iv	IV
5	v	V
6	vi	VI
7	vii	VII
8	viii	VIII
9	ix	IX
10	x	X

The most common prefixes for the units of measure are listed in Table 7-2. The prefixes in the table are added to the base unit to describe the measurement. For example, the prefix "kilo-" means "thousands of"; when it is added to "grams," the result is "kilograms," or 1,000 grams. When the prefix "deci-," which means "1/10 of" a unit, is added to "liter," the result is "deciliter," or 1/10 of a liter. Each prefix provides a hint about the unit of measure. Dosage calculations do not usually involve very large or very small numbers. In Check Up 7.4, determine how many units are in 1 gram. Use Table 7-2 for reference.

Dosage calculations predominantly use the base units of liters and grams because they are the units of weight and volume. Rarely is a unit of length needed when giving medication. For instance, a syringe is calibrated so that 1 cubic centimeter (cc) of space holds 1 mL of fluid.

If a syringe is narrow (smaller circumference), more length is needed to form the area needed to make up 1 cc of fluid. If a syringe is wide, the plunger does not need to be pulled back as far to fill the syringe with 1 cc (Check Up 7.5).

TABLE 7.2 Common Metric Units of Measurement

Prefix	Level of Measurement
Deci-	Tenths
Centi-	Hundredths
Milli-	Thousandths
Micro-	Millionths
Kilo-	Thousands

CHECK UP 7.4: GRAMS

Number the following measurements in order, from the smallest (1) to the largest (4).

gram _____   kilogram _____

microgram _____   milligram _____

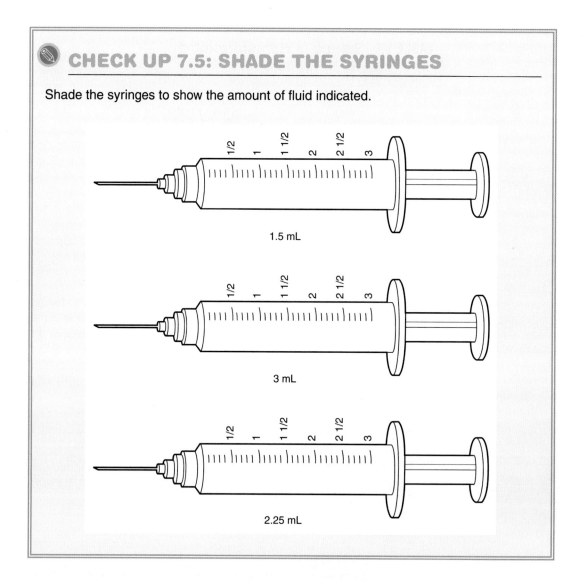

CHECK UP 7.5: SHADE THE SYRINGES

Shade the syringes to show the amount of fluid indicated.

1.5 mL

3 mL

2.25 mL

Converting units within the metric system is a common task when administering medications. For instance, if a prescriber orders a medication that uses grams in the order, could you convert this order to milligrams, which is how the label usually states the drug amount? The following examples show what an order may contain and ways to convert the units to ascertain the correct dosage. Table 7-3 summarizes whether you need to multiply or divide when converting from one type of unit to another.

Example 1: A prescriber orders 0.2 gram; think of this as 0.200. Milligrams are 1/1,000 gram, so multiply 0.200 by 1,000.

$$0.200 \times 1,000 = 200 \text{ mg}$$

Example 2: Sometimes it is helpful to use fractions or ratios for the conversion.

$$\frac{0.500 \text{ gram}}{? \text{ mg}} = \frac{1 \text{ gram}}{1,000 \text{ mg}}$$

You can cross-multiply to find the answer.

$$1 \times ? = 0.500 \times 1,000$$
$$? = 500 \text{ mg}$$

In Check Up 7.6, determine whether you need to multiply or divide to solve the problems. Use Table 7-3 for reference. How did you do? If you have trouble with this, it may help to create a chart, as shown in Box 7-2.

TABLE 7.3   Simple Unit Conversions

Conversion	Multiply/Divide
Grams to kilograms	Divide by 1,000
Grams to milligrams	Multiply by 1,000
Kilograms to grams	Multiply by 1,000
Milligrams to grams	Divide by 1,000
Liters to milliliters	Multiply by 1,000
Milliliters to liters	Divide by 1,000

CHECK UP 7.6: CONVERSIONS

0.200 gram to milligrams _____   0.5 L to kilograms _____

200 mg to grams _____   1 kg to grams _____

2 grams to kilograms _____

Convert the following orders into milligrams.

0.35 gram _____   0.125 gram _____

0.5 gram _____

BOX 7.2 Converting from One Unit to Another

Kilo-	$\times 1,000$ to get to unit $\rightarrow$ 1 km = 1,000 meters
Centi-	$\div 100$ to get to unit $\rightarrow$ 100 cm = 1 meter
Milli-	$\div 1,000$ to get to unit $\rightarrow$ 1,000 mm = 1 meter
Micro-	$\div 1,000,000$ to get to unit $\rightarrow$ 1,000,000 mcm = 1 meter

The prescriber may order a drug in grams or milligrams of weight, but this number must be converted into fluid volume, in milliliters, so the correct amount can be injected. In other words, a prescriber may order a dose of medication, but the medication comes in different sizes, strengths, and forms. It is up to you to find the correct medication and convert the order to the correct amount and form of the drug. For example, a physician may order 100 mg ampicillin to be given intramuscularly (IM). You go to the cabinet and find that you have a vial of ampicillin, but in powder form, which cannot be used "as is." Information on the label of the drug vial states exactly what and how much liquid to mix with the powder to transform the drug into an appropriate form. In addition, the label states the concentration of the resulting liquid if the directions are followed correctly. For the ampicillin example, the label on the vial states that 100 mg of drug is dispersed in 1 mL of fluid. To draw up 100 mg of the drug, you would need to fill the syringe with 1 mL of fluid, so you would pull back the syringe to 1 cc.

Once you have calculated the milliliters to administer, recall that 1 cc of space in the syringe is equal to 1 mL of fluid, so you do not need to convert to cubic centimeters.

CRITICAL THINKING

Do you have trouble seeing the decimal point? Do you think pharmacists ever do? How can you be sure that a patient is given 0.5 gram instead of 5 grams?

If you prefer to use words to visualize concepts, you may find this story helpful. There was once a farmer named Gram. He had 1,000 employees, called milligrams. He owned 15 grain fields (apothecary). In each grain field, 60 milligrams worked.

Repeat this story, and learn to draw the picture (conversion triangle) in Figure 7-1. The words in the story can help you understand whether to use 1/15 or 15 in the triangle.

You can also memorize these equivalents:

$$1 \text{ gram} = 1,000 \text{ mg}$$
$$1 \text{ gram} = 15 \text{ grains}$$
$$1 \text{ grain} = 60 \text{ mg}$$

Keeping in mind the story and triangle, consider the following more difficult example. Farmer Gram has 1,000 milligrams. Each milligram is 1/1,000 of his workforce. If a milligram is sick one day, 1/60 of the workforce in one field is missing, because 60 milligrams work in each grain field. If Gram gives away one grain field to his child as a wedding gift, he will give away 1/15 of his fields. Refer to Figure 7-2 as a guide.

As an alternative to relating conversions to the farmer Gram story, you can also memorize the conversions.

$$1 \text{ mg} = 1/1,000 \text{ gram (g)} \qquad 1 \text{ g} = 1,000 \text{ mg}$$
$$1 \text{ grain} = 1/15 \text{ gram (g)} \qquad 1 \text{ g} = 15 \text{ grains}$$
$$1 \text{ mg} = 1/60 \text{ grain (gr)} \qquad 1 \text{ gr} = 60 \text{ mg}$$

You must know these conversions to calculate drug dosages safely while keeping in mind that a grain in the apothecary system is equivalent to anywhere from 60 to 65 mg.

In Check Up 7.7, use the previous story and triangle or memorization tables to answer the questions.

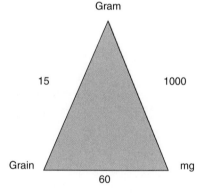

FIGURE 7-1: Farmer Gram's conversion triangle. Following the words of the story, there is one farmer (gram) who has 1,000 employees (milligrams). The farmer owns 15 grain fields (grains). Each grain field (grain) has 60 employees (milligrams) working them. Thus, 1 gram = 1,000 mg, 1 gram = 15 grains, and 1 grain = 60 mg.

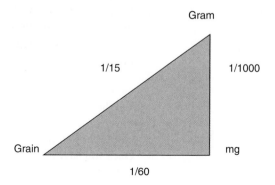

FIGURE 7-2: Farmer Gram's fractional conversion triangle. Following the words of the story, there is one farmer (gram) who has 1,000 employees (milligrams). The farmer owns 15 grain fields (grains). Each grain field (grain) has 60 employees (milligrams) working them. If one worker (milligram) is sick, the farmer is missing 1/1,000 of his work force, and the grain field (grain) is missing 1/60 of its workforce. If the farmer (gram) gives away one grain field (grain), he is giving away 1/15 of his fields. Thus, 1 mg = 1/1,000 gram, 1 mg = 1/60 of a grain, and 1 grain = 1/15 of a gram.

CHECK UP 7.7: FARMER GRAM CONVERSIONS

1. How many employees did Farmer Gram have? _____

2. How many milligrams are in a gram? _____

3. How many grain fields did Farmer Gram have? _____

4. How many grains are in a gram? _____

5. How many milligrams worked in each field? _____

6. How many milligrams are in a grain? _____

7. If Farmer Gram gives away 1 grain field, what fraction of his wealth has he given away? _____

8. A grain is _____ of a gram.

9. Each milligram is what fraction of his workforce? _____

10. A milligram is _____ of a gram.

11. A milligram is sick today. What fraction of the workers in the field is out sick?

    _____

12. A milligram is _____ of a grain.

● ● ○ SUMMARY

- This chapter describes the four measurement systems: avoirdupois, apothecary, household, and metric.
- The avoirdupois system is often used in weight measurements and is based on the pound.
- The apothecary system, which is the oldest, is seldom used today. It uses fractions instead of decimals.
- The household measurement system is based on the apothecary system and is the system with which patients are most comfortable and familiar. Because of inadequate standardization of measurements, however, it is not the safest method to use for medication administration.
- The most accepted measurement system is the metric system; it is the most accurate and is based on units of 10. The base units of measure are grams, meters, and liters. Prefixes are added to the base unit to create multiples of the units of 10.
- Converting units within the metric system is a common task when administering medications.

Activities

To make sure that you have learned the key points covered in this chapter, complete the following activities.

Fill in the blanks to show what you have learned.

1. 1 juice glass = _____ oz

2. 1 teacup = _____ oz

3. 1 cc = _____ mL

4. 1 kg = _____ lb

5. 1 oz = _____ t

6. 1 lb = _____ kg

7. 1 dr = _____ minims

8. 1 oz = _____ dr

9. 1 pint = _____ oz

10. 1 oz = _____ mL

11. 1 quart = _____ pints

12. 1 oz = _____ gtt, minims, or grains

13. 1 gallon = _____ quarts

14. 1 oz = _____ gtt

15. 1 T = _____ t

16. 1 cup = _____ oz

17. 1 kg = _____ gram

18. 1 gram = _____ mg

19. 1 grain = _____ mg

20. 1 gram = _____ grain

21. 1 glass = _____ oz

22. 1 oz = _____ grain

23. 1 oz = _____ T

24. 8 oz = _____ mL

25. 2 T = _____ dr

26. 1,000 mL = _____ oz

27. 12 oz = _____ mL

Write Roman numerals two ways for the numbers 1 through 10.

1. _____

2. _____

3. _____

4. _____

5. _____

6. _____

7. _____

8. _____

9. _____

10. _____

Define the following.

kilo- _____

micro- _____

deci- _____

milli- _____

centi- _____

Application Exercises

Respond to the following scenarios.

1. Faith calls the medical office. The label on the over-the-counter cough syrup she is using lists the dose as 30 mL. She wants to know how many teaspoons to take. How would

   you respond? _____

   _____

2. Charlie weighs 110 lb. How many kilograms is this? _____

   _____

3. Doug has a fluid restriction of 1,000 mL/day. He has had 40 oz to drink today. Has he

   exceeded his restriction? Show your calculations. _____

   _____

4. Nancy is calculating a drug dose. The doctor ordered 0.500 gram. She calculates that as

   500 mg. Is she correct? _____

   _____

5. Jaquan calls from the pharmacy. The physician ordered 1/15 gram, and he was given 2 grains. He wants to know whether he received the correct dose. Did he? Show your work. _____

_____

Internet Research

1. Use your preferred search engine and search for "apothecary in Williamsburg." Read the information about what it was like to work as an apothecary in Colonial Williamsburg.

2. Use your preferred search engine and search for the U.S. Metric Association. Write down one interesting fact about the metric system.

8

Dosage Calculations

Now that you have reviewed and learned the mathematical principles necessary to calculate dosages safely and the systems of measurement, this chapter identifies four methods by which to calculate dosages. The four methods are the ratio and proportion method, the formulation method, dimensional analysis, and the fraction method. Each method is independent of the others, so try them all and select the one you prefer and perhaps another to check your work. Always check your answer to be sure it is accurate and reasonable. In this chapter, you will learn dosage calculations for special circumstances, such as for the pediatric and geriatric patient, as well as calculations for parenteral medications and for dosages based on weight and body surface area. You will also learn how to reconstitute solutions and how to help patients calculate their intake and output.

LEARNING OUTCOMES

At the end of this chapter, you should be able to:

8.1 Define key terms.
8.2 Learn and understand the four methods for calculating drug dosages.
8.3 Explain why certain calculations are considered special and which populations are affected.
8.4 Explain how to reconstitute powdered medication and calculate the desired dosage.
8.5 Discuss the factors to consider when calculating the dosages of parenteral medications and the two ways intravenous medications are administered.
8.6 Explain the calculation process for determining fluid intake.

KEY TERMS

Available dose	Desired dose	Diluent	Ordered dose
Body surface area (BSA)	Dimensional	Formula	Reconstitute
Conversion factor	analysis	Infiltrate	

■ METHODS FOR CALCULATING DRUG DOSAGES

When approaching mathematical problems, you may use multiple methods to find the correct answer. Some methods will be easier for you than others; decide which works best and stick with it. There are four methods by which to calculate drug dosages for the nonparenteral (oral) route of administration:

1. Ratio and proportion

2. Formulation

3. Dimensional analysis

4. Fractions

The ratio and proportion method uses two ratios (comparisons between two things) and a proportion (statement saying those two ratios are equal). The formulation method involves inserting numerical values into a **formula** (rule prescribing how to calculate a dosage) to arrive at the correct dosage. Dimensional analysis is a method based on the premise that any number can be multiplied by 1 without changing its value. The fraction method uses two equivalent proportions to find the answer.

Regardless of the method chosen, you follow the same basic steps. First, you must accurately read the drug label. Second, convert the numbers to the same unit of measurement. Third, using the preferred method, write the problem on paper. Finally, check and check again to confirm that your calculations are correct. You may choose one method of calculation and use another to check the accuracy of your results.

Figure 8-1 shows a sample drug label. The quantity is sometimes in tablets, capsules, milliliters, or another unit, and each label has its own equivalents. As discussed in Chapter 5, the manufacturer, lot number, and expiration dates are included on the label, as well as the name, dosage, form, and route of the drug. Most of this information is needed to calculate the dosage. The prescriber usually states the number of milligrams (or other unit of measurement) of a medication to administer, but unless you know what is in the container holding the ordered medication, you will not have the necessary numbers for the calculations. Now you are ready to learn how to calculate dosages.

Ratio and Proportion Method

The ratio and proportion method uses ratios, which are comparisons between two objects (numbers in this case). For example, if you have four pieces of pepperoni pizza and three pieces of cheese pizza, the ratio would be written as 4:3, or it may be written as 4/3. A proportion is a statement saying that two ratios are equal and, in this case, would be written as 4:3::8:6 or 4/3 = 8/6.

Example: The medication order is for 400 mg. The available medication is 300 mg in 1 mL.

Step 1: Write the ratio that you know (what is available).

$$\frac{300 \text{ mg}}{1 \text{ mL}}$$

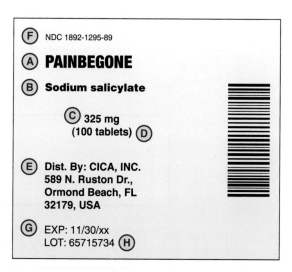

FIGURE 8-1: Sample drug label. The drug label should include (A) the brand (trade) name, (B) generic name, (C, D) drug strength and drug form, route of administration if other than oral, total amount of medication in the container, directions for reconstitution if necessary, (E) manufacturer, (F) National Drug Code (NDC), (G) expiration date, and (H) lot number.

(F) NDC 1892-1295-89

(A) **PAINBEGONE**

(B) **Sodium salicylate**

(C) 325 mg
(100 tablets) (D)

(E) **Dist. By: CICA, INC.
589 N. Ruston Dr.,
Ormond Beach, FL
32179, USA**

(G) EXP: 11/30/xx
LOT: 65715734 (H)

Step 2: Write the ratio that you need to solve for.

$$\frac{400 \text{ mg}}{? \text{ mL}}$$

Step 3: Write the proportion.

$$\frac{300 \text{ mg}}{1 \text{ mL}} = \frac{400 \text{ mg}}{? \text{ mL}}$$

Step 4: Cross-multiply to discover what ? equals.

$$300 \text{ ?} = 400$$

Step 5: Divide both sides by 300 to isolate ?.

$$\frac{300?}{300} = \frac{400}{300}$$
$$? = 1.25 \text{ mL}$$

Use the means and extremes method discussed in Chapter 6 as a shortcut to solve problems if you prefer. Figure 8-2 illustrates the following calculation using the means and extremes method.

Example: The medication order is for 100 mg. The medication label reads "200 mg/mL."

Step 1: Write what is on the label.

$$200 \text{ mg: 1 mL}$$

Step 2: Write what you need to solve.

$$100 \text{ mg: ? mL}$$

Step 3: Write the whole proportion statement. Both sides of the equation should have the same units (e.g., mg-mL or mg-tablets).

$$200 \text{ mg:1 mL::100 mg:? mL}$$

Step 4: Using means and extremes, multiply the inner (means) numbers and outer (extremes) numbers.

$$1 \text{ mL} \times 100 = 200 \times ?$$
$$00 = 200 \text{ ?}$$

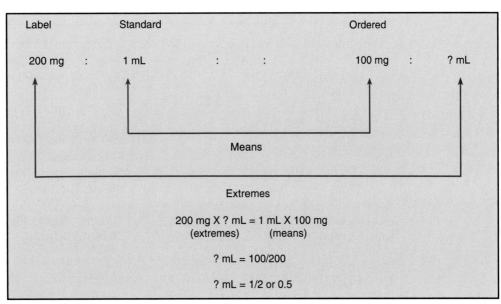

FIGURE 8-2: Means and extremes. To calculate, multiply the means (inner units) and relate them to the extremes (outer units).

Step 5: To isolate ? and discover the correct amount to administer, divide both sides of the equation by 200.

$$\frac{100}{200} = \frac{200?}{200}$$
$$0.5 \text{ mL} = ?$$
$$200 \text{ mg:1 mL::100 mg:? mL}$$
$$\text{mL} \times \text{mg (means)}$$
$$\text{mg} \times \text{mL (extremes)}$$

Setting the calculation up in one of these two ways should help you determine ratios correctly (Check Up 8.1).

The Formulation Method

The formulation method involves stacking units that are the same and multiplying by the unit requested. In this formula, D is the desired dose, H is the on-hand or available amount in ordered units, and Q is the quantity of liquid, tablets, capsules, etc. containing the available units. The **desired dose** is the dosage that has been ordered, or **ordered dose.** This dose must be in the same units as the **available dose** (the dosage on hand). The following is an example of a calculation using the formulation method.

Example 1: If the physician orders 200 mg, and the label reads "200 mg = 1 tablet," you would give one tablet when following the formula.

Step 1: Set up the D/H × Q formula with known values.

$$\frac{D}{H} \times Q = \frac{200 \text{ mg (order)}}{200 \text{ mg (label)}} \times 1 \text{ tablet}$$

Step 2: Solve the formula.

$$\frac{200 \text{ mg}}{200 \text{ mg}} \times 1 \text{ tablet}$$
$$1 \times 1 \text{ tablet} = 1 \text{ tablet}$$

🖊 CHECK UP 8.1: RATIO AND PROPORTION

Using ratio and proportion, calculate the dosage amount that must be administered.

1. $\dfrac{400 \text{ mg}}{1 \text{ mL}} = \dfrac{200 \text{ mg}}{? \text{ mL}}$ _____

2. $\dfrac{250 \text{ mg}}{1 \text{ mL}} = \dfrac{750 \text{ mg}}{? \text{ mL}}$ _____

3. $\dfrac{200 \text{ mg}}{2 \text{ mL}} = \dfrac{100 \text{ mg}}{? \text{ mL}}$ _____

4. $\dfrac{50 \text{ units}}{1 \text{ mL}} = \dfrac{150 \text{ units}}{? \text{ mL}}$ _____

5. $\dfrac{100 \text{ mg}}{1 \text{ tablet}} = \dfrac{200 \text{ mg}}{? \text{ tablets}}$ _____

6. 400 mg:1 mL::200 mg:? mL _____

7. 250 mg:1 mL::750 mg:? mL _____

8. 200 mg:2 mL::100 mg:? mL _____

9. 50 units:1 mL::150 units:? mL _____

10. 100 mg:1 tablet::200 mg:? tablets _____

Example 2: The physician's order is for 400 mg. The label reads "200 mg/mL."

Step 1: Set up the D/H × Q formula with known values.

$$\frac{400 \text{ mg}}{200 \text{ mg}} \times 1 \text{ mL}$$

Step 2: Solve the formula.

$$\frac{400 \text{ mg}}{200 \text{ mg}} \times 1 \text{ mL}$$
$$2 \times 1 \text{ mL} = 2 \text{ mL}$$

Often, ordered units do not match the units on the drug's label. Here is how to proceed in such a case:

Example 1: The medication order is for 0.25 gram, but the label has "250 mg/mL."

Step 1: Convert grams to milligrams.

$$0.25 \text{ g} \times 1{,}000 \text{ mg (the number of milligrams in 1 g)} = 250 \text{ mg}$$

Step 2: Set up the D/H × Q formula.

$$\frac{250 \text{ mg (order)}}{250 \text{ mg (label)}} \times 1 \text{ mL}$$

Step 3: Solve the formula.

$$1 \times 1 \text{ mL} = 1 \text{ mL}$$

Example 2: The medication order is for gr X (10 grains), but the label states "300 mg per tablet" (Check Up 8.2).

Step 1: Convert grains to milligrams.

$$1 \text{ grain} = 60 \text{ mg; therefore, } 10 \text{ grains would be } 10 \times 60 \text{ mg} = 600 \text{ mg}$$

Step 2: Set up the D/H × Q formula.

$$\frac{600 \text{ mg}}{300 \text{ mg}} \times 1 \text{ tablet}$$

Step 3: Solve the formula.

$$2 \times 1 \text{ tablet} = 2 \text{ tablets}$$

Dimensional Analysis

Dimensional analysis uses the ordered amount of a drug to multiply with two equal quantities in different dimensions (units of measurement) to derive the answer. The physician or practitioner always includes both a quantity and a dimension in each medication order. If you focus on the dimension rather than the numbers, you can create a template to use for every problem.

Dimensions (or units) vary depending on the circumstance. They may be tablets, capsules, bottles, milliliters (mL), ounces (oz), tablespoons (T), milligrams (mg), grams, grains, or something else. Calculating the dimension analysis can be done in four steps:

Step 1: Write the *units* of the dose ordered. For example, if the ordered dose is milligrams, write "mg" in the first position of the equation. If the order is in grams, write "grams." An order for 500 mg would be "mg."

Step 2: Write the *units* that are on the label and the *unit* that you plan to give to the patient. For instance, if a label shows that a drug is available in *milligrams*, and you want to give the drug in *milliliters,* you would place the unit of the ordered dose on the bottom of the **conversion factor** (formula to change from one unit of measurement to another). In this way, if you found that this unit of the ordered dose was mg, putting it on the bottom of

CHECK UP 8.2: FORMULATION METHOD

Calculate these dosages.

1. Physician's order: 500 mg
   Label: 250 mg/mL
   What would you give in milliliters? _____

2. Nurse practitioner's order: 100 mg
   Label: 200 mg/scored tablet
   How many tablets would you give? _____

3. Physician's order: 500 mg
   Label: 500 mg/capsule
   What would you give in capsules?

4. Physician assistant's order: 200 mg
   Label: 1 oz = 100 mg
   What would you give in ounces? _____

5. The patient weighs 100 lb. How many kilograms is this? _____

6. D = 1,000 units   H = 10,000 units   Q = 10 mL
   Milliliters to be given? _____

7. D = 200 mg   H = 400 mg   Q = 1 tablet
   Tablets to be given? _____

8. D = 250 mg   H = 500 mg   Q = 2 mL
   Milliliters to be given? _____

9. D = 700 mg   H = 0.35 gram   Q = 1 tablet
   Tablets to be given? _____

10. D = 1,000 mg   H = 1 gram   Q = 2 bottles
    Bottles to be given? _____

this formula would cancel out the mg in the first position and leave you with the unit that is on the top. Cancelling is simply removing a unit if it appears in both the numerator and the denominator of a fraction. The desired unit is the unit that you want to give and is placed on the top of the conversion factor.

$$\frac{\text{mg (ordered)} \times \text{mL}}{\text{mg from label (ordered)}} = \text{mL (desired)}$$

The conversion factor effectively multiplies the other units by $\frac{1}{1}$ because the two values are equal but in different units. The answer to this equation is the desired dose.

Therefore, if 250 mg = 1 mL (from the label), then

$$\frac{250 \text{ mg}}{1 \text{ mL}} = \frac{1}{1}$$

Can you find equivalents?

$$\frac{1 \text{ oz}}{? \text{ mL}} = \frac{1}{1} \qquad \frac{1 \text{ gram}}{? \text{ mg}} = \frac{1}{1}$$

Step 3: Now fill in the numbers for each unit and cancel the ordered units.

$$\frac{500 \text{ mg} \times 1 \text{ mL}}{250 \text{ mg (from label)}} = 2 \text{ mL}$$

Note: 1 mL = 250 mg (from label)

Check each label carefully; different vials may have different equivalents. Sometimes a label may not have a conversion of 1 mL; it may read "250 mg = 2 mL." You can reduce this fraction to be 125 mg = 1 mL or leave it as 250 mg = 2 mL for calculations. Both are equivalents.

Step 4: Check your work for accuracy and sense.

Would you inject 2 mL? Yes, OK.

What if your calculations resulted in an answer of 20 mL? Would you inject that much fluid? No.

If no, then you would go back and check your calculations again. Are these values equivalents?

$$\frac{500 \text{ mg}}{2 \text{ mL}} = \frac{250 \text{ mg}}{1 \text{ mL}}$$

Yes.

In Check Up 8.3, try calculating drug amounts based on medication orders.

Dimensional analysis can be used to convert between measurement systems. For example, the nurse practitioner orders a 1,000-mL fluid restriction for Clark C. Clark drank 50 oz of fluid today. Did he exceed the restriction?

Step 1: mL (units in which the fluid restriction is ordered)

Step 2:

$$\frac{\text{oz}}{\text{mL}}$$

mL $\times$ = oz (units for the fluid he drank)

Step 3:

$$1,000 \text{ mL} \times \frac{1 \text{ oz}}{30 \text{ mL}} = 33.3 \text{ oz}$$

Thus, 33.3 oz is less than 50 oz. If he drank 50 oz, he exceeded the 33.3-oz restriction.

Step 4: Check for common sense. Think of 1 liter (1,000 mL) as approximately a quart, which is 32 oz. Fifty ounces is larger than a quart. You may need to teach Clark not to drink more than a quart a day because he may not know what a liter looks like.

 CHECK UP 8.3: DIMENSIONAL ANALYSIS I

Using the information in the box, calculate the amount in milliliters of drug you would give according to the following orders.

> Generic cough syrup
> 100 mg/1 mL
> For oral use only

1. 100 mg

2. 200 mg

3. 50 mg

4. 300 mg

5. 250 mg

Dimensional analysis can also be used when dosages given are not in the unit on the label—if equivalent conversion units are used.

Example 1: The physician orders 1/2 gram of medication. The label says "250 mg = 1 capsule."

Step 1: Convert to the same unit of measure.

$$1/2 \text{ gram} = 0.5 \text{ gram}$$

Step 2: Use the dimensional analysis equation.

$$g \times \frac{mg}{grams} = capsule$$

Step 3: Plug in known values.

$$0.5 \text{ gram} \times \frac{1,000 \text{ mg}}{1 \text{ gram}} = 500 \text{ mg}$$

$$500 \text{ mg} \times \frac{1 \text{ capsule}}{250 \text{ mg}} = 2 \text{ capsules}$$

Step 4: Does a two-capsule dose make sense? Yes.

Example 2: Suppose you weighed a patient in pounds but needed to know the weight in kilograms to calculate a dosage. Could you use dimensional analysis? The patient weighs 70 lb. What is the equivalent in kilograms?

Step 1: Convert pounds to kilograms.

Step 2: Use the dimensional analysis equation.

$$lb \times \frac{kg}{lb} = kg$$

Step 3: Plug in known values.

$$70 \text{ lb} \times \frac{0.45 \text{ kg}}{1 \text{ lb}} = 31.5 \text{ kg}$$

Step 4: Does this answer make sense? If a pound is approximately 1/2 kg, the amount of kilograms should be approximately half of the number of pounds.

$$70 \text{ lb} \times 1/2 = 35 \text{ kg}$$

Is 31.5 approximately 35 kg? Yes (Check Up 8.4).

The Fraction Method

To use the fraction method for calculating dosages, the ordered dose and units given must be in the same proportion as the amount on the label. This method uses two equivalent proportions (the label and the desired dose) to find the missing number.

$$\frac{\text{Dosage on hand}}{\text{Dosage unit}} = \frac{\text{Desired dose}}{\text{Dose given}}$$

Example: If the label reads "200 mg of a drug is in 1 mL of fluid," the correct dosage must maintain that proportion.

$$\frac{100 \text{ mg}}{0.5 \text{ mL}} = \frac{200 \text{ mg}}{1 \text{ mL}} = \frac{300 \text{ mg}}{1.5 \text{ mL}} = \frac{400 \text{ mg}}{2 \text{ mL}} = \frac{500 \text{ mg}}{2.5 \text{ mL}} = \frac{600 \text{ mg}}{3 \text{ mL}} = \frac{700 \text{ mg}}{3.5 \text{ mL}}$$

All these proportions are the same. Sometimes you may even be able to cancel to obtain a lower number. This is fine as long as you maintain the same proportion.

CHECK UP 8.4: DIMENSIONAL ANALYSIS II

Using dimensional analysis, try solving the problem.

A mother calls your office from home and says that she does not know how many teaspoons to give her child because the directions on the medication bottle read "Give 15 mL."

Step 1: Write the units ordered.

Step 2: Write the known equivalent (hint: teaspoons to milliliters).

Step 3: Calculate.

Step 4: Does the answer make sense?

If you worked out the answer like this, congratulations!

$$15 \text{ mL} \times \frac{1 \text{ teaspoon}}{5 \text{ mL}} = 3 \text{ teaspoons}$$

Suggestion: Make sure your patient uses a properly calibrated teaspoon, such as a measuring spoon or medication spoon, because teaspoons that we eat with can vary in size.

Example: If the label reads "100 mg/tablet," what dose would be given if 200 mg is ordered?

Step 1: To find the desired proportion, write the label ratio on one side, and the same units on the other.

$$\underset{\text{On hand}}{\frac{\text{mg}}{\text{tablets}}} = \frac{\text{mg}}{\text{tablets}} \quad or \quad \underset{\text{Desired}}{\frac{\text{mg desired}}{\text{mg on label}}} = \frac{\text{tablets desired}}{\text{tablets on label}}$$

Step 2: Write the same units on the other side of the equal sign.

$$\frac{\text{mg}}{\text{tablets}} = \frac{\text{mg}}{\text{tablets}}$$

Step 3: Insert the numbers.

$$\frac{100 \text{ mg}}{1 \text{ tablet}} = \frac{200 \text{ mg}}{? \text{ tablets}}$$

Step 4: Perform the calculation.

$$\frac{100 \text{ mg}}{1 \text{ tablet}} = \frac{200 \text{ mg}}{2 \text{ tablets}}$$

Step 5: Check for sense. Would it make sense to give two tablets? Yes (Check Up 8.5 and 8.6).

CHECK UP 8.5: FRACTION METHOD

Solve the problems using fractions.

1. $\dfrac{1 \text{ mL}}{200 \text{ mg}} = \dfrac{? \text{ mL}}{100 \text{ mg}}$

4. $\dfrac{1 \text{ capsule}}{200 \text{ mg}} = \dfrac{? \text{ capsules}}{400 \text{ mg}}$

2. $\dfrac{1 \text{ tablet}}{250 \text{ mg}} = \dfrac{? \text{ tablets}}{500 \text{ mg}}$

5. $\dfrac{1 \text{ bottle}}{1,000 \text{ mL}} = \dfrac{? \text{ bottles}}{500 \text{ mL}}$

3. $\dfrac{1 \text{ oz}}{300 \text{ mg}} = \dfrac{? \text{ oz}}{150 \text{ mg}}$

 CHECK UP 8.6: FRACTION METHOD TO VERIFY RESULTS

Using the fractions, check to see whether these dosage calculations are correct. You may reduce or cross-multiply. Write true or false next to each calculation.

1. $\dfrac{250 \text{ mg}}{1,000 \text{ mg}} = \dfrac{1 \text{ mL}}{3 \text{ mL}}$

4. $\dfrac{700 \text{ mg}}{350 \text{ mg}} = \dfrac{1 \text{ mL}}{2 \text{ mL}}$

2. $\dfrac{100 \text{ mg}}{200 \text{ mg}} = \dfrac{1 \text{ mL}}{2 \text{ mL}}$

5. $\dfrac{300 \text{ mg}}{100 \text{ mg}} = \dfrac{3 \text{ mL}}{1 \text{ mL}}$

3. $\dfrac{500 \text{ mg}}{250 \text{ mg}} = \dfrac{2 \text{ mL}}{1 \text{ mL}}$

 CRITICAL THINKING

Does it make a difference if you align like units on one side and desired units on the other? Explain.

■ SPECIAL CIRCUMSTANCES

Special calculations often include the special populations of pediatric and geriatric patients because their body systems are either immature (pediatric) or weakened by the aging process (geriatric). Special calculations use the patient's weight or body surface area (BSA) to calculate for the correct dosage. For example, an order may be for a drug in milligrams per kilogram per day (mg/kg/day), which would require you to convert the patient's weight from pounds to kilograms and multiply that number by the number of milligrams to determine the daily dosage.

Calculating Pediatric Dosages

In the **pediatric** (infants and children) population, weight is frequently used to calculate dosages because the body systems of a child have not matured. In addition, the total body water content is higher in a child than in an adult, and thus medication is absorbed differently and at a different rate. Children's bodies simply cannot tolerate an adult dose. Most drug references list a pediatric dosage for drugs approved for use in children. If a dose is not listed, the drug may not be indicated for children, and the reference will often state that the drug has not been approved for pediatric use. Consult with the physician who wrote the order or the pharmacist if you have any question regarding the safety of a prescribed medication for a child.

A pediatric dosage can be calculated as follows.

Example: The physician orders a drug that has a recommended dosage of 30 mg/kg/*day*. How much would you give a 100-lb child each *day*?

Step 1: Convert 100 lb to kilograms.

$$100 \text{ lb} \times \frac{0.45 \text{ kg}}{1 \text{ lb}} = 45 \text{ kg}$$

Step 2: Multiply weight in kilograms by the order for 30 mg/*day*.

$$45 \text{ kg} \times \frac{30 \text{ mg/}day}{1 \text{ kg}} = 1,350 \text{ mg/}day$$

Note: If the drug is given bid (twice daily), divide the *daily* dose by 2.

$$\frac{1,350 \text{ mg}}{\text{day}} \div 2 = \frac{675 \text{ mg}}{\text{dose}}$$

If the dose is labeled qid (four times daily), divide the *daily* dose by 4. If the dose is labeled tid, which is three times daily, divide by 3.

CRITICAL THINKING

Some dosages may be numbers that are difficult to decide how to administer. For example, when the dose is 337 mg/dose and the medication comes in 200-mg tablets, what would you do? How many tablets will you give? Whom do you ask for advice?

Sometimes the ordered dose is given in milligrams per kilogram per *dose* (mg/kg/dose). To determine the total daily dose, multiply by the times per day the dosage is given.

Example: The patient weighs 100 lb. What is the total *daily dose* of a drug ordered as 20 mg/kg/*dose* to be given bid?

Step 1: Convert to kilograms.

$$100 \text{ lb} \times \frac{0.45 \text{ kg}}{1 \text{ lb}} = 45 \text{ kg}$$

Step 2: Plug in the known values. Solve.

$$45 \text{ kg} \times 20 \text{ mg/}dose = 900 \text{ mg/}dose$$

Step 3: To determine the total daily dosage and solve for bid, multiply by 2.

$$900 \text{ mg} \times 2 = 1,800 \text{ mg/}day$$

Other frequencies would change the total daily dose:

■ tid (three times daily): 900 mg × 3 = 2,700 mg/day

■ qid (four times daily): 900 mg × 4 = 3,600 mg/day

If the drug was available in 500-mg tablets, what would you give for each dose (Check Up 8.7)?

CHECK UP 8.7: PEDIATRIC DOSAGES

Answer these questions about pediatric dosages.

1. If a drug is ordered at 10 mg/kg/day, how much would a 20-lb patient need each day? _____ mg/day

2. If the drug in question 1 is given tid, what would be the milligrams per dose? _____ mg/dose

3. If a different drug is ordered at 20 mg/kg/day for the same patient, how much would he or she need each day? _____ mg/day

4. If the 20 mg/kg/day drug is to be given qid, what would be the milligrams per dose? _____ mg/dose

5. If a drug is ordered bid, how many doses do you give per day?

6. If the drug is ordered at 10 mg/kg/dose for a 50-lb patient, how much is given per dose? _____ mg/dose

7. If the drug in question 6 is given tid, how much is given per day? _____ mg/day

8. If the drug is ordered at 20 mg/kg/dose for a 50-lb patient, how much is given per dose? _____ mg/dose

9. If the drug in question 8 is given qid, how much is given per day? _____ mg/day

Calculating Geriatric Dosages

Geriatric (aged) patients also need medications calculated very carefully because of the high risk for toxicity resulting from their aging body systems, particularly the renal (kidneys), hepatic (liver), and circulatory systems. The most common adjustments that must be made are to reduce the dosage. Unfortunately, no magic "formula" exists for safe administration of medications to geriatric patients. Thus, changes in adult dosage are made on an individual basis by the physician after evaluating the patient's organ function and body weight. In addition, each elderly individual reacts slightly differently (e.g., mental confusion, lack of appetite) to each medication and therefore must be assessed after each medication is begun or changes to doses implemented.

Another confounding factor is the complicated health of many elderly patients. These patients may be seeing a multitude of practitioners, each of whom treats a different health issue, as well as self-medicating with vitamins and herbal medications. Unless the primary care physician is keeping close watch on all drugs taken by the patient, the common problem of drug interactions, with unwanted and sometimes dangerous reactions in the patient, may occur. For example, a patient who is given two different medications that lower blood pressure may suffer a significant drop in blood pressure and risk falling.

Calculation Using Body Surface Area

In some situations, knowing the exact size of a patient, both weight and height, is necessary. **Body surface area (BSA)** uses height and weight and a formula or nomogram to calculate the total surface area of the human body. This method is used most commonly in children, and it may also be used for administering chemotherapy to adults when dosage accuracy is critical. A patient's BSA is calculated by the prescriber and pharmacist to verify dosage. The health professional's role is primarily to obtain accurate measurements of the patient.

To find a patient's BSA, use the chart in Figure 8-3.

- Find the patient's height on the left side of the chart, and put a ruler or piece of paper at that point.

- Find the patient's weight on the right side (be sure to find it in kilograms or pounds, depending on how it was measured), and place the other side of the ruler or piece of paper at that point.

- The ruler or paper cuts across the chart. The intersection point indicates the patient's BSA (Check Up 8.8).

RECONSTITUTING POWDERS

Powdered medications occasionally must be converted to liquid form to be administered. This process is called **reconstituting.** After adding a specified amount of sterile water or saline solution, use the conversion ratio on the drug label to calculate the dosage. You are looking for the concentration of the resulting solution (i.e., how much medication is contained in how much liquid). The amount of fluid, called the **diluent,** used to reconstitute the formula adds to the powder's volume, so the final solution (powder and fluid) may be greater than the volume of the diluent. Directions are on the label.

Example 1: A drug label indicates that you should mix 9 mL sterile water with 500 mg powder, which makes a total of 10 mL. To calculate the dosage after reconstituting, use the ratio 500 mg/10 mL.

If you had an ordered dose (D) of 300 mg, available dose (H) of 500 mg in quantity (Q) 10 mL:

$$\frac{300 \text{ mg}}{500 \text{ mg}} \times 10 \text{ mL} = 6 \text{ mL}$$

Example 2: A drug label indicates you should mix 74 mL of diluent to powder. After reconstitution, the resulting solution will provide 250 mg of medication in every teaspoon (5 mL). Therefore, the ratio for calculating the dosage is 250 mg/5 mL.

If you had an ordered dose of 200 mg:

$$\frac{200 \text{ mg}}{250 \text{ mg}} \times 5 \text{ mL} = 4 \text{ mL}$$

Example 3: A drug label indicates that you should add 3.4 mL diluent to powder containing 1 gram of antibiotic. The resulting solution will provide 250 mg medication per mL. Thus, the ratio for dosage calculations is 250 mg/1 mL (Check Up 8.9).

If you had an ordered dose of 300 mg:

$$\frac{300 \text{ mg}}{250 \text{ mg}} \times 1 \text{ mL} = 1.2 \text{ mL}$$

PARENTERAL CALCULATIONS

Calculating dosages for parenteral (intravenous [IV]) administration is not as difficult as it would seem, but you must understand the equipment and the therapy, covered in Chapter 10. Dimensional analysis is the best way to calculate an IV drip rate because this method uses ratios as conversion factors and reduces the possibility of errors.

The laws related to IV therapy vary from state to state. Check with your state board of medicine to determine your legal responsibilities in terms of the scope of practice for your profession and what you are allowed to handle with parenteral therapy. Parenteral therapy policies also vary among organizations. Regardless of the scope of your responsibilities, you must know how IV dosages are calculated so you can double-check other health-care workers' calculations.

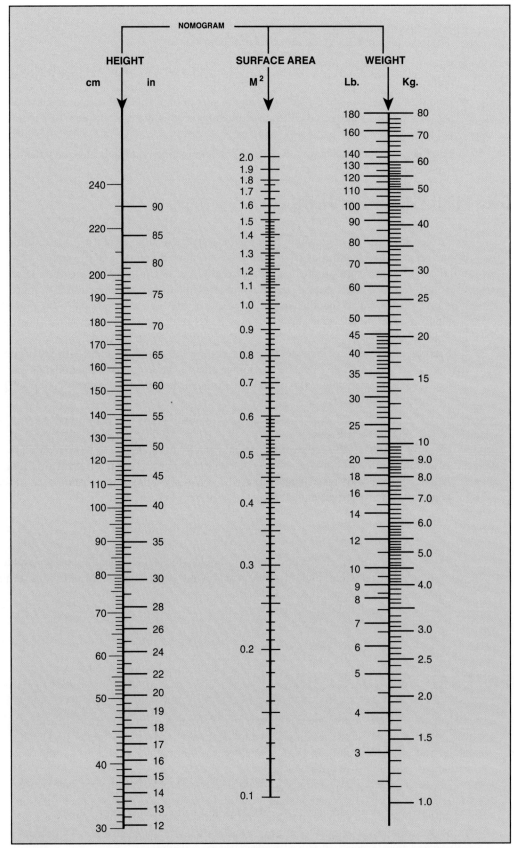

FIGURE 8-3: Body surface area (BSA) chart. This nomogram is used to determine the BSA of a patient. The chart is used primarily with medications that are particularly caustic, such as chemotherapy agents.

CHECK UP 8.8: BODY SURFACE AREA (BSA)

Using the BSA chart (see Fig. 8-3), determine the BSA of the patient. Be sure to note the dimensions (cm, kg, inches, lb).

1. 50 cm and 6 kg
2. 45 inches and 36 lb
3. 80 cm and 25 lb
4. 14 inches and 7.5 lb
5. 58 cm and 9 kg

 CHECK UP 8.9: RECONSTITUTION
OF POWDERED MEDICATIONS

Add 4 mL of sterile water. Resulting solution will contain 250 mg of medication/5 mL.

1. What amount of sterile water would you add to the vial?

2. What conversion factor would you use to calculate the dosage?

Add 1.7 mL diluent. Resulting solution contains 250 mg medication/1 mL.

3. What amount of diluent will you add to the vial?

4. What conversion factor would you use to calculate the dosage?

Add 33 mL diluent. Resulting solution will contain 500,000 units/mL.

5. How much diluent will you add to the vial?

6. What conversion factor would you use to calculate the dosage?

Add 19 mL of sterile water for injection. Resulting solution contains 10 mg/mL of medication.

7. How much diluent will you add to the vial?

8. What conversion factor would you use to calculate the dosage?

Electronic Regulator Pumps

Electronic regulator pumps are machines that deliver and monitor IV fluids at a set rate. These pumps allow the health-care professionals to perform other tasks and will alert health-care professionals if a problem arises. The physician or practitioner writes an order in milliliters to be infused over a certain period of time (e.g., 1,000 mL over 2 hours or 400 mL over 8 hours). The IV tubing, which is specific to the type of pump, is run through an electronic regulator; someone needs to program the rate for the regulator. The rate is expressed as follows:

$$\frac{\text{Total mL ordered}}{\text{Total time ordered in hours}} = \text{mL/hour (rounded to a whole number)}$$

Example: If the physician ordered 1,000 mL to be administered over 2 hours:

Step 1: Divide total fluid (mL) to be administered by time (hr).

$$\frac{1,000\,\text{mL}}{2\,\text{hours}} = \frac{500\,\text{mL}}{1\,\text{hour}}$$

Step 2: Does this seem reasonable? Cross-multiply to double-check (Check Up 8.10).

CHECK UP 8.10: IV ELECTRONIC MILLIGRAMS PER HOUR

What is the electronic milligrams per hour for the following?

1. 1,000 mL over 3 hours _____ mL/hr

2. 500 mL over 2 hours _____ mL/hr

3. 1,000 mL over 4 hours _____ mL/hr

4. 250 mL over 1 hour _____ mL/hr

5. 150 mL over 3 hours _____ mL/hr

Sometimes a patient wants to know when the infusion will be finished. If the physician orders an amount over a certain number of hours, it is easy to calculate the completion time.

For example, a patient arrives at 10 a.m., and the physician orders 1,000 mL of IV fluid to be given over 3 hours:

$$10:00 + 3 \text{ hours} = 13:00, \text{ or } 1 \text{ p.m. } (13:00 - 12:00 = 1 \text{ p.m.})$$

At noon, the patient asks whether the infusion will be done on time. You see there are still 500 mL to be infused. The physician ordered 500 mL/hour.

$$\frac{500 \text{ mL}}{500 \text{ mL}} \times 1 \text{ hour} = 1 \text{ hour}$$

You can tell the patient that the infusion will be finished in 1 hour.

$$\text{Noon} + 1 \text{ hour} = 1 \text{ p.m.}$$

Suppose you looked up at noon and there were 750 mL left? When would the patient be finished?

$$\frac{750 \text{ mL}}{500 \text{ mL}} \times 1 \text{ hour} = 1.5 \text{ hours}$$
$$\text{Noon} + 1.5 \text{ hours} = 1:30$$

Not only will your patient be disappointed, but something may have malfunctioned. If the flow rate is not constant and correct, report it to your supervisor. Do not change the flow rate because the change may cause the fluid or medication to be infused too quickly, or the patient's IV may be **infiltrated** (leakage of IV fluid or medication into the surrounding tissue). In either case, you could cause damage by increasing the flow rate.

 CRITICAL THINKING

In the foregoing case, in which the flow rate has not been consistent, you see that the IV insertion site is swollen. Would you increase the flow rate to make up the difference? What would you do?

A CLOSER LOOK: Military Time

Some facilities use military time, which is based on a 24-hour clock. The hours pass from 0100 to 1200 and then continue the next sweep from 1300 (1 p.m.) to 2400 (12 midnight). To return to the 12-hour clock, simply subtract 1200 from the number: 1300 − 1200 = 1. Complete the following for 24-hour times.

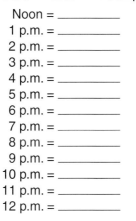

Noon = _____
1 p.m. = _____
2 p.m. = _____
3 p.m. = _____
4 p.m. = _____
5 p.m. = _____
6 p.m. = _____
7 p.m. = _____
8 p.m. = _____
9 p.m. = _____
10 p.m. = _____
11 p.m. = _____
12 p.m. = _____

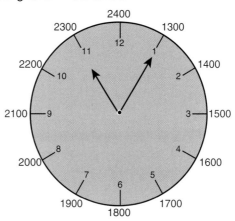

Manual IV Sets

Manual IV sets use gravity to infuse a solution at a set rate. This means that you need to know the drop factor. The drop factor is the number of drops in 1 milliliter of IV fluid (gtt/mL) and is stated on the package of the IV tubing. IV tubing has either a microdrip or a macrodrip chamber. The microdrip is 60 gtt/mL, and the macrodrip is either 10 or 15 gtt/mL, again as stated on the tubing packaging. (The drop factor is built into electronic pumps because the tubing matches the pump.)

The health-care professional who starts the IV infusion establishes the rate by hanging the bag or bottle at a certain height and adjusting the number of drops per minute with the roller clamp. The IV set must not be moved higher or lower in relation to the patient; doing so could change the drip rate. If the bag is moved, the drip rate must be readjusted.

The formula for the IV flow rate is:

$$\frac{\text{Total volume (V) to be infused (mL)}}{\text{Total time in minutes}} \times \frac{\text{Drop factor (D) (gtt)}}{\text{mL}} = \frac{\text{Rate of flow (R) (gtt)}}{\text{min}}$$

or, more simply,

$$\frac{V}{T} \times D = R$$

Example: The prescriber has ordered 500 mL to be infused over 4 hours. You have on hand 15 gtt/mL tubing. You need to determine the desired drip rate.

Step 1: Convert hours to minutes, and set up the equation.

$$60 \text{ minutes} \times 4 \text{ hours} = 240 \text{ minutes}$$

Step 2: Plug known values into the equation.

$$\frac{500 \text{ mL}}{240 \text{ minutes}} \times 15 \text{ gtt}$$

Step 3: Solve the equation.

$$\frac{32 \text{ gtt}}{\text{minute}}$$

If you were the health-care professional starting this infusion, you would count the drips in the drip chamber and adjust until you reached 32 gtt in 1 minute.

CRITICAL THINKING

When you receive an order to infuse fluid and are using manual drip tubing, which would drip faster at the same hourly rate, macrodrip or microdrip tubing? Explain your answer (see Check Up 8.11).

■ CALCULATING FLUID BALANCE

Fluid balance is vital for life. Pediatric and geriatric (elderly) patients can easily suffer from dehydration, overhydration, or electrolyte imbalances because of the differences in their immature or aging kidneys. Calculating a patient's input and output of fluids can help you determine his or her fluid status and can guide treatment planning.

Fluid output is determined by measuring, in milliliters, either urine or emesis (vomit) caught in a special container that includes the unit of measure. Measuring or calculating fluid intake presents more of a challenge. Patients may comply easily with urinating into a plastic device placed on the toilet that allows correct calculation of output. However, because part of measuring input relies on a patient's remembering to complete a log of ingested fluids, it is more difficult to calculate, especially if a patient is cognitively impaired. Instruct patients on the importance of keeping an accurate log of both intake and output.

In addition, education of patients about fluid intake should clarify that coffee, caffeinated sodas, and beer have a diuretic effect on the kidneys, meaning that they increase urination. Although consumption of these fluids counts as hydration, these drinks are not the best choices when intake and output are important to the patient's health.

The physician's order will usually indicate fluid intake restrictions or goals in milliliters, so you may need to teach the patient how to convert household measurements into milliliters to measure input and output or to use metric tools. Because some patients forget how to do conversions, you must be able to convert household measurements to metric measurements.

Example 1: Nita P., who presents with dehydration, is required to drink 1,500 mL/day. Her fluid intake is as follows:

One 20-oz soda
One 8-oz glass of water
One 4-oz glass of orange juice
One 8-oz cup of milk

CHECK UP 8.11: MANUAL IV RATE CALCULATIONS

Calculate the following in drops per minute to use with a manual setup:

1. 1,000 mL NS over 24 hours. Tubing: 15 gtt/mL

2. 250 mL over 3 hours. Tubing: 10 gtt/mL

3. 50 mL penicillin IV over 1 hour. Tubing: 60 gtt/mL

4. 750 mL RL over 8 hours. Tubing: 15 gtt/mL

5. 40 mEq KCL in 100 mL NS over 1 hour. Tubing: 10 gtt/mL

Step 1: Add all fluid in ounces: 40 oz.

Step 2: Set up the equation with known values.

$$40 \text{ oz} \times \frac{30 \text{ mL}}{1 \text{ oz}}$$

Step 3: Calculate the answer: 1,200 mL.

Step 4: Compare amounts to determine whether Nina met her requirement of 1,500 mL.

$$1,200 \text{ mL} < 1,500 \text{ mL}$$

No, she did not achieve 1,500 mL of fluid intake.

 CRITICAL THINKING

What instructions would you give to a child's parents about increasing the child's fluid intake to counteract dehydration?

Example 2: Jeremy J. is in heart failure and is restricted to a 1,000-mL fluid intake. Did he meet this requirement?

Step 1: Calculate total number of ounces of intake.

Two 6-oz cups of herbal tea: $2 \times 6 = 12$
One 8-oz bowl of milk in cereal: $1 \times 8 = 8$

One 4-oz glass of prune juice: $1 \times 4 = \dfrac{4}{32 \text{ oz}}$

Step 2: Set up the equation with known values. Remember, 30 mL = 1 oz.

$$32 \text{ oz} \times \frac{30 \text{ mL}}{1 \text{ oz}}$$

Step 3: Multiply and solve the equation.

$$32 \text{ oz} \times \frac{30 \text{ mL}}{1 \text{ oz}} = 960 \text{ mL}$$

Step 4: Compare amounts to determine whether Jeremy met his restriction of 1,000 mL.

$$960 \text{ mL} < 1,000 \text{ mL}$$

Yes, Jeremy should be praised (Check Up 8.12).

 ## CHECK UP 8.12: INTAKE CALCULATIONS

Solve these problems.

1.   John E. has a 1,000-mL fluid restriction. He drank two 10-oz lemon-lime sodas, one 8-oz glass of milk, and one 8-oz cup of decaffeinated coffee. Did he exceed his restriction? Show your work.

2.   Kathy T. is dehydrated. Her physician ordered her to drink at least 1,200 mL/day. Did she achieve this goal if she drank two 12-oz decaffeinated sodas, one 8-oz cup of decaffeinated coffee, and one 8-oz glass of water? Show your work.

● ● ● ○ **S U M M A R Y**

- Calculating dosages is instrumental in providing quality care to your patients.
- The four methods for calculating dosages are the ratio and proportion method, the formulation method, dimensional analysis, and the fraction method.
- The ratio and proportion method uses two ratios and a proportion.
- The formulation method involves inserting numerical values into a formula to arrive at the correct dosage.
- Dimensional analysis is based on the premise that any number can be multiplied by one without changing its value.
- The fraction method uses two equivalent proportions to find the answer.
- Pediatric and geriatric medication dosages are calculated differently from the average adult dose. Infants and children are given medications based on their body weight, whereas older adults are given medication after evaluation by their physician on an individualized basis depending on numerous factors (e.g., organ function, individual reactions to medications, body size).
- Body surface area (BSA) is a ratio of height to weight or the total surface area of the human body.
- Reconstitution is the process of converting powdered medications to liquid form. The concentration of the resulting solution is the amount of medication contained in a given amount of much liquid.
- Dimensional analysis is the best way to calculate an IV drip rate. The drop factor is the number of drops in 1 milliliter of IV fluid (gtt/mL).
- Electronic regulator pumps are machines that deliver and monitor IV fluids at a set rate. Manual IV sets use gravity to infuse a solution at a set rate
- Calculating a patient's input and output of fluids can help determine his or her fluid status and can guide treatment planning.

Activities

To make sure that you have learned the key points covered in this chapter, complete the following activities.

Using ratio and proportion, calculate the following.

1. 100 mg:1 tablet::200 mg:? tablets

2. 1,000 units:1 mL::10,000 units:? mL

3. 1 gram:1,000 mL::500 mg:? mL

4. 1 oz:30 mL::? oz:90 mL

5. 2 T:1 oz::? oz:90 mL

6. 1 oz:8 drams::3 oz:? drams

7. 4 oz:1 oz::? mL:30 mL

8. 250 mg:500 mg::? mL:1 mL

9. 1,000 units:10,000 units::? mL:1 mL

10. 500 mg:250 mg::? mL:1 mL

Use the formulation method to calculate the following.

D	H/Q
1. 1.5 g	500 mg/capsule
2. 290 mL	30 mL/oz
3. 200 mg	100 mg/tablet
4. 0.5 g	1,000 mg/bottle
5. 160 mg	80 mg/tablet
6. 600 mg	100 mg/capsule
7. 200 mg	100 mg/tablet
8. 750 mg	250 mg/tablet
9. 125 mg	250 mg/mL
10. 25 mg	100 mg/mL

Calculate the following using dimensional analysis.

1. Order: 100 mg   Label: 50 mg/mL

2. Order: 2 oz   Label: 1 oz/30 mL

3. Order: 10,000 units   Label: 1,000 units/mL

4. Order: 500 mg   Label: 250 mg/tablet

5. Order: 300 mg   Label: 100 mg/capsule

6. Order: 125 mg   Label: 250 mg/mL

7. Order: 125 mg   Label: 75 mg/mL

8. Order: 250 mg   Label: 1,000 mg/bottle

9. Order: 250 mg   Label: 125 mg/mL

10. Order: 1 g   Label: 500 mg/capsule

Calculate the following using fractions.

Order	Label
1. 200 mg	100 mg/2 mL
2. 250 mg	500 mg/tablet
3. 160 mg	80 mg/capsule
4. 350 mg	70 mg/mL
5. 75 mg	150 mg/mL
6. 1,000 units	500 units/mL
7. 250 mg	125 mg/mL
8. 25 mg	50 mg/tablet
9. 0.5 g	500 mg/mL
10. 1 gram	500 mg/tablet

Give the flow rate for an IV solution that is being infused through an electronic pump.

1. 50 mL over 2 hours

2. 2,500 mL over 4 hours

3. 1,000 mL over 8 hours

4. 500 mL over 3 hours

5. 1,000 mL over 2 hours

Give flow rates in gtt/minute for a solution that is being infused through a manual IV setup.

1. 100 mL D5RL over 8 hours   set: 15 gtt/mL

2. 500 mL NS over 4 hours   set: 10 gtt/mL

3. 1,500 mL RL over 6 hours   set: 60 gtt/mL

4. 2,500 mL NS over 10 hours   set: 15 gtt/mL

5. 1,000 mL D5 and 1/2 NS over 6 hours   set: 60 gtt/mL

6. 90 mL NS over 1 hour   set: 15 gtt/mL

7. 50 mL over 40 minutes   set: 10 gtt/mL

8. 200 mL NS over 2 hours   set: 10 gtt/mL

9. Kefzol 0.5 gram in 50 mL D5W over 30 minutes   set: 60 gtt/mL

10. 250 mL 1/2 NS over 5 hours   set: 60 gtt/mL

Application Exercises

Respond to the following situations.

1. Dr. McCauley orders 400 mg. The label reads "100 mg per 1 mL." How many cubic centimeters (cc) do you inject? _____

_____

2. Dr. Palmer orders 10,000 units of a drug. On hand you have 1,000 units. The quantity is 1 mL. How many milliliters do you give? _____

_____

3. Dr. Seiler orders 500 mg. The label says "250 mg/mL." What do you give? _____

_____

4. The examination question says:

   100 mg:1 mL::250 mg:? mL

   What is your answer? _____

_____

5. You are asked to make a large quantity of 10% bleach solution. If you need 20 mL of total solution, how much bleach do you need? _____

_____

6. Emily weighs 44 lb. If the doctor orders a medication for 10 mg/kg/day, how much should she receive per day? _____

_____

7. If the patient in question 6 was ordered a drug for 20 mg/kg/dose with two doses per day, how much would she receive per day? _____

_____

8. When Maria goes to the drug cabinet, she notes that there is 1 gram of medication in a bottle. She adds 4 mL of sterile water. This yields 250 mg/mL. If the ordered dose is 500 mg, what should she give? _____

_____

9. Mr. Belcher calls to try to understand how to compute his child's fluid intake. All he has at home are regular cups, glasses, and mugs. What would you suggest? _____

_____

10. Matthew has a 1,000-mL fluid restriction. Does he exceed it if he drinks two 20-oz sodas, one 8-oz glass of milk, and one 4-oz glass of orange juice? Show your work. _____

_____

11. You notice that a nurse has not set the correct IV drip dose for an electronic pump. What would you do or say? _____

_____

12. Kathy is having an infusion. She needs to pick up her children by 4:30 p.m. at the day-care center. If the infusion begins at 10 a.m. at 125 mL/hour and she needs 750 mL, will she be able to pick up her children on time? Show your work. _____

_____

13. Gloria is having an IV infusion. She is supposed to be finished in 2 hours at 150 mL/hour, and the infusion bag has 450 mL left. Is it infusing correctly? Show your work. _____

_____

Internet Research

1. Use your preferred search engine and find a tutorial on dimensional analysis. Print the information, and use it for practice.

2. Use your preferred search engine and search for a site to instruct patients on pediatric dosages. Print a teaching tool, and bring it to class to share.

3. Find three websites that manufacture IV tubing, and see what is used as the gtt factor. Use each of these drip factors to solve the problems in Check Up 8.11 on manual IV rates.

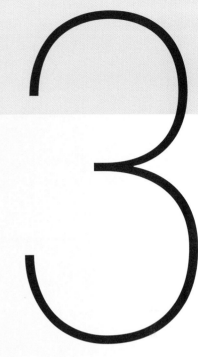

Administration
of Medications

9

Enteral Medications and Administration

*B*uilding *on the review of basic calculations and an understanding of the methods for correct dosage calculation, you are ready to learn the different routes of administration and the medications associated with them. This chapter discusses those medications forms associated with the enteral route and covers oral, buccal, sublingual, and rectal medications, their uses, and procedures for administering them to patients. Each of these routes and forms of medication has specific considerations related to administration.*

LEARNING OUTCOMES

At the end of this chapter, you should be able to:

9.1   Define all key terms.

9.2   List the forms in which medications are manufactured for the enteral route.

9.3   Differentiate how the different forms of drugs affect the body.

9.4   Describe the possible enteral routes for administering medications.

9.5   Describe how to administer oral medications safely.

9.6   Discuss the methods for administering medications through nasogastric or gastric tubes.

9.7   Explain why prescribers choose certain forms and routes over others.

KEY TERMS

Buccal	Enema	Sublingual
Buffered	Enteric-coated	Timed-release
Delayed action	Mortar and pestle	

■ ENTERAL MEDICATIONS

Enteral medications include any medications that involve the gastrointestinal tract, such as capsules, tablets, enemas, suppositories, and many others. The most common enteral route of administration is the oral route. Most common medications are given orally and include antibiotics, antacids, and antihypertensives to treat infections, heartburn, and hypertension, respectively, as well as vitamins to supplement the diet. Although absorption is slower compared with the parenteral route, oral administration is less invasive and is well tolerated by patients. In addition, because it requires little to no equipment, it is one of the least expensive routes of medication administration. For these reasons, the oral route is preferred. These are some of the advantages. Disadvantages include the risks of choking and possible aspiration of the medication into the lungs, thus leading to infections or even death. Another disadvantage is that stomach acid destroys or inactivates many medications. The most common medication that cannot be given by mouth is insulin. The stomach acid destroys insulin and renders it useless to the body. In addition, the patient's cooperation is necessary for this route to work.

Medications given via the oral route are absorbed at different points in the digestive tract. Some medications are absorbed directly from the mucosa of the stomach. Others are coated to protect them from stomach acid or to allow timed released and thereby eliminate the need for frequent doses. Many medication-related considerations arise with regard to food. Sometimes, it is important to take a medication on an empty stomach to ensure the most rapid action. Certain other medications are very irritating to the gastric mucosa and lead to nausea and vomiting, so patients are advised to take these medications with a glass of milk or food. Sometimes, patients are advised to take medications with a full glass of water, which will also prevent stomach irritation. In other instances, plenty of water is indicated to prevent dehydration. The guiding principles are familiarity with the medication and an awareness of dietary guidelines to teach the patient.

Contraindications to the oral route include nausea, vomiting, and difficulty swallowing. In addition, the oral route should not be used for medications that become inactivated by stomach acids or in patients who are not conscious and alert. Precautions include close monitoring of any patient with difficulty swallowing or a questionable level of consciousness. In addition, care must be taken to make sure that patients actually swallow the medication and do not hide it or throw it away.

Oral Solid Medications and Administration

Oral medications can be either solid or liquid. Solid forms include tablets and capsules. Tablets are disks of compressed medication in distinctive shapes and colors (Fig. 9-1). Oral drugs are frequently poured out of a bulk (multiple-dose) bottle first into the cap of the bottle and then into a medicine cup (Fig. 9-2). Frequently, pills come prepackaged in individual doses, referred to as unit-dose. A group of unit-doses may be contained in a blister pack, which must be opened gently by pressing on the tablet so that the pill falls into the medicine cup. Always wash your hands before administering medications, and avoid touching the pill to prevent transfer of microbes to the patient.

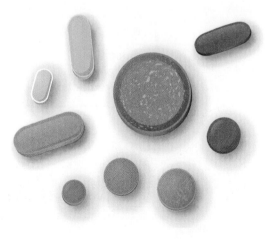

FIGURE 9-1: Tablets. Tablets come in a variety of sizes, colors, and shapes. Oblong tablets are known as caplets.

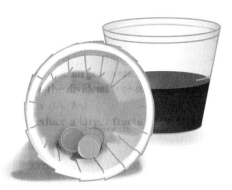

FIGURE 9-2: Medication cup. Both liquid and solid medications are placed in a cup for the patient.

Sometimes, a tablet must be crushed before it is administered; these tablets can be mixed with food or a liquid to make it easier for patients to swallow. A pair of devices called **mortar and pestle** is used to crush pills and tablets (Fast Tip 9.1).

Because tablets can be difficult to swallow given their chalk-like consistency, some medications are also available as gelatin-coated capsules (Fig. 9-3). These capsules can be easily pulled apart to mix the drug into food for patients with difficulty swallowing pills. This should be done only if approved by the pharmacy, and the contents of a capsule should be mixed only with small amounts of soft, thick food, such as ice cream or applesauce, to ensure that the entire dose is consumed.

Tablets can be coated to improve swallowing or prevent release in the stomach. **Enteric-coated** drugs are released not in the stomach but in the intestines; they are especially useful for patients with stomach ulcers or sensitivity. **Buffered** tablets have added antacids to prevent stomach irritation. Tablets can be scored (grooved in halves) for easy separation if half of a tablet is needed (Fig. 9-4). Caplets (see Fig. 9-1) are similar to tablets but may be easier for some patients to swallow because of the oblong shape.

A capsule can be in a **timed-release** or **delayed action** form that prevents it from being broken down in the acidic environment of the stomach. Instead, the capsule breaks down in the more alkalotic environment of the small intestine. Adderall XR is an extended-release capsule used to treat attention-deficit hyperactivity disorder. This medication is given only one time, in the morning, and the timed-release action allows the patient to take it less often. Timed-released capsules cannot be opened or crushed because doing so releases the drug all at once, causing an overdose. Steps for administering solid oral medications are outlined in Procedure Box 9-1.

 Fast Tip 9.1   Pills that Shouldn't be Crushed

Not all pills can be crushed. For example, pills coated to slow the release of the drug (enteric-coated tablets) and timed-release capsules should not be crushed. If in doubt, contact a pharmacist or check drug resources to see whether a tablet can be crushed.

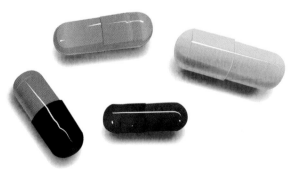

FIGURE 9-3: Capsules. Capsules are available in variety of sizes and colors.

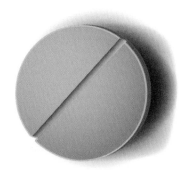

FIGURE 9-4: Scored tablets. Tablets are marked to allow for easy splitting.

Procedure Box 9-1 *Administration of Solid Medications*

- Observe the seven "rights" of medication administration.
- Read the medication order, and compare it with the medication container.
- Wash hands.
- Compare the medication order with the container a second time. Check the expiration date.
- Assemble equipment needed: medication, medication cup, order, and cup of water to help swallow medication.
- Identify the patient, and explain what you will be doing.
- Compare the order and container a third time.
- Without touching the medication, gently tap the correct amount into the cap of the container.
- If the medication is scored and must be cut, place it (without touching it) into a pill-splitting device, and cut correctly.
- Place solid medication in a medicine cup.
- Give the medication to the patient with a glass of water.
- Instruct the patient to swallow the medication completely. (Never leave until you witness the patient taking medication.)
- Assess the patient for any negative response (e.g., choking).
- Wash hands.
- Document medication administration and the patient's response.

Example:
11/15/2012 8:15 a.m: 500 mg ampicillin given PO. No problems noted. CJ Watkins RN, MSN

Oral Liquid Medications and Administration

At times, solid medication is not the best option for oral medication administration. Patients may have difficulty swallowing solid medication, or the medication needs to start working sooner than the solid form allows. Liquid medications are easier to swallow and are more quickly absorbed than are solid forms, and they are available in a variety of compositions (Fig. 9-5). For instance, effervescent salts are granules or coarse powders containing one or more medicinal agents, as well as tartaric acid or sodium bicarbonate. When dissolved in water or other liquids, effervescent salts produce carbonation. An example is Alka-Seltzer, which is a medication used for heartburn. The advantage of taking it in effervescent salt form is that the medication is already dissolved and does not have to wait for the stomach to dissolve it before the medication begins to work. Disadvantages of this form are the same as those of most other medications. Because of possible allergy to inactive ingredients, patients must read the ingredient list carefully before using this form of liquid medication.

Another form of liquid medication is an elixir, named because it contains alcohol (ETOH) in the preparation. The alcohol helps to dissolve the medication and makes it more palatable. Dimetapp Elixir used for cold symptoms is an example. Elixirs must be kept tightly capped to prevent evaporation of the alcohol because this would change the concentration of the medication in the elixir, and dosing

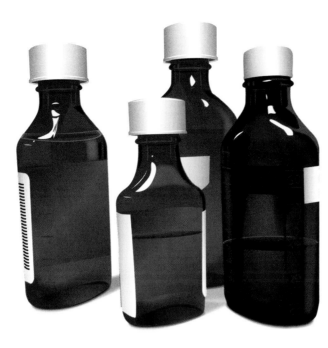

FIGURE 9-5: Liquid medication. Liquid medications are easiest for most patients to swallow and are more rapidly absorbed than are solid medications.

errors could occur. Elixirs are used less often because of the detrimental effects of alcohol, the potential for interaction with many other medications, and the development of new medication delivery systems. Elixirs should not be given to children or to anyone suffering from alcoholism or diabetes (the liver converts alcohol to sugar). Other liquid forms include the following: emulsions, which are liquid drug preparations that contain oils and fats in water; magmas, which are liquid and fine particles in water, such as Milk of Magnesia; and powders, which are finely ground forms of an active drug, sometimes given for pain relief. Goody's powder, for example, is placed on the tongue and absorbed into the bloodstream for pain relief. Other powders, such as bulk laxatives, are added to large amounts of liquid and are taken orally.

Occasionally, oral liquid medications are given as a solution. This means that the medication is evenly distributed throughout a liquid and will not separate. For this reason, solutions do not need to be shaken. The first milliliter in the bottle should contain the identical amount of medication as the last milliliter. An example is normal saline solution (NSS) used to irrigate eyes. Conversely, suspensions are medications dispersed in a liquid, but because the medication may not have been evenly distributed, it must be shaken before it is administered. Read the directions to help you tell the difference. Additionally, a suspension separates into different layers of liquid, thus indicating the misdistribution of medication. An example of a suspension that must be shaken before administration is Pepto-Bismol, which is used for stomach discomfort.

Syrups are medications added to highly sweetened liquids, and they are popular with children. Robitussin cough syrup is an example. Medications that are made more appealing to children can encourage these young patients to consume more than the recommended dose and can lead to an overdose; therefore, all medications must be removed from a child's reach.

To administer a liquid medication, a calibrated medicine cup is used. It is important to place the medicine cup on a flat surface and pour the liquid into the cup to ensure accurate dosing. The cup must be at eye level for reading the measurement. The patient may need some water after swallowing a thick or bad-tasting medication; however, if the medication is used to coat the throat, do not offer water.

If the patient is a small child or has trouble swallowing a liquid medication, the medication can be drawn up into a syringe (without a needle) and injected slowly and gently into the buccal pouch (cheek). This helps to prevent aspiration if the medication were injected directly toward the back of the throat. The infant should also be in a semireclined position, not flat on the back, for this reason.

Procedure Box 9-2 outlines the necessary equipment and steps to take to administer liquid oral medications safely.

Procedure Box 9-2 *Administration of Liquid Medications*

- Observe the seven "rights" of medication administration.
- Read the medication order, and compare it with the medication container.
- Wash hands.
- Compare the medication order with the container a second time. Check the expiration date.
- Assemble equipment needed: medication, order, calibrated medication cup.
- Identify the patient, and explain what you will be doing.
- Shake the bottle if needed.
- Compare the order and the container a third time.
- With the container on a flat surface, pour the correct amount of medication. The top of the fluid (meniscus) should be at the calibration line ordered. If you pour too much, you must dispose of the excess. Do not return the excess to the stock bottle.
- Give the patient the liquid medication.
- Instruct the patient to swallow the medication completely. (Never leave until you witness the patient taking medication.) If medicine is thick or tastes bad, offer patient water afterward.
- Assess the patient for any negative response (e.g., choking).
- Wash hands.
- Document medication administration and the patient's response.

Example:
03/02/2013 3:45 p.m.: 125 mg Tylenol drops given PO. Patient tolerated well. CJ Watkins RN, MSN

Nasogastric Tube Medications and Administration

Most liquid oral forms of medications can be administered through a nasogastric (NG) tube, which leads from the nose to the stomach, or a gastric tube, which a surgeon places directly into the patient's stomach under sterile conditions (Procedure Box 9-3). These tubes are used for patients who, for various reasons, have trouble swallowing or ingesting an adequate diet for optimal health.

Only liquids or tablets that have been crushed and mixed in water can be delivered through the tube. Before the drug is given, the NG tube must be checked to ensure proper placement. NG tubes may become displaced, with the tip in the respiratory system, and this can lead to aspiration pneumonia or death if fluid is administered by this route. Be sure to flush the tube with NSS before and after medications are administered to keep the tube patent (Fast Tip 9.2).

Procedure Box 9-3 *Administration of Medications by Nasogastric or Gastric Tube*

- Observe the seven "rights" of medication administration.
- Read the medication order, and compare it with the medication container.
- Wash hands.
- Compare the medication order with the container a second time. Check the expiration date.
- Assemble equipment needed: syringe, medication, flushing fluid, order.
- Compare the order and the container a third time.
- Identify the patient, and explain what you will be doing.
- Elevate the patient's head.
- Hold end of tube up, and remove the clamp, plug, or adapter.
- Attach an empty syringe (without a needle) to the port.
- Verify the tube is in the stomach (see Fast Tip 9.2).
- Use the syringe to flush the tube with NSS.
- Use the syringe to administer medications.

Procedure Box 9-3 *Administration of Medications by Nasogastric or Gastric Tube—cont'd*

- Place more critical medications into the tubing first so it is less likely that a crucial medication will be vomited out of the tube.
- After medication has been administered, flush the tubing with NSS.
- Clamp the tube with your fingers by pinching it.
- While the tube is closed, remove the syringe and reattach the securing device.
- Assess the patient.
- Wash hands.
- Document medication administration and the patient's response.

Example:
12/01/2012 12:25 p.m.: 15 mg Reglan liquid administered via NG. Tube placement checked ×2. Patient tolerated well. CJ Watkins RN, MSN

 Fast Tip 9.2   Checking Tube Placement

You can check that the nasogastric (NG) tube is in the stomach either by injecting air into the tube while listening with a stethoscope for the sound of air in the stomach or by drawing back on a syringe attached to the tube and checking whether stomach contents flow backward into the syringe.

The Buccal Route of Medication Administration

The **buccal** pouch, or cheek, is a good route for applying medication in the mouth or throat to ease local inflammation. Troches (lozenges) can be held in the cheek. They are usually pleasant tasting and melt slowly over time, coating the throat and mouth. For patients with a sore throat, this route is ideal. It is important to tell the patient not to swallow or bite the buccal medication because it will not work as planned. In addition, liquid medication may be used to coat the interior of the mouth and cheeks. The patient is instructed to swish the medication around and then spit it out. One example is nystatin, used for fungal infections. Another example is a lidocaine solution, which is used in patients who are receiving chemotherapy and have resulting lesions in the mouth. The patient may need to refrain from drinking for 15 to 20 minutes after taking the buccal medication, to maximize the effect and prevent the medication from being washed away.

The Sublingual Route of Medication Administration

Sublingual means under the tongue. The many capillaries under the tongue provide a rich blood supply for quick absorption of a medication. For that reason, nitroglycerin, which improves heart function, is placed sublingually for immediate relief of chest pain or during a heart attack. Although slower than an injection into a vein, the sublingual route delivers medication quickly without having to pass completely through the digestive system.

Rectal Medications and Administration

Some medications, such as suppositories, enemas, suspensions, or ointments, must be administered rectally. This route is sometimes necessary because the patient has severe nausea or vomiting or is not alert enough to swallow. Some may ask why the medication cannot be given by the intravenous (IV) route. The reason is that some medications do not come in parenteral forms (e.g., Tylenol), or the patient may not have IV access. Many medications, such as Tylenol (fever, pain) and Phenergan (nausea and vomiting), are available as suppositories. They have a glycerin or cocoa butter base containing the medication. Because suppositories soften when warm to release the medication, they must be kept cool before administration. Be sure to insert a rectal suppository immediately after opening it or it will melt in your hand. **Enemas** are liquids administered through the rectum to soften stool, cleanse bowels, or deliver medication. Enemas are rarely given in the ambulatory setting, but many patients must administer them at home as a preparation for bowel procedures or surgery or as treatment for constipation. For these reasons, patients must be taught how to use them. To administer a rectal suppository or enema, follow the instructions in Procedure Box 9-4.

Other medications that may be given rectally include rectal suspensions (e.g., mesalamine, used as a gastrointestinal anti-inflammatory medication) and ointments (e.g., Preparation H, used to treat hemorrhoids). Both types of medications are usually administered through an applicator tip placed into the rectum.

 CRITICAL THINKING

Why is the gastrointestinal a popular route for taking medication?

Procedure Box 9-4 *Rectal Administration*

This procedure can be used for a rectal suppository or an enema.
- Observe the seven "rights" of medication administration.
- Read the medication order, and compare it with the medication container.
- Wash hands.
- Compare the medication order with the container a second time. Check the expiration date.
- Identify the patient, and explain what you will be doing.
- Compare the order and the container a third time.
- Have the patient remove his or her underwear.
- Assist the patient to lie on the left side.
- Place waterproof sheeting under the patient.
- Drape the patient for privacy.
- Put on gloves.
- Open the suppository wrapping, or remove the cover from the enema bottle.
- Gently separate the patient's buttocks.
- Apply a water-based lubricant to the tip of the enema bottle or suppository.
- Insert the suppository with one finger into the patient's rectum, or insert the tip of the enema bottle past the anal sphincter, and squeeze contents slowly into the rectum.
- Remove your finger or the tip of bottle from the patient's rectum.
- Assess the patient.
- Ask the patient to lie still for approximately 30 minutes.
- Clean the patient and the patient's area.
- Remove gloves.
- Wash hands.
- Document medication dosage and the patient's response.

Example:
04/5/2013 3:30 p.m.: temperature 103.2 rectal. grV Tylenol PR. Patient tolerated procedure well. CJ Watkins RN, MSN
04/5/2013 4:00 p.m.: temperature now 100.2 rectal. CJ Watkins RN, MSN

● ● ○ S U M M A R Y
This chapter covers the following concepts:

■ There are many different ways to give enteral medications:

   ■ Oral

   ■ Buccal

   ■ Sublingual

   ■ Rectal

■ Forms that enteral medications come in include:

   ■ Tablets

   ■ Capsules

   ■ Liquids

   ■ Troche

   ■ Suppository

   ■ Spray

■ Knowing which medication form can be given by which route is an important concept to master

Activities

To make sure that you have learned the key points covered in this chapter, complete the following activities.

True or False

Write true if the statement is true. Beside the false statements, write false, and correct the statement to make it true.

1. Sublingual is the most common enteral route used by patients. _____

   _____

2. A troche is a lozenge that is placed in the cheek (buccal pouch) and allowed to dissolve.

   _____

   _____

3. Patients should be instructed to rinse the mouth after being given a buccal medication.

   _____

   _____

4. Patients should be encouraged to lie quietly for 30 minutes after being given a suppository.

   _____

   _____

5. Insulin is a common medication given by mouth (oral). _____

   _____

6. A suspension never needs to be shaken. _____

   _____

7. Elixirs contain alcohol and therefore should not be given to children. _____

   _____

8. Effervescent salts must be mixed with carbonated water to create bubbles. _____

   _____

9. Solutions never need to be shaken. _____

   _____

10. A troche should be chewed completely within 5 minutes for maximum effect. _____

    _____

Multiple Choice

Choose the best answer for each question.

1. Which of the following is an example of a GI route?

   A. IV

   B. Nasal

   C. Oral

   D. ID

2. Suppositories are administered through which of the following routes?

A. IV

B. Inhalation

C. ID

D. Rectal

3. Which of the following contains alcohol?

A. Capsule

B. Magma

C. Emulsion

D. Elixir

4. Which must be added to a liquid before administering?

A. Effervescent salts

B. Magmas

C. Foams

D. Troches

5. Which of the following is given orally?

A. Syrups

B. Emulsions

C. Suspensions

D. All of the above

6. Which of the following is a term that means a tablet can be easily divided into two parts?

A. Scored

B. Divided

C. Marked

D. None of the above

7. A blister pack is _____.

A. Bubble wrap to ship medication

B. The way that effervescent salts are packaged

C. A common way that individual medication doses are packaged together

D. None of the above

8. The reason NG tube placement must be checked before the administration of medication is to verify that the tip is correctly placed in the _____.

A. Lung

B. Esophagus

C. Bowel

D. Stomach

9. **Medications that may be administered via an NG tube include** _____.

   A. Liquid medication

   B. Tablets that are crushed and mixed with water

   C. Both of the above

   D. None of the above

10. **What type of oral medication consists of a gelatin coating containing a powdered form of medication?**

   A. Capsule

   B. Tablet

   C. Caplet

   D. None of the above

Application Exercises

Respond to the following situations.

1. To aid your memory, complete the following table to help you remember the content of this chapter. Use books and resources as needed to complete the chart.

Reference Guide for Routes

Route	When Used	Example
Buccal		
Oral		
Rectal		
Sublingual		

2. Your patient does not understand why his medication cannot be given orally. Discuss the advantages and disadvantages of the gastrointestinal route. _____

_____

3. Your physician has asked you to assemble the following drugs in case of an emergency and store them in the crash cart. By what route is each drug given, and for what is it used?

   A. acetaminophen _____

   _____

   B. aspirin _____

   _____

   C. diphenhydramine _____

   _____

   D. Compazine _____

   _____

E. digoxin _____

_____

F. furosemide _____

_____

G. nitroglycerin _____

_____

4. You notice that your colleagues at work do not wear gloves when handling medications. For what routes must gloves be worn? Defend your answer. _____

_____

5. You need to give a dose of liquid Tylenol to a 3-month-old baby. Explain how you would accomplish this and what equipment you would need. _____

_____

Parenteral Medications and Administration

This chapter describes the routes known as parenteral, the forms of medication used, the supplies needed, and the proper procedures for administering medication. The parenteral routes include transdermal or topical, nasal, inhaled, ophthalmic, otic, and vaginal. The medications come in many different forms and compositions. Some are ready to administer immediately, whereas others require you to prepare them for use. The types of injectable medications are intramuscular (IM), subcutaneous (SC), intradermal (ID), and intravenous (IV). In this chapter, you will also learn the multiple factors that determine the route of administration, including chemicals used, necessary response time, and desired effect (whether local or systemic). A big part of each procedure is to always observe the seven "rights" of safe medication administration (right patient, right drug, right dose, right time, right route, right documentation, and right technique).

LEARNING OUTCOMES

At the end of this chapter, you should be able to:

10.1 Define all key terms.

10.2 Describe how to apply transdermal patches and other topical medications correctly.

10.3 Indicate how to administer ophthalmic, otic, and nasal medications correctly.

10.4 Describe how to insert vaginal medications safely.

10.5 List precautions for the safe administration of inhalation therapy.

10.6 Choose the correct needle and syringe for parenteral injections.

10.7 Indicate how to inject IM, SC, and ID medications safely.

10.8 Indicate how to prepare the patient for IV therapy.

10.9 Distinguish among the solutions used in IV therapy.

> ### KEY TERMS
>
> | | | |
> |---|---|---|
> | Ampule | Intradermal (ID) | Subcutaneous (SC) |
> | Calibrated | Intramuscular (IM) | Topical |
> | Emboli | Lumen | Thrombus |
> | Gauge | Parenteral | Vial |
> | Infiltration | Phlebitis | |

■ PARENTERAL MEDICATIONS

Parenteral medications include all medications that are not ingested or introduced into the gastrointestinal system. They include topical, ophthalmic, otic, vaginal, nasal, inhaled, and injectable (intradermal [ID], intramuscular [IM], subcutaneous [SC], and intravenous [IV]) medications. The reasons for choosing a particular route, the forms of medication that can be administered parenterally, and the correct procedure for each parenteral route are discussed. When giving any medication, you must wash your hands, observe the seven "rights" of medication administration (right patient, right drug, right dose, right time, right route, right documentation, and right technique), compare the order with the container three times, and document the administration of the drug. The patient needs to know what the procedure entails before you administer the medication. Safely administering medications requires strict adherence to the protocols listed in this chapter or in your facility's procedure manual.

■ TOPICAL MEDICATIONS AND ADMINISTRATION

Topical medications are applied directly to the skin as a patch, ointment, cream, lotion, or gel and are absorbed transdermally (through the skin). Topical medications are sometimes used if patients have difficulty swallowing or cannot take oral medications because of severe nausea. In addition, many conditions of the skin are treated by directly applying medication to the affected areas. Some medications are applied topically to achieve a systemic effect by maintaining continuous release of therapeutic doses of the drug.

Semisolid Preparations

Topical drugs come in several types of preparations. Semisolid preparations include creams, ointments, gels, and plasters and are applied to the surface of the skin. Ointments are petroleum based and work to keep the medication in contact with the skin. For this reason, before additional doses are applied, the remaining ointment should be wiped away to avoid cumulative effects of medication (overdose). Common ointments include antibiotic ointments such as Bactroban placed on a wound and hydrocortisone used for itchy skin patches.

Creams are medications in a water base that absorb into the skin and disappear. Kwell (lindane) is a prescription cream used for the treatment of lice and scabies. Another cream is Oxy 10 Balance medicated cream, used on existing blemishes.

Gels are semisolid suspensions. This means that particles of drug are suspended in a thickened water base. An example is MetroGel for acne.

Plasters are medicated preparations that adhere to the skin with materials such as paper, linen, moleskin, or plastic. Examples include salicylic acid plaster, which is used for warts, and bandages that are saturated with antibiotics. These plasters are used to hold the medication directly against the lesion or wound to be treated. Other plasters are used to administer pain medication for arthritis or diabetic neuropathy and must be placed on healthy, intact skin only. Examples of these types of plasters are capsaicin plaster and 5% lidocaine medicated plaster.

Most of the previously mentioned medicated preparations contain significant doses of medication, and care must be taken when they are combined with oral medications so that overdosage does not occur. In addition, ingredients must be checked carefully to avoid exposing patients to allergens.

Liniments (or salves) and lotions are also semisolid preparations. Liniments are rubbed on the skin. They have an ingredient (usually camphor, wintergreen, or alcohol) that irritates the skin. This irritation (patients feel burning or pain) causes blood flow to increase to the affected area and decreases pain. Examples are Bengay and Icy Hot, used for sore muscles.

Lotions are used externally for skin disorders, such as the itchy skin associated with chickenpox or poison ivy. Lotions are similar to creams in that they are water based. Creams are basically 50% water and 50% oil, whereas lotions contain more water than oil, thus making them lighter and less greasy. They are patted on, not rubbed into, the skin, to allow the medication to stay on the target area and not absorb into the skin. An example is calamine lotion, which must be shaken and applied with a cotton ball or other applicator because of its thin consistency.

Solid Preparations

Topical medications are also available in solid form, such as a powder or patch. Powders are often applied to the skin to treat fungal disease or reduce moisture. One example is Desenex (miconazole nitrate), a powder to put on toes to prevent or treat athlete's foot. Gold Bond Extra Strength Medicated Powder is used to reduce moisture anywhere on the body, but most commonly the feet and toes.

A transdermal patch holds a specific amount of medication over a specific area and delivers medication over time (Fig. 10-1). Patches are often used to relieve nausea, provide pain relief, alleviate nicotine addiction, and control angina, as well as provide hormonal treatment such as birth control and hormone replacement therapy.

Advantages of using the transdermal patch include ease of application and removal, effectiveness over time, and reliable results based on even drug distribution in the body. Disadvantages include difficulty keeping the patch in place. Some patients' skin is not ideal because of excessive dryness or oiliness, which can cause the patch to fall off. Failure to wipe away leftover medication at the site when changing patches can lead to medication overdose. If patches are not disposed of properly, pets finding the patches in the garbage may be exposed to the medication and become very sick. In addition, this medication route may have a slow onset.

An example of a transdermal patch is NicoDerm (nicotine patch), which delivers very small amounts of nicotine through the skin to help curb nicotine cravings when a person is trying to quit smoking. Another example is nitroglycerin, which is used to treat and prevent angina (chest pain caused by decreased blood flow to the heart). Nitroglycerin is a vasodilator that helps the coronary blood vessels open up and allows more efficient blood flow to the heart.

Most patches come from the manufacturer ready for administration. Wear gloves so medication from the patch does not enter your body. Remove the sticky backing on the patch, and apply the patch to an appropriate location on the body (Fig. 10-2). Be sure the area is free of tattoos, scarring, and redness because these features may alter absorption of the medication. Teach the patient to rotate sites to prevent skin irritation.

To remove the patch, apply gloves to avoid contact of the remaining medication with your own skin. Then fold the patch inward, and dispose of it carefully so that children or pets are not inadvertently exposed to the medication. See Procedure Box 10-1 for administration of a transdermal patch.

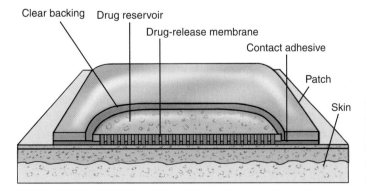

FIGURE 10-1: Transdermal administration. In a transdermal delivery system, the medication is contained in a drug reservoir, which is released through a membrane when the patch is applied to the skin by an adhesive backing.

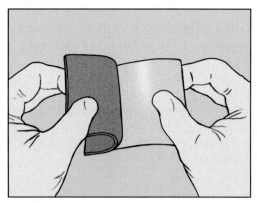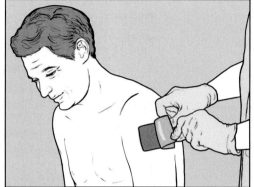

FIGURE 10-2: Applying a transdermal patch. Remove the sticky backing on the transdermal patch, and apply it to an appropriate location on the body.

Procedure Box 10-1 *Transdermal Patch Administration*

Safety Precautions: Avoid touching medication to bare skin. Care should be taken when disposing of an old patch or wrapping of a current patch to avoid exposure of housekeepers, children, or animals to medication.

Supplies: Order, patch, gloves, teaching materials

Steps:

1. Observe the seven "rights" of medication administration.
2. Read the order, and compare it with the label on the medication container. Check the expiration date.
3. Wash hands.
4. Compare the medication order with the container a second time.
5. Identify the patient, and explain what you will be doing.
6. Compare the order and the container a third time.
7. Put on gloves.
8. Inspect the application site, and make sure that it is clean, dry, and free of lesions.
9. Carefully remove the adhesive backing from the patch.
10. Place the patch on the selected site, and make sure that all edges of the adhesive adhere securely to skin.
11. Remove gloves and wash hands.
12. Document medication dosage, location, and the patient's response.

Example:

02/20/2013 6:45 p.m: fentanyl 25 mcg/hr patch placed to left upper quadrant of abdomen. Patient advised to be cautious with change of positions to avoid falls. Pt. states understanding of side effects to report and activities to avoid. CJ Watkins RN, MSN

There are still a few patches that you may have to prepare on your own. The most common patch you will need to make is nitroglycerin, although the use of these patches has declined in favor of commercially prepared patches. To make a transdermal patch, take an empty patch that marks the area of measurements on the application area. The medication order will be for centimeters or inches. Squeeze the tube of medication to place a specified measure on the ruled area. The more slowly you squeeze and move the tube, the thicker the line of medication will be. Therefore, the amount given is variable.

 CRITICAL THINKING

What would be the effect of cutting a transdermal patch? Is it advisable?

■ OPHTHALMIC MEDICATIONS AND ADMINISTRATION

Ophthalmic medications are placed directly in the eye for infections, for glaucoma treatment and prevention, and to facilitate examination and treatment. These medications can be given as drops or ointments. Eye drops may be used to lubricate the eye or treat other conditions through absorption in the inner canthus of the eye. Ophthalmic ointments are thickened drug solutions that are applied to the inside lower eyelids. Ocular inserts are small transparent membranes that contain medication. These inserts have the advantage of prolonging contact of the medication with the surface of the eye. One reason for using this method would be to treat chronic dry eye with an insert such as Lacrisert® (hydroxypropyl cellulose). Inserts are also in different stages of development for the treatment of infections and glaucoma. They are placed between the eye and lower conjunctiva and release medications over a period of time. Always keep ophthalmic preparations sterile, to avoid infection (Procedure Box 10-2).

Many patients are anxious about having medicine dropped into their eyes, so be sure to keep the patient informed at all times. When placing medication in a patient's eye, wear gloves and be careful not to touch the dropper to the eye or eyelid itself, to avoid the spread of infection or contamination. Have the patient look upward as you drop in the exact number of drops ordered (Fig. 10-3). After the drops are instilled, have the patient close his or her eyes. This helps prevent the medication from entering a tiny tube called the nasolacrimal duct, which runs from the inside corner of the eye to the nose. Applying light pressure with a finger on the inner part of the closed eyelid after administration of the medication also helps to keep the drug from leaking into the nasolacrimal duct.

Some eye medications come in the form of an ointment, which is applied to the inside of the bottom eyelid or conjunctival sac. Pull down on the lower eyelid and apply the ointment stream from the inner (nasal) to outer aspect. You may need to use a twisting motion to break the ointment stream. Be sure not to touch the tip of the tube to the eye or eyelid. If you have orders to administer both eye drops and ointment, always administer the drops first because ointment forms a barrier that will not allow drops to penetrate.

Procedure Box 10-2 *Administration of Ophthalmic Medication*

Safety Precautions: Maintain sterility of applicator tips to avoid infection. Be sure to have assistance for uncooperative children, to avoid injury to the eye.

Supplies: Medication, order, gauze, gloves, teaching materials

Steps:

1. Observe the seven "rights" of medication administration.
2. Read the medication order, and compare it with the medication container. Check the expiration date.
3. Wash hands.
4. Make sure that the medication is at room temperature, not cold.
5. Compare the medication order with the container a second time.
6. Put on gloves.
7. Identify the patient, and explain what you will be doing.
8. Compare the order and the container a third time.
9. Ask the patient to look upward.
10. Drop the medication by dropper into the affected eye, or apply ointment by placing a line of ointment on the inner (nasal) to outer aspect of the lower eyelid (conjunctival sac), as ordered. REMEMBER: Drops BEFORE ointment if both are ordered.
11. Assess the patient.
12. Remove gloves and wash hands.
13. Document dosage, site of placement, and the patient's response.

Example:

03/21/2013 09:30 a.m.: 2 drops gentamicin ophthalmic solution administered to left eye. Patient tolerated procedure well. CJ Watkins RN. MSN

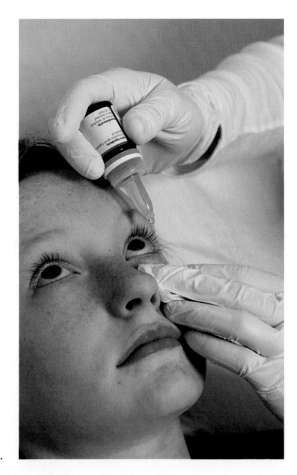

FIGURE 10-3: Ophthalmic administration.

OTIC MEDICATIONS AND ADMINISTRATION

Otic medications are placed directly into the ear canal to treat infections of the external ear canal and middle ear, and for the treatment of cerumen (ear wax) impaction. Cerumen is treated with Debrox (carbamide peroxide). To decrease discomfort, ear medications should be at room temperature before they are given. Instill the exact number of drops ordered. Although ear medications do not leak as easily as ophthalmic medicines, the patient must keep the affected ear upright for a few minutes to allow maximum absorption of the medication.

Pull on the outer ear (pinna) to adjust the ear canal for best access (Fig. 10-4). Adults should pull the pinna up and back; the outer ear should be pulled down and back in children, to straighten the ear canal for best absorption. See Procedure Box 10-3 for administration of otic medications.

VAGINAL MEDICATIONS AND ADMINISTRATION

Vaginal medications are usually used for a local effect and are available in several forms: foams, gels, jellies, and lotions. Foams deliver medications via aerosolized foam. An example is VCF (vaginal contraceptive foam), which is sold over the counter. Gels and jellies are solid particles of medication in viscous (thick) suspensions. The thickness of the suspension keeps the medication from leaking. An example is metronidazole vaginal gel, used to treat bacterial infections of the vagina. Creams (lotions), jellies, and gels are all products that can release hormones for contraceptive purposes. Antifungal creams are often used to treat yeast infections and are delivered via an applicator inserted high up into the vagina. An intrauterine device (IUD) is a contraceptive device implanted into the uterus by an advanced practitioner; some devices are coated with and release the hormone progesterone.

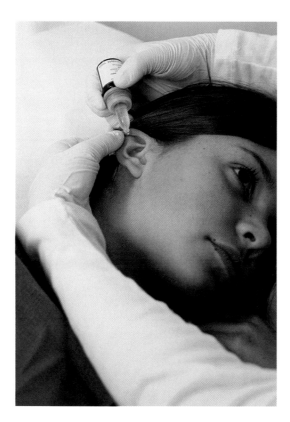

FIGURE 10-4: Otic administration.

Procedure Box 10-3 *Administration of Otic Medication*

Safety Precautions: Have patient remain lying down after administration, to avoid balance issues.

Supplies: Medication, order, cotton ball, gloves, teaching materials

Steps:

1. Observe the seven "rights" of medication administration.
2. Read the medication order, and compare it with the medication container. Check the expiration date.
3. Wash hands.
4. Make sure that the medication is at room temperature, not cold.
5. Compare the medication order with the container a second time.
6. Assess the patency of the ear dropper.
7. Identify the patient, and explain what you will be doing.
8. Compare the order and the container a third time.
9. Put on gloves.
10. Ask the patient to place his or her head on a counter or to lie down on the examination table with the affected ear upward.
11. Pull the pinna in the proper direction (up and back for adults, down and back for children).
12. Drop the medication by dropper into the affected ear.
13. Ask the patient to remain still for a few minutes.
14. Assess the patient.
15. Remove gloves and wash hands.
16. Document dosage, site of placement, and the patient's response.

Example:

8/10/2012 3:10 p.m.: 3 drops of Ciprodex otic drops to right ear as ordered. Patient tolerated with complaints of minimal pain. CJ Watkins RN, MSN

Vaginal medications such as suppositories and foams are often self-administered and do not require a health-care workers' assistance unless the patient is young or impaired. The patient should wash her hands and lie on her left side to make it easier to insert the foam or suppository. See Procedure Box 10-4 for administration of a vaginal medication.

NASAL ROUTE OF MEDICATION ADMINISTRATION

Nasal medications are used to treat conditions such as seasonal allergies, asthma, congestion due to colds, and other sinus conditions. Nasal medications can be in the form of a spray, inhaler, or instillation. Nasal sprays are fine droplets inhaled from droppers (Fig. 10-5) or small spray bottles. If a patient

Procedure Box 10-4 *Vaginal Administration*

Safety Precautions: Assist patient on and off the examination table, to avoid falls.

Supplies: Medication, order, gloves, teaching materials

Steps:

1. Observe the seven "rights" of medication administration.
2. Read the medication order, and compare it with the medication container. Check the expiration date.
3. Wash hands.
4. Compare the medication order with the container a second time.
5. Identify the patient, and explain what you will be doing.
6. Compare the order and the container a third time.
7. Put on gloves.
8. Ask the patient to assume a relaxed, supine position with legs spread apart.
9. Drape the patient for privacy.
10. Remove the medications from the container.
11. Use a water-based lubricant to lubricate the applicator or medication as needed.
12. Use the applicator (if needed) or fingers to insert the medication into the vagina.
13. Remove the applicator or fingers from the vagina after the medication is inserted.
14. Ask the patient to close her legs and remain still for several minutes.
15. Assess the patient.
16. Remove gloves and wash hands.
17. Document dosage, site of placement, and the patient's response.

Example:

04/06/2013 7:15 p.m.: miconazole 200 mg vaginal suppository administered. Patient tolerated procedure well. CJ Watkins RN, MSN

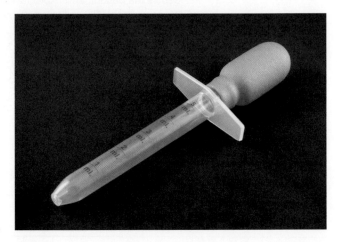

FIGURE 10-5: Medication dropper.

requires nasal drops, perhaps to clear out the nose or sinuses, you may need to help the patient administer these drops with a dropper or spray mist (Procedure Box 10-5). Instruct the patient to blow the nose before giving nasal drops because this clears the mucosa for maximum absorption. Administer according to the order in the correct nostril or both nostrils. Instruct the patient to tilt the head backward to facilitate absorption (Fig 10-6). Be sure that the dropper is patent, and rinse the dropper afterward.

The same technique is used with a spray inhaler, except instead of drops, mist is sprayed into the nose via a pump. You do not rinse spray bottles, and you never use them for more than one patient.

Procedure Box 10-5 *Nasal Administration*

Safety Precautions: Assist patient on and off the examination table, to avoid falls.

Supplies: Medication, order, gloves, teaching materials

Steps:

1. Observe the seven "rights" of medication administration.
2. Read the medication order, and compare it with the medication container. Check the expiration date.
3. Wash hands.
4. Compare the medication order with the container a second time.
5. Assess the patency of the nose dropper.
6. Identify the patient, and explain what you will be doing.
7. Compare the order with the container a third time.
8. Put on gloves.
9. Ask the patient to tilt his or her head backward.
10. Draw up medication into the dropper, as ordered.
11. Insert the dropper with medication into the nostril, as ordered.
12. Squeeze the dropper.
13. Ask the patient to maintain head tilt while you squeeze the nostril for a few moments, to prevent medication from leaking.
14. Assess the patient.
15. Remove gloves and wash hands.
16. Document dosage, site of placement, and the patient's response.

Example:

07/14/2012 2:20 p.m: Nasonex 50 mcg nasal spray 1 spray administered to each nostril as ordered. Patient tolerated procedure well and verbalizes understanding of procedure. CJ Watkins RN, MSN

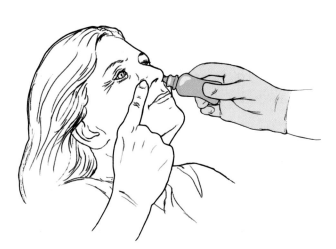

FIGURE 10-6: Nasal administration.

■ INHALED MEDICATIONS AND ADMINISTRATION

Administering medications through inhalation into the respiratory system is a quick and effective way to access blood vessels. Techniques for administration include cannulas, masks, and a continuous positive airway pressure (CPAP) machine, as well as inhalers and nebulizers.

Sometimes a medication must be applied directly to the lungs or absorbed directly into the body through the lungs. Patients who have asthma especially benefit from inhaled medications because parts of their lungs are inflamed, and inhaling a medication directly into their lungs relieves this inflammation. Special devices, such as metered-dose inhalers (MDIs), are used to ensure that as the patient inhales, the medicine enters the lungs. Powders are more easily inhaled if sterile water or sodium chloride is added to be aerosolized with the medication.

Metered-Dose Inhalers

MDIs are used to deliver specific doses of medication through a hand-held inhalation device. Some medications are prescribed for respiratory system conditions because these drugs are easily inhaled and begin working almost immediately at the site of distress. This rapid method of administration is ideal for delivering certain kinds of drugs that break up congestion in the lungs, such as Mucomyst (acetylcysteine), and other medications, such as albuterol, that dilate the airways to assist a patient in breathing. Hand-held inhalers fit into a patient's pocket or purse. Spacers are used to allow the patient some control over when the medication is inhaled (Fig. 10-7). A spacer is an extension tunnel that attaches to an inhaler and allows the medication to be held and administered whenever the patient can inhale, rather than escaping into the air if the patient exhales instead of inhaling. Spacers are especially useful for children and for adults who are cognitively impaired or disabled.

Patients should have their own inhalers for administering a specific dose of medication. Be sure to instruct the patient to take the medication exactly as ordered. The prescribed medication should be inserted into the plastic inhaler so that the opening on the prescription is inserted into the hole in the bottom of the chamber. Instruct the patient to put his or her mouth around the plastic inhalation device opening and depress the medication vial as he or she inhales for the number of puffs prescribed (see Fig. 10-7). Patients should not use another person's inhaler. Besides being unsanitary, the prescription dosages may be different. The plastic inhaler mouthpiece (not the prescription bottle) can be cleaned with soap and water after each use, to prevent infection (Procedure Box 10-6).

Nebulizers

Sometimes powders or drugs in solution are added to special equipment called a nebulizer. This equipment introduces the medication by using compressed air or oxygen to aerosolize or suspend medication into small particles in a fine mist for inhalation into the lungs through a face mask or mouthpiece. This form of treatment is common among asthmatic patients to help ease their breathing by administering medicine that, when inhaled, opens and relaxes the air passages to the lungs. Patients with cystic fibrosis

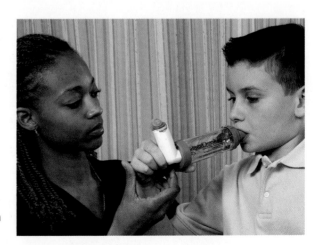

FIGURE 10-7: Metered-dose inhaler with an attached spacer/chamber.

Procedure Box 10-6 *Administration of Medication by Metered-Dose Inhaler*

Safety Precautions: Monitor the patient for elevation in heart rate, and report significant elevations to the physician.

Supplies: Medication, order, teaching materials

Steps:

1. Observe the seven "rights" of medication administration.
2. Read the medication order, and compare it with the medication container. Check the expiration date.
3. Wash hands.
4. Compare the medication order with the container a second time.
5. Identify the patient, and explain what you will be doing.
6. Compare the order and the container a third time.
7. Insert medication in the inhaler.
8. Gently shake the inhaler to ensure that the medication is aerosolized.
9. Ask the patient to exhale.
10. Instruct the patient to inhale slowly and deeply through mouth.
11. Insert the inhaler into the patient's mouth; depress the container when the patient inhales, and instruct the patient to hold his or her breath for approximately 10 seconds, to allow medication to reach the airway.
12. If more than one puff of medication is ordered, wait 1 to 5 minutes between puffs to allow for full distribution of medication.
13. Assess the patient.
14. Wash hands.
15. Document dosage, site of placement, and the patient's response.

Example:

06/14/2013 11:15 a.m.: Atrovent MDI 2 puffs administered. Patient instructed on proper use and care of inhaler. Patient states understanding of instructions. Patient states relief of symptoms 5 minutes after administration. CJ Watkins RN, MSN

also use this treatment method to deliver medication to break up the abnormally thick secretions in their lungs and allow them to be exhaled. Nebulizers are fairly portable (Fig. 10-8). Place the liquid medication in the chamber attached to the nebulizer tubing and pump. Once the pump is turned on, the mist will start to form, and the patient can begin to inhale the aerosol, as prescribed, through a special mouthpiece or mask. Procedure Box 10-7 explains the proper way to administer a medication via nebulizer.

Not as portable as a nebulizer or MDI is a CPAP machine, which forces room air or oxygen into the lungs, even when the patient forgets to breathe. A CPAP machine is ideal for patients with sleep apnea, in which the patient stops breathing for short periods of time while asleep. Oxygen from a tank or out of a special wall port is considered a medication and requires an order from a doctor or other licensed health-care professional for the number of liters to be delivered each minute. This order is usually written as "L/minute."

Oxygen can be given to the patient through a nasal cannula or a mask (see Fig. 10-9). The prongs of the nasal cannula fit into a patient's nose. Although a nasal cannula is more comfortable for a patient than a mask, only lower concentrations (levels) of oxygen can be delivered. A mask is used to deliver high concentrations of oxygen, but it can be frightening to small children and patients who are disoriented and do not know where or who they are. These patients may feel like they are being suffocated. Teaching the patient what to expect or placing the mask near, but not on, the face may help ease the fear.

The use of CPAP, a nasal cannula, and a mask over periods of time requires the air to be moisturized to avoid drying out the skin and mucosa. Patients should add distilled water to special chambers

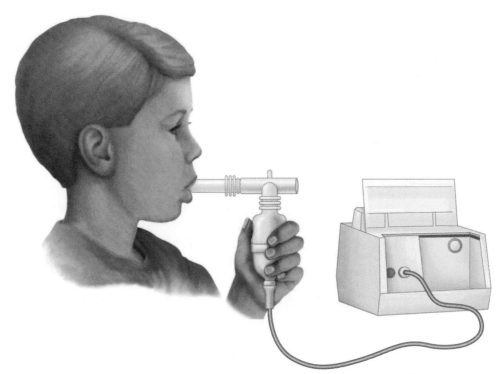

FIGURE 10-8: Nebulizer. This machine is used to administer aerosolized medication to patients.

Procedure Box 10-7 *Nebulizer Administration*

Safety Precautions: Observe the patient for elevation in heart rate, and report significant elevations to the physician.

Supplies: Medication, nebulizer machine, order, teaching materials

Steps:

1. Observe the seven "rights" of medication administration.
2. Read the medication order, and compare it with the medication container. Check the expiration date.
3. Wash hands.
4. Compare the medication order with the container a second time.
5. Identify the patient, and explain what you will be doing.
6. Compare the order and the container a third time.
7. Place the liquid medication in the chamber of the nebulizer tubing.
8. Turn on the nebulizer machine, and wait for mist to begin forming.
9. Place a mouthpiece in the patient's mouth (or put on a face mask), and instruct the patient to breathe slowly and deeply through the mouth.
10. Wait 1 to 5 minutes between puffs to allow for full distribution of medication.
11. Assess the patient during treatment.
12. Wash hands.
13. Document dosage, site of placement, and the patient's response.

Example:

04/28/2013 07:45 a.m.: 10 mg albuterol via nebulizer treatment. Patient tolerated procedure well. Pulse ox reading 99% 15 minutes after completion of treatment. Patient resting comfortably. CJ Watkins RN, MSN

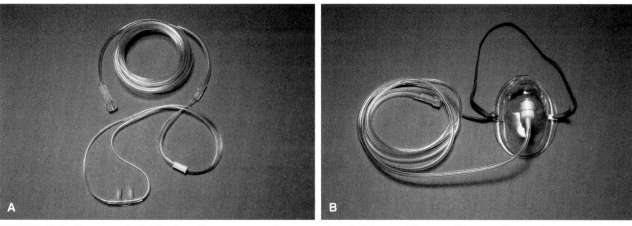

FIGURE 10-9: Oxygen administration. Oxygen is most commonly administered through (A) a nasal cannula or (B) a face mask.

in the CPAP machine to humidify the air. Unlike tap water, distilled water does not add chemicals to the machine.

CRITICAL THINKING

What should you teach the patient about cleaning and/or replacing their mask and tubing?

INJECTABLE MEDICATIONS

Injectable medications are available from the manufacturer in liquid or powder form. Powders must be mixed with sterile water or bacteriostatic sodium chloride solution. Liquids, however, may be diluted in this way or given as is. The medication is administered via needle and syringe and is drawn up from ampules or vials.

Types of Injectable Medications

Four different routes of administration can be used with injectable medications: intradermal, intramuscular, subcutaneous (Fig. 10-10), and intravenous.

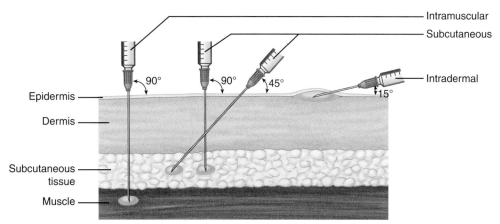

FIGURE 10-10: Standard angles of insertion for intramuscular, subcutaneous, and intradermal injections.

The **intradermal (ID)** site is just below the epidermis, in the dermis itself. ID injections are used for tuberculosis (TB) and allergy testing, so they need to be given immediately under the epidermis for easy evaluation.

The health-care worker selects the proper needle length and gauge and adjusts the angle of injection to reach the appropriate tissue level. The usual sites for ID injections are the inner aspect of the forearm and the upper back (Fig. 10-11). After preparing the site with an alcohol swab, the health-care professional holds the skin taut and inserts the needle just under the epidermis at a 10° to 15° angle. Typically, a short, small-gauge (diameter) needle is used. If the injection is administered properly, a wheal will form (Fig. 10-12).

Procedure Box 10-8 outlines ID injection protocol. At a 10° to 15° entry angle, be sure you gently push the needle just under the skin. Do not aspirate for blood return. Instead, slowly inject the medication,

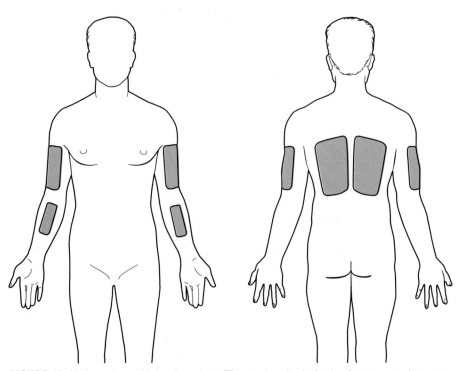

FIGURE 10-11: Intradermal injection sites. These sites include the forearm and upper back.

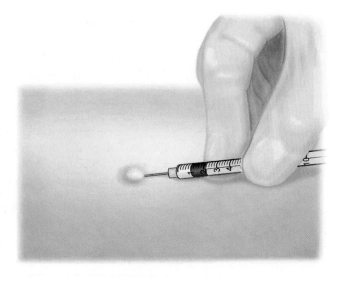

FIGURE 10-12: Wheal. If the medication is administered properly, a wheal will form on the skin.

Procedure Box 10-8 *Administration of Intradermal Injections*

Safety Precautions: Immediately dispose of sharps after administration.

Supplies: Medication in appropriate syringe with appropriate needle, alcohol wipe, cotton ball, gloves, order, teaching materials, sharps container

Steps:

1. Observe the seven "rights" of medication administration.
2. Read the medication order, and compare it with the medication container. Check the expiration date.
3. Wash hands.
4. Compare the medication order with the container a second time.
5. Identify the patient, and explain what you will be doing.
6. Compare the order and the container a third time.
7. Put on gloves.
8. Position the patient comfortably.
9. Locate the site.
10. Clean the selected site with a disinfectant wipe in a circular motion.
11. Allow disinfectant to dry.
12. Pull the skin taut.
13. Insert a needle at a 10° to 15° angle, bevel up, for about 1/4 inch.
    Note: Do not aspirate for blood, because it would traumatize tissue.
14. Slowly inject all medication to produce a wheal (slight elevation under the skin).
15. Remove the needle and syringe quickly at the same angle of insertion, and place a cotton ball at the insertion site.
16. Do not massage the site.
17. Dispose of the needle and syringe immediately in a sharps container. **Do not recap.**
18. Remove gloves and wash hands.
19. Observe the patient for reaction for 15 minutes, because allergic reactions are more likely with ID wheals than with other types of drug administration.
20. Document dosage, site of placement, and the patient's response.

Example:

03/01/2013 9:50 a.m: Tuberculin PPD (Mantoux) 0.1 mL to left inner forearm with wheal formation. Patient tolerated procedure well. CJ Watkins RN, MSN

thus forming a **wheal** (slight elevation of the skin). Gently remove the needle, and do not massage the site. If some of the medication leaks or a wheal does not form, you will have to repeat the procedure.

 CRITICAL THINKING

Can you think of a way to make it more pleasant for a child to receive an ID injection?

Intramuscular (IM) injections allow medications to be absorbed quickly into the bloodstream because of the plentiful blood supply to muscles. For example, if a patient presents with a serious streptococcal throat infection, the physician may order a dose of Rocephin (ceftriaxone), an antibiotic, to be administered as an injection to start the healing process rapidly. The patient may then continue on an oral antibiotic regimen at home. This type of injection is also preferred for vaccinations and pain medications. The onset of drug action usually occurs within 10 to 15 minutes. IM injections are inserted at a 90° angle into a muscle. Although the injection may hurt when the needle is inserted, the patient does not usually experience great pain at the injection site if care is taken to select the correct site and the solution is injected slowly. Sites for IM injections must be identified accurately. Damage to major blood vessels, bones, and nerves can occur if an inappropriate site or improper technique is used. In addition, sites should be rotated to avoid damaging the muscle.

Sites for IM injections depend on the viscosity of the liquid, the size and development of the muscle, and, to a certain extent, the patient's preference. Be sure not to inject into a scar or tattoo because the tissue under these areas may have an inadequate blood supply. In addition, any injection site should be healthy (free of rashes, lesions, or other injuries). The following is a list of possible IM injections sites.

■ Deltoid: The deltoid is a triangular muscle in the upper arm that is usually well developed and easily accessible (Fig. 10-13A). Because the deltoid tends to be small, the general rule of thumb is that 1 mL is the maximum amount of fluid to inject, and the length of the needle should not exceed 1 inch.

■ Ventrogluteal: The ventrogluteal site is used when the patient cannot stand and, instead, lies on his or her side. This site is not as commonly used, but it is considered safe for all patients older than 2 years. To locate this site, place the heel of the hand over the greater trochanter of the patient's hip with your thumb pointing toward the patient's umbilicus. Your index finger should be on the patient's anterior iliac spine. Spread your middle finger back as far as possible. The injection is then given in the center of the triangle formed by your index and middle fingers (Fig. 10-13B).

■ Vastus lateralis: The deltoid muscle is not well developed in infants and small children, so a better site is the vastus lateralis thigh muscle. As the name suggests, it is a large muscle on the side of the thigh. This site can be used in all age groups and is the site of choice in infants and small children. To locate this site properly, place one hand on the patient's upper thigh (just below the greater trochanter) and the other hand on the patient's lower thigh (just above the knee). The injection is given between your hands and the slightly lateral (toward the outer edge) aspect of the muscle (Fig. 10-13C). The procedure for IM injections is described in Procedure Box 10-9.

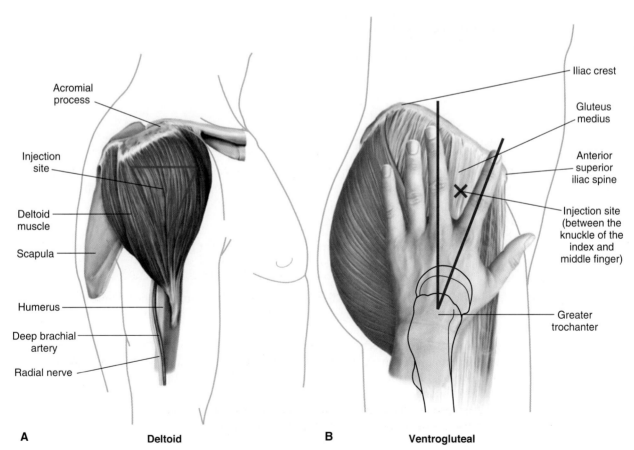

A　　　　**Deltoid**　　　　**B**　　　　**Ventrogluteal**

FIGURE 10-13: Intramuscular injection sites: (A) deltoid, (B) ventrogluteal.

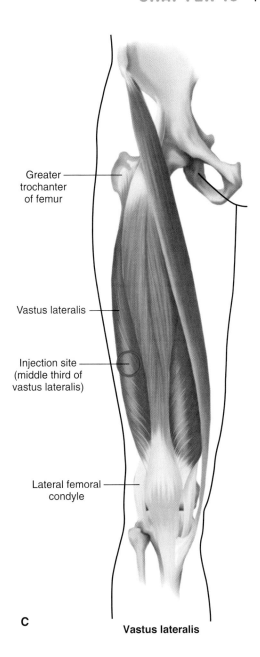

Greater trochanter of femur

Vastus lateralis

Injection site (middle third of vastus lateralis)

Lateral femoral condyle

C

Vastus lateralis

FIGURE 10-13—cont'd: (C) vastus lateralis.

Procedure Box 10-9 *Administration of Intramuscular Injections*

Safety Precautions: Immediately dispose of sharps after administration. Use extreme care in locating landmarks for injection sites to avoid injury to muscles, nerves, and bones.

Supplies: Medication in appropriate syringe with appropriate needle, alcohol wipe, cotton ball, adhesive bandage, gloves, order, teaching materials, sharps container

Steps:
1. Observe the seven "rights" of medication administration.
2. Read the medication order, and compare it with the medication container. Check the expiration date.
3. Wash hands.
4. Compare the medication order with the container a second time.
5. Identify the patient, and explain what you will be doing.

(continued)

Procedure Box 10-9 *Administration of Intramuscular Injections—cont'd*

6. Compare the order and the container a third time.
7. Put on gloves.
8. Position the patient comfortably.
9. Locate the site using appropriate landmarks.
10. Clean the selected site with disinfectant wipe with circular motion.
11. Allow disinfectant to dry.
12. Remove the needle cover by pulling straight up.
13. Hold the skin taut at the selected, cleansed site (Fig. 10-14).
14. Use a dart-like motion to insert the needle at a 90° angle completely to the hub.
15. Release the skin.
16. Aspirate for blood return (accidental placement in a blood vessel) by pulling backward on the plunger if agency policy requires.
17. If no blood is noted, gently and slowly inject all medication. (If blood is noted, withdraw the needle, discard the syringe and needle, and start the procedure over with clean needle/syringe.)
18. Remove the needle and syringe quickly at the same angle of insertion, engage the needle safety feature, and place a cotton ball at the insertion site.
19. Massage the site if the organization's policy suggests massage, or ask the patient to move a muscle.
20. Dispose of the needle and syringe immediately in a sharps container. **Do not recap**.
21. Assess the patient and injection site.
22. Cover the wound with an adhesive bandage.
23. Remove gloves and wash hands.
24. Document dosage, site of placement, and the patient's response.

Example:

07/10/2012 3:15 p.m.: 200 mg Rocephin IM to left vastus lateralis. Patient tolerated procedure well. CJ Watkins RN, MSN

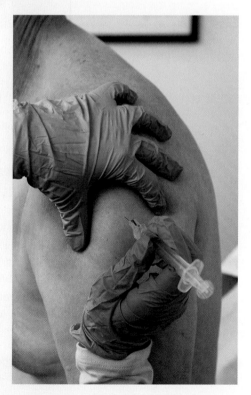

FIGURE 10-14: Holding the skin taut.

A different method is used when a medication is very irritating to the skin or may cause skin discoloration and in fact is now the recommendation for all adult IM injections. This is called the **Z-track** method (Fig. 10-15). If a health-care professional does not use the Z-track method with a medication such as Imferon, the patient may have permanent discoloration of the skin at the site. It is important to follow the directions for Z-tracking closely, or the needle may break in the skin (Procedure Box 10-10).

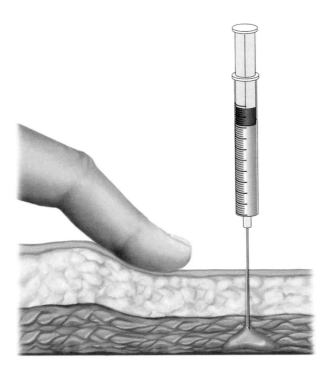

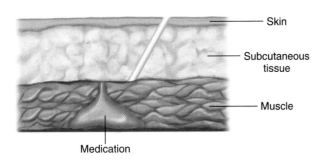

Skin

Subcutaneous tissue

Muscle

Medication

FIGURE 10-15: Z-track method. This method is used to administer medications that are caustic or will stain the skin.

Procedure Box 10-10 *Z-Track Administration*

Safety Precautions: Immediately dispose of sharps after administration. Use extreme care in locating landmarks for injection sites, to avoid injury to muscles, nerves, and bones.

Supplies: Medication in appropriate syringe with appropriate needle, alcohol wipe, cotton ball, adhesive bandage, gloves, order, teaching materials, sharps container

Steps:
1. Follow all steps from Procedure Box 10-9 up until actually inserting the needle.
2. Before inserting the needle, pull the skin laterally 1 inch away from the injection site (see Fig. 10-15).
3. Insert the needle at 90°, as for all IM injections.

(continued)

Procedure Box 10-10 *Z-Track Administration—cont'd*

4. Aspirate for blood return (accidental placement in a blood vessel) by pulling backward on the plunger if agency policy requires.
5. If no blood is noted, gently and slowly inject all medication. (If blood is noted, withdraw the needle, discard the syringe and needle, and start the procedure over with a clean needle and syringe.)
6. Wait 10 seconds before removing the needle, to allow medication to be absorbed deeply.
7. Remove the needle and syringe quickly at the same angle of insertion engaging the needle's safety device and place a cotton ball at the insertion site.
8. Quickly release traction on the Z-track position (see Fig. 10-15). This prevents medication from leaking back into more superficial tissues.
9. Dispose of the needle and syringe immediately in a sharps container. **Do not recap.**
10. Assess the patient and the injection site.
11. Cover the wound with an adhesive bandage.
12. Remove gloves and wash hands.
13. Document dosage, site of placement, and the patient's response.

Example:

01/25/2013 8:30 a.m.: iron dextran 25 mg IM given via Z-track method to right ventrogluteal. Patient tolerated procedure well. CJ Watkins RN, MSN

A **subcutaneous (SC)** injection may be prescribed if the medication must be absorbed more slowly than it does with an IM injection. The SC route places the medication into the fat under the skin. SC injection enters the fatty layer of the skin (Fig. 10-16), where medications are absorbed more slowly than when administered by the IM route. Insulin is one example of a medication that is administered by the SC route. Because fat does not have as generous a blood supply as muscle and also has fewer nerve endings, patients rarely complain of pain at the site, which rarely bleeds after injection. The most common medications given by this route are insulin and heparin.

Commonly used areas for SC injections include the fleshy part of the upper arm, the abdomen, and the thigh. If the patient is to receive regular injections, such as of insulin, the sites must be rotated so the medication does not accumulate in one area (Fig. 10-17). In the office or clinic setting, you may choose the back of the upper arms (not the deltoid muscle). Procedure Box 10-11 explains how to administer an SC injection. The needle is injected at a 45° angle. You do not need to aspirate to check for blood return because SC tissue has few blood vessels. You will also bunch up the tissue instead of holding it taut before injections as you would for an IM injection. Fast Tip 10.1 provides teaching tips for these patients.

Intravenous Medications and Administration

Finally, the IV route, which involves injecting the drug directly into a vein, is the most rapid method for administering medication into the bloodstream. IV medications are immediately absorbed and available for the body to use. The advantages of the IV route are not only rapid absorption, but also

FIGURE 10-16: Subcutaneous injections. These injections are administered into the subcutaneous fatty tissue.

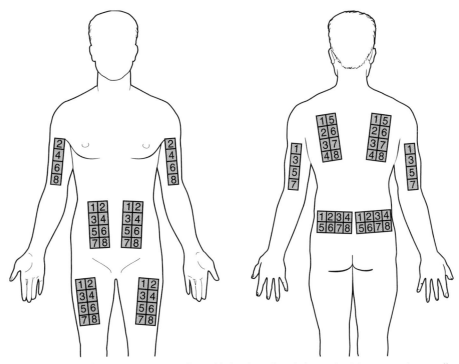

FIGURE 10-17: Site rotation. Rotation of injection sites is important to prevent complications such as abscesses.

Procedure Box 10-11 *Administration of Subcutaneous Injections*

Safety Precautions: Immediately dispose of sharps after administration.

Supplies: Medication in appropriate syringe with appropriate needle, alcohol wipe, cotton ball, adhesive bandage, gloves, order, teaching materials, sharps container

Steps:

1. Observe the seven "rights" of medication administration.
2. Read the medication order, and compare it with the medication container. Check the expiration date.
3. Wash hands.
4. Compare the medication order with the container a second time.
5. Identify the patient, and explain what you will be doing.
6. Compare the order and the container a third time.
7. Put on gloves.
8. Position the patient comfortably.
9. Locate the injection site.
10. Clean the selected site with a disinfectant wipe with circular motion.
11. Allow disinfectant to dry.
12. Remove the needle cover by pulling straight up.
13. Bunch the skin between thumb and fingers at the selected site.
14. Use a dart-like motion to insert the needle at a 45° angle completely to the hub.
    Note: It is not necessary to aspirate for blood return because fat has few blood vessels.
15. Slowly inject all medication.
16. Remove the needle and syringe quickly at the same angle of insertion, and place a cotton ball at insertion site.
17. Do not massage the site.
18. Dispose of the needle and syringe immediately in a sharps container. **Do not recap.**

(continued)

Procedure Box 10-11 *Administration of Subcutaneous Injections—cont'd*

19. Assess the patient and the injection site.
20. Cover the wound with an adhesive bandage.
21. Remove gloves and wash hands.
22. Document dosage, site of placement, and the patient's response.

Example:

01/27/20xx 7:25 a.m.: 40 mg Lovenox (enoxaparin) SC to left lower abdomen. Patient tolerated procedure well. CJ Watkins RN, MSN

 Fast Tip 10.1　Rotating Sites for Regular SC Injections

Be specific when you instruct the patient to rotate sites. For example, you could draw a chart: Sunday, above the naval; Monday, right thigh; Tuesday, below the navel; Wednesday, left thigh; Thursday, right side of the navel; Friday, left side of the navel; Saturday, back of the left arm. There are more than enough injection sites to provide variety.

---

quick relief of symptoms. This route is the fastest method in an emergency. IV fluids and medications are administered directly into a vein to treat illness, to prevent illness, as part of a diagnostic procedure, or to provide nutrition and hydration. State and organizational policies differ on which health professionals can start IV infusions, so you may not be asked to perform this procedure. It is likely, however, that because so many patients are discharged from the hospital with IV lines in place, and because so many patients are receiving long-term infusion therapy, you may be asked to assess these patients and be familiar with IV supplies in case you are asked to help prepare them. These supplies include special bags filled with solutions that may or may not contain additives (medications, electrolytes, and vitamins), tubing, and IV catheters.

A CLOSER LOOK 10.1: **Advantages and Disadvantages of IV Therapy**

Advantages

- It provides several options for medication and fluid delivery: direct injection or continuous or intermittent infusion.
- Patients can avoid multiple injections.
- An indwelling (in the vein) catheter with tubing or a port can be used. Ports are more comfortable for patients.

Disadvantages

- Medications may be incompatible. The health-care provider should check compatibility before combining any drugs in an IV line.
- A risk of complications exists, such as infiltrations, embolus, and infection.
- It costs more than other types of parenteral administration.
- Clots can form in an IV catheter or port, thus making it useless.

Sometimes a patient just needs fluids, and at other times the patient may need additives, total parenteral nutrition (TPN), or blood. The three main types of fluids or solutions are as follows:

1. Dextrose: A dextrose solution is a sugar and water solution. Dextrose 2.5% in water (D2.5W), 5% in water (D5W), and 10% in water (D10W) are the most popular. Dextrose can also come in combinations of 20% to 70%, but these are for patients with extremely low blood glucose levels, such as diabetic patients, infants, and severely malnourished patients, and are given only under very controlled circumstances, usually in an emergency room or intensive care unit.

2. Saline: If sugar is not needed, a saline, or sodium chloride (salt), solution may be prescribed. Sodium is a vital electrolyte for the body because it helps cells function normally along with other electrolytes such as potassium and magnesium. The usual solution, 0.9% sodium chloride (NaCl), is called normal saline solution (NSS). Also available is 1/2 NSS, which is 0.45% NaCl. NSSs can be added to dextrose solutions, such as D5NS, or D10/0.45 NaCl.

3. Lactated Ringer's: Lactated Ringer's solution was created by Sidney Ringer, an English physiologist who mixed dextrose, potassium chloride, sodium, lactate, and calcium to form an especially healthful mixture for patients. Other names for these mixtures include Ringer's lactate (RL) and dextrose 5% in lactated Ringer's (D5LR).

These three solutions are examples of crystalloids, which are simple solutions used to increase fluid volume when a patient is dehydrated or possibly in shock from bleeding. All these solutions are usually stored in dark cabinets because they can deteriorate if exposed to light for long periods of time. IV solutions look similar, so it is important to check the label against the order three times, as for any other medication.

Drugs administered by the IV route are given in one of three ways: infusion, piggyback line, or IV push. Infusion is slow IV administration of a large volume of fluid. The solution can contain additives such as medications, electrolytes, or minerals. IV fluid is usually packaged in a 250- to 1,000-mL bag or bottle. The health professional hangs the bag on a pole that is raised higher than the patient's heart. The fluid then flows into the vein by gravity or via an infusion pump. Some pumps strictly monitor the infusion rate, whereas others push the fluid into the patient's vein while regulating the infusion rate and the pressure it takes to infuse the fluid. Patient-controlled analgesia (PCA) pumps allow patients to push a button and receive medication, usually pain medication (such as morphine or Demerol), on demand within parameters ordered by the physician. Typically, licensed health professionals program these pumps and then lock them.

The possible complications of IV therapy are many, and as a health professional, you should be comfortable recognizing a problem, even if you are not responsible for implementing and administering the IV therapy. In some states and some facilities, health professionals can insert IV lines, hang IV fluids, disconnect IV lines, or flush indwelling ports. In other facilities and localities, these tasks are considered solely nursing functions. Become familiar with your state and facility parameters for your role so that you do not practice out of your permitted area. However, it is helpful to understand IV therapy, and you should be prepared to assess patients for signs and symptoms of infection and other problems associated with their IV lines.

A CLOSER LOOK 10.2: Dialysis: Not for Veins

An IV solution treatment option for patients who have kidney problems is dialysis. If you work at a dialysis clinic, you need to understand the process. Dialysis refers to the passage of small particles through membranes. Electrolytes and drugs move from areas of high concentration to areas of lower concentration (osmosis). During this process, waste products are removed from the blood and then from the body. Normally, the kidneys perform this function, but when they are not working correctly, a machine must be used.

Dialysis solutions are never put directly into patients' veins, but they can be placed in a dialysis machine or across a membrane such as the peritoneum. If the patient lacks the electrolyte needed, it crosses from the solution into the blood. If the patient has too much of an electrolyte, it crosses from the blood into the dialysis solution.

Sometimes a patient needs medications or electrolytes several times per day over short periods of time. In such cases, a piggyback solution is used. A piggyback solution consists of a separate IV bag and tubing connected to the primary IV tubing. The piggyback may contain, for example, an antibiotic or potassium that is given every 4 hours in 100 mL of fluid. Vitamins can be added to IV solutions, especially when patients are unable to process vitamins in their gastrointestinal system.

An IV push refers to quick delivery of a small amount of medication in a syringe. An IV push cannot be used for drugs that can potentially irritate the vein, for drugs that may be fatal if given too quickly, or for a large amount of medication. Only a licensed health-care professional can administer IV push medication.

TPN is given when the patient's digestive system needs a complete rest. This treatment is also known as hyperalimentation. TPN is a nutritional solution infused (flowed) directly into the veins to give the patient complete nutrition. The solution is placed directly into a large vein because of the risk of damage to the vein or tissues surrounding a peripheral vein. TPN provides the patient with a well-rounded supply of fluid and electrolytes, in addition to calories from fats, protein, and vitamins. TPN fluids require the use of special long-term IV catheters placed by a physician, usually in the subclavian vein. The end of the catheter lies in the superior vena cava.

A CLOSER LOOK 10.3: Types of IV Lines

Peripheral lines are IV lines placed in veins in the arms, hands, or sometimes the feet or scalp of a small child. Central lines are IV lines inserted in large veins such as the subclavian vein or internal jugular vein. These catheters terminate in the superior vena cava; that is, the tip of the catheter lies in the superior vena cava, just above the heart, to allow the medication and fluids to mix with a larger amount of blood. Central lines are used to give additives that irritate small veins, such as total parenteral nutrition. Peripherally inserted central catheter (PICC) lines are similar to central lines in that they terminate in a large vein close to the heart, but they are inserted from a peripheral site such as the lower arm.

Lipids, or fats, may also be added to IV solutions. Commercial lipid solutions contain substances such as soybean or safflower oil, which is added to water, glycerin, and egg yolks. These lipids increase the caloric source for patients who need it. Lipids, like TPN, usually require a special line.

Blood and blood products can be administered through an IV line. A licensed health-care professional administers blood, but everyone on the team must understand the types of blood products. Whole blood provides complete correction of blood loss in that it restores not only the fluid volume lost, but also the components, such as platelets and white blood cells, that were depleted. One unit of whole blood is 500 mL. Blood products provide various portions of whole blood based on a patient's needs. Patients with hemophilia, for example, require only clotting factors and platelets, not whole blood.

Before blood or a blood product is given, the patient's blood type must be checked against what is to be administered. This process, called "type and cross," ensures that patients do not have a transfusion reaction to blood that does not match their own.

A transfusion reaction is a serious negative response to the administration of blood or blood products. Signs and symptoms of a reaction include a rapid change in vital signs, dyspnea, restlessness, fever, chills, blood in the urine (hematuria), and pain in the chest, back, or flank. To discontinue a blood transfusion, the health-care worker first clamps the line infusing the blood and opens the line infusing NSS that is hung like a "Y" with the blood (Fig. 10-18). You should closely watch the patient's vital signs, including pulse, temperature, respiratory rate, and blood pressure, when transfusing blood products.

Injectable Medication Supplies

Ampules, vials, needles, and syringes, as well as IV-related items, including bags or bottles of solutions, tubing, needles, and catheters, comprise some of the equipment you will need to know how to use if you are preparing an injection for administration or will be administering one.

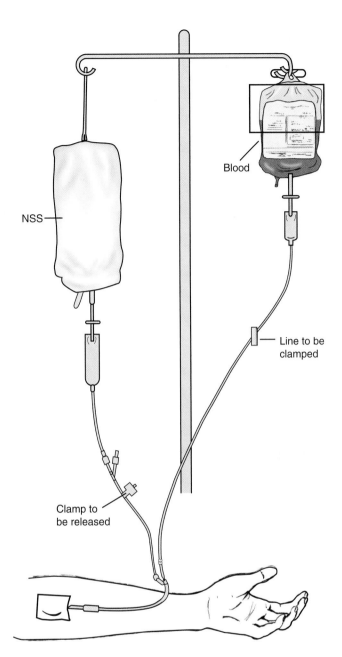

NSS

Blood

Line to be clamped

Clamp to be released

FIGURE 10-18: Blood administration setup. To discontinue a blood transfusion, the health-care professional first clamps the line infusing blood and opens the line infusing normal saline solution, which is hung like a "Y" with the blood.

An **ampule** is a small glass container that holds only one dose of a medication in solution for injections (Fig. 10-19). The ampule is broken by placing gauze around the neck of the container, to protect the hand and to keep glass from falling into the medicine. It is best to draw the solution from the ampule into a syringe with a filtered needle (needle with a filter built into it) and then change to a different needle to inject the solution into the patient; this reduces the chance that broken glass will enter the patient.

Most injectable solutions are supplied in vials instead of ampules. **Vials** are glass or plastic containers sealed on top with rubber stoppers. This makes the inside of the container sterile because it does not have to be opened or broken. Occasionally, the vial contains powder, and fluid (e.g., bacteriostatic sodium chloride or water) is added to reconstitute (mix) the solution. Once the solution is reconstituted, the vial should be used fairly quickly, according to the drug manufacturer's instructions, because the powder is more durable when it is stored without the fluid.

Vials are either multiple-dose or unit-dose. Multiple-dose vials contain several doses. After the first dose, the top of the stopper should be cleaned with an alcohol swab or other disinfecting swab before a needle is inserted into the vial for another dose. Multiple-dose vials should also be discarded within

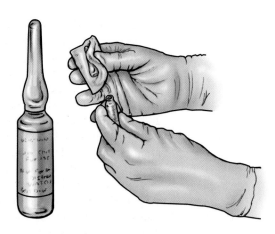

FIGURE 10-19: Ampule. This small glass container holds only one dose of medication.

a specified time period after use, according to the manufacturer's recommendation, and labeled with the time and date of first use. Unit-dose vials contain just one dose of medicine and are discarded after use.

 CRITICAL THINKING

Why do you think vials are used more than ampules?

Needles and Syringes

When an injection is given, needles are used to puncture the skin and underlying layers, to deliver medication to the desired location. When an IV infusion is started, a needle is used to puncture the skin and place a plastic catheter. The needle is then removed, and the plastic catheter is left in place to deliver the IV fluid or medication. Choosing a needle is based on two measurements: length and circumference. Needle length ranges from 3/8 inch to 2 inches (Fig. 10-20). A shorter needle is used for ID injections, and a longer one is used for IM injections. Typically, a small needle is used in children or in adults with small muscles. Longer needles are used in large adults or in patients with large muscles.

The needle's **gauge** is determined by the width or circumference of the **lumen,** the inside of the needle (Fig. 10-21). Gauges vary from 14 (largest) to 27 (smallest): the higher the number, the smaller the lumen. The viscosity (thickness) of the fluid given determines the gauge. Drug resources or the instructions

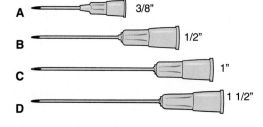

A 3/8"
B 1/2"
C 1"
D 1 1/2"

FIGURE 10-20: Various needle lengths: (A) 3/8 inch, (B) 1/2 inch, (C) 1 inch, (D) 1 1/2 inch.

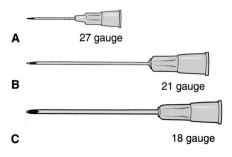

A 27 gauge
B 21 gauge
C 18 gauge

FIGURE 10-21: Various gauges of needles: (A) 27 gauge, (B) 21 gauge, (C) 18 gauge.

that come with the medications help determine the proper gauge of needle for viscous fluid. Thin fluid can pass through a 27-gauge needle, whereas a 20-gauge needle may be needed for thick fluid (e.g., blood).

Safety devices are frequently attached to needles because the Occupational Safety and Health Administration (OSHA) of the Department of Labor requires that employers protect employees from accidental needle sticks. These devices make needles more costly, but safer. Accidental needle sticks can result in the transfer of blood-borne pathogens (bacteria and viruses) from the patient to the person administering the medication.

Needle protectors either retract the needle before it is pulled out of the patient or cover the needle after use (Fig. 10-22). The easiest way to become familiar with the various types of needle protectors is to practice with them on a mannequin. Ideally, a needle is never recapped by hand. After the injection, the needle and syringe should be thrown away immediately in a biohazard sharps container (Fig. 10-23). However, after medication has been prepared, the needle may be recapped so it can be taken to the patient for administration of the medicine. The safest procedure is called the "scoop" method, in which you lay the cap on a flat surface and scoop it onto the needle.

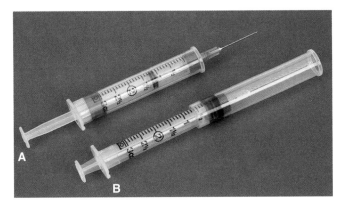

FIGURE 10-22: (A) Safety syringe. (B) The syringe has a needle protector covering the needle after use.

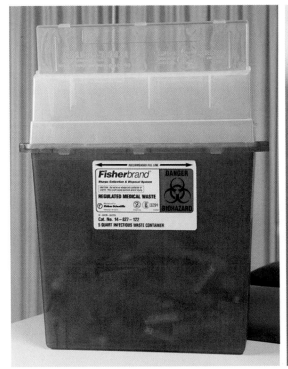
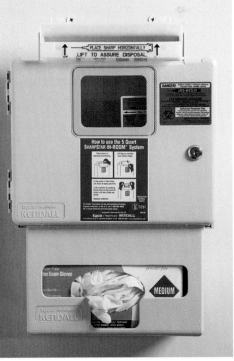

FIGURE 10-23: Biohazard sharps containers. Dispose of used needles, syringes, or any other sharp object such as a broken medication vial in a biohazard sharps container. When placing a needle into a sharps container, always place the dirty tip of the needle down.

The last item to prepare for injection is the syringe, which holds the fluid to be administered. A syringe has the following parts: barrel, tip, and plunger (Fig. 10-24). The barrel is the hollow part of the syringe that holds the liquid medication and through which the plunger passes. The needle is attached to the tip of the syringe. Finally, the plunger is the part that pushes the medication through the barrel and the needle to deliver the medication to its intended site.

The three basic types of syringe are tuberculin (TB), insulin (Fig. 10-25), and standard hypodermic (see Fig. 10-24). For TB testing or other ID injections, little fluid is injected, and therefore a narrow, finely **calibrated** (divided into accurate measurements) syringe known as a **tuberculin** syringe is used. Tuberculin syringes are calibrated to a hundredth of a milliliter (0.01 mL). These syringes are frequently used for newborns and children because doses of medicine for these patients are small.

An insulin syringe is calibrated in units instead of milliliters (Fig. 10-26). It can hold no more than 1 mL. The standard U-100 insulin syringe has 100 units calibrated on the barrel, and each line usually equals 2 units. Insulin syringes are also available with 30- and 50-unit capacity, used primarily for small children or when small amounts of insulin are needed. Because this insulin syringe has less capacity, each mark equals 1 unit, not 2. All insulin syringes are used solely for insulin because an error in measurement can be fatal. No other syringe should ever be used to administer insulin. Regardless of manufacturer, these syringes generally have orange in the coloring (usually the needle cap) to identify them as insulin syringes. Facilities may have a policy that all insulin doses must be checked by two people before the injection is administered.

Standard, or **hypodermic,** syringes are available in sizes ranging from 3 to 60 mL. Even if the needle is attached or packaged together with the syringe, a different gauge or length needle may be necessary, especially if the patient is small or is a child. Prepackaged needles can be replaced with smaller needles in most cases. The calibration of these syringes depends on the size. Syringes holding 3 mL are calibrated in 0.1-mL increments, whereas larger syringes are calibrated in 0.2-mL increments.

Syringes can be purchased without needles, so separate needles can be attached according to the length and gauge desired for the specific task. Syringes are available without needles to deliver medication into the mouth. The various types of syringes are summarized in Table 10-1. Table 10-2 summarizes the different types of injections and the needles and syringes used for them. Procedure Box 10-12 explains how to draw up medication by using the information you have learned regarding ampules, vials, needles, and syringes.

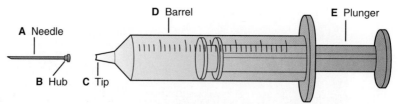

FIGURE 10-24: Parts of a syringe: (A) needle, (B) hub, (C) tip, (D) barrel, (E) plunger.

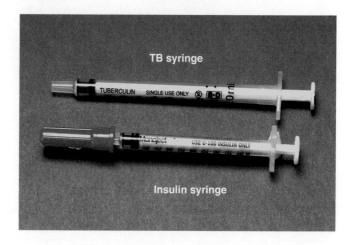

FIGURE 10-25: (A) tuberculin syringe (TB), (B) insulin syringe.

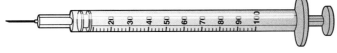

One side of U-100 insulin syringe

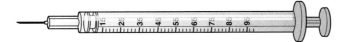

Other side of U-100 insulin syringe

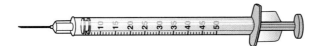

U-50 insulin syringe

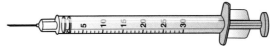

U-30 insulin syringe

FIGURE 10-26: Insulin syringes are available in the following sizes: U-100, U-50, and U-30.

TABLE 10.1   Syringes and Uses

Syringe Type	Calibration and Capacity	Sample Use

Tuberculin	One line = 0.01 mL
	    Capacity = 1 mL
		Tuberculin testing or other ID injections
		    Newborn and pediatric dosages

Insulin	One line = 2 mL Capacity = 100 units	Insulin administration
Standard	Varies with size	IM injections

TABLE 10.2   Parenteral Injections

Type	Depth	Injection Volume	Usual Needle Size	Angle
IM (deltoid)	Muscle	0.5 to 1 mL	23 to 25 gauge 5/8 inch	90°
IM (ventrogluteal)	Muscle	1 to 2 mL	18 to 23 gauge 1 1/4 to 3 inch	90°
IM (vastus lateralis in adult)	Muscle	1 to 2 mL	20 to 23 gauge 1 1/4 to 1 1/2 inch	90°
IM (vastus lateralis in child)	Muscle	0.5 to 1 mL (Maximum 1 mL in infants and 2 mL in child)	23 to 25 gauge 5/8 inch to 1 inch	90°
IM (dorsogluteal)	Muscle	1 to 2 mL	18 to 23 gauge 1 1/4 to 3 inch	90°
SC (various sites)	Subcutaneous tissue	Up to 1 mL	25 to 29 gauge 5/8 inch	45°
ID (various sites)	Under the epidermis	0.1 to 0.2 mL	25 to 27 gauge 5/8 inch	10° to 15°

Note: this information addresses the typical patient. Make adjustments based on individual patient assessment.

Procedure Box 10-12 *Drawing Up Medication*

Safety Precautions: Maintain sterility of the equipment. Work in a quiet, well-lit area free of distractions.

Supplies: Medication, alcohol wipe, appropriate syringe, appropriate needle, order

Steps:

1. Observe the seven "rights" of medication administration.
2. Read the medication order, and compare it with the medication container. Check the expiration date.
3. Wash hands.
4. Calculate the dosage correctly.
5. Compare the order and the container a second time.
6. Compare the order and the container a third time.
7. Remove the cap from the vial. If the vial has been used before, check for a discard date, and wipe with a disinfectant wipe. If using an ampule, break it carefully by using a piece of gauze.
8. Remove the cover from the needle by pulling it straight off.
9. If the drug is in an ampule, insert the needle into the ampule, and draw up the fluid into the syringe. Make sure to use a filtered needle. Change the needle after drawing up the medication.
10. If a vial is used, draw up an amount of air equal to the amount of fluid to be withdrawn. The air you inject will help to prevent a vacuum from occurring when you withdraw medication. Insert the needle into the vial, and inject the air (Fig. 10-27).
11. Turn the vial upside down, and withdraw the ordered amount of medication into the syringe. If bubbles appear, tap the syringe with your fingernail, or pull the plunger down farther and then push it back to the ordered calibration to push air above the medication and back into the vial.
12. Remove the needle and syringe from the vial, and carefully recap the needle using the scoop method.
13. You are now ready to inject the medication into the patient. Immediately proceed to administer the medication. Do not leave the medication sitting unattended.

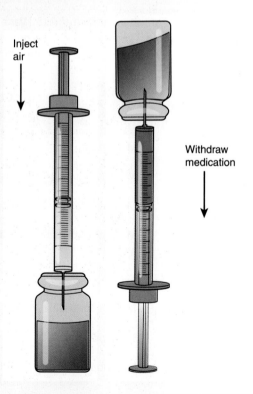

Inject air

Withdraw medication

FIGURE 10-27: Drawing medication from a vial.

During an emergency, there is little time to prepare medication for injection. To expedite receipt of necessary medication and to ensure accuracy in a critical situation, some drugs are available in a prefilled cartridge that can quickly be attached to a special cartridge holder (Fig. 10-28). After the cartridge is used, do not throw the holder away. Simply dispose of the glass or plastic cartridge, and retain the holder for future use.

 CRITICAL THINKING

Why is it dangerous to recap a needle? With so many safety devices available, why may there continue to be problems with needle sticks?

Intravenous Setup

Most IV lines and setups have the basic components illustrated in Figure 10-29. The health-care worker *spikes* the IV bag or bottle and attaches it to the IV tubing. He or she does this by inserting the end of the tubing into the outlet port of the bag or bottle. The cap on the spike section of the IV tubing is removed just before it is inserted into the IV container, to keep the spike sterile. An IV bottle may have an air vent located below the spike. The health-care worker must remove a diaphragm to let air in and release the vacuum. The vent allows air to enter the bottle as fluid flows out of it. Bags collapse as the solution flows out, and therefore venting is not an issue. Bottles maintain their shape as they empty. Calibration marks on the bag or bottle show how much IV solution has been administered and how much is left.

Below the spike (allows tubing to puncture the IV fluid container) is a drip chamber. The drip chamber allows the flow of fluid from the bag after it has been primed (emptied of air) by squeezing it. The purpose of the drip chamber is to encourage any air in the line to remain in the chamber while only the solution flows down to the patient. The flow rate is set by counting the drops entering the drip chamber.

On the IV tubing, the flow regulator adjusts the flow through the line. The ports in various places along the line allow IV medications to be infused through them. The IV needle enters the patient's vein but is usually removed, thus leaving a flexible catheter in the vein. A protective cap covers the needle until it is ready for use.

The length of the IV tubing varies from 6 to 120 inches, depending on need. The amount of fluid needed for priming (filling the tubing with fluid and removing air) the tubing varies, depending on the length of the tubing. A filter may be present to capture any air bubbles or particles or dirt or debris present in the IV fluid.

IV sets are individually wrapped and sterilized, to ensure a sterile pathway for the fluids. Damaged packages are not used because sterility may be compromised. Rigid parts of the IV set are made from plastic or polymerized chloride. Only plastic sets may be used for nitroglycerin, which interacts with polymerized chloride.

The most common needle sizes for IV infusions are 14 (largest) to 24 (smallest) gauge. The needle can be the winged "butterfly" type (Fig. 10-30) or a straight needle within a catheter, called an Angiocath (Fig. 10-31). Table 10-3 compares the two types of needles.

To begin IV therapy, the health-care worker assembles the necessary equipment, including a bag or bottle of the IV solution ordered, IV tubing, and a needle and cannula set to insert into the vein. Placing the IV needle and cannula into the patient is similar to drawing blood, and only an indwelling cannula

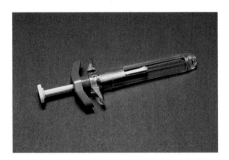

FIGURE 10-28: Prefilled medication cartridge. Many commonly used medications are available in prefilled cartridges and are placed into a cartridge holder such as this.

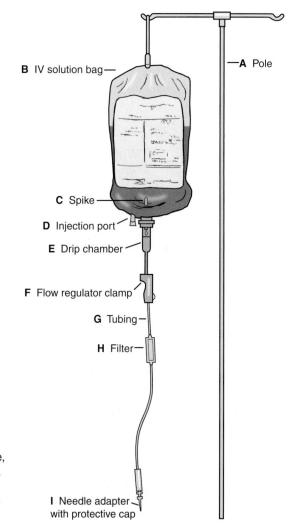

B IV solution bag

A Pole

C Spike

D Injection port

E Drip chamber

F Flow regulator clamp

G Tubing

H Filter

I Needle adapter with protective cap

FIGURE 10-29: IV lines and setup: (A) pole, (B) IV solution, (C) spike, (D) injection port, (E) drip chamber, (F) flow regulator clamp, (G) tubing, (H) filter, (I) needle adapter with protective cap.

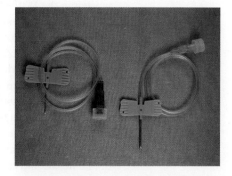

FIGURE 10-30: Butterfly needle. These IV needles are used for small and fragile veins. The metal needle remains in place.

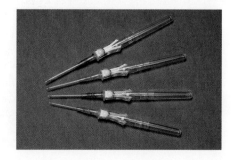

FIGURE 10-31: Angiocath. The IV needle is removed, leaving a flexible plastic catheter in place.

TABLE 10.3 Comparison of Winged and Straight IV Needles

Winged	Straight
Short-term use	Long-term use
Easy to insert	More difficult to insert
More likely to lead to infiltration (leakage of fluid from the vein into the tissue)	Inadvertent vein puncture less likely
Uncomfortable	More comfortable once placed

is left in the patient when the needle is removed. Procedure Box 10-13 shows how to insert an IV line. Never insert an IV line unless you are legally authorized to do so. See Fast Tip 10.2 for more information on the use of a tourniquet. After inserting the IV line, the following information must be documented:

- Size and type of device
- Date and time inserted
- Site location
- Type of solution
- Name of health-care provider who inserted the IV catheter or hung an IV bag
- Any additives added to the IV solution
- Flow rate
- Number of attempts at insertion (successful and unsuccessful)
- Complications, if any, and your interventions
- Patient teaching

Procedure Box 10-13 *Insertion of an IV Line*

Safety Precautions: Maintain sterility of the equipment. Dispose of the needle as soon as possible after an attempt is made.

Supplies: Tourniquet, needle and catheter, IV bag and tubing, disinfectant swab, adhesive tape

Steps:

1. Observe the seven "rights" of medication administration.
2. Read the medication order, and compare it with the medication bag.
3. Wash hands.
4. Compare the order and the bag a second time. Check the expiration date.
5. Identify the patient, and explain what you will do.
6. Compare the order and medication bag a third time.
7. Assess the appropriate site.
8. Apply gloves.
9. Place a tourniquet 6 to 8 inches proximal to the site to be used.
10. Ask the patient to close his or her fist four to six times; if necessary, gently tap the vein.
11. Cleanse the site with circular motion, and use a disinfecting swab, either povidone-iodine or alcohol.
12. Stabilize the vein by stretching skin 1 inch from the insertion site.
13. Insert the IV needle and catheter with the bevel upward at a 30° to 45° angle directly into the selected vein; then advance the catheter, and remove the needle.
    Note: Advance the catheter (without a needle) into a vein at a 10° to 15° angle.
14. Connect the IV tubing that has been primed (fluid runs out of the end to flush air out).
15. Turn on the IV infusion using the flow regulator or slide clamp.

(continued)

Procedure Box 10-13 *Insertion of an IV Line—cont'd*

16. Secure the site with an occlusive, waterproof dressing and tape.
17. Some organizations require certain information be written on the dressing, such as your initials and the date and time.
18. Assess the patient.
19. Remove gloves and wash hands.
20. Document medication administration and the patient's response.

Example:

06/21/2012 10:00 a.m.: #22 Angiocath placed to left hand after 1 unsuccessful attempt. D5LR started at 75 mL/hr as ordered. Patient tolerated procedure well. Patient advised of signs and symptoms to report to staff and states understanding. CJ Watkins RN, MSN

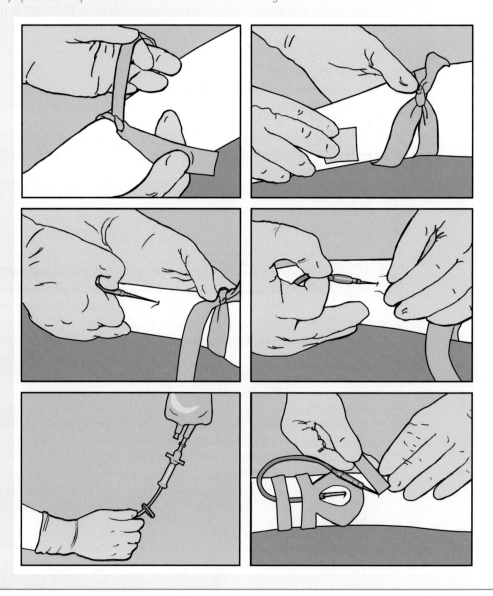

Health professionals are sometimes allowed to stop IV therapy. To do so, put on gloves and then loosen the securing tape. Gently pull out the needle or catheter, and properly dispose of it. Apply pressure to the site with a sterile 2 × 2 gauze pad until the bleeding stops. Be sure to assess the patient and document the removal, including the time and date. Follow your organization's policy for assessing the site, changing sites, flushing, and changing tubing.

● *Fast Tip 10.2* Tourniquets

Wrapping a constricting band (tourniquet) around the arm helps the vein become more visible. The tourniquet should never be placed on the patient for more than 2 minutes. If it takes longer to find a suitable site, release the tourniquet and begin elsewhere. Check your organization's policy, and call for assistance if you cannot insert the IV line after two attempts.

Health-care professionals may be asked to flush an indwelling IV device that is not attached to a running IV line. Follow the organization's policy by flushing with heparin or NSS as ordered and at the frequency specified. Also make sure that your agency's policy allows you to do this procedure. Clean the port with an antiseptic wipe, and enter the port with the needleless adapter and syringe drawn up with the ordered flush solution following your agency's procedure manual. Even if you are not allowed to flush a line, you should assess the patient who has an indwelling port for signs and symptoms of infiltration, infection, and other problems.

As a health-care professional, you must observe the IV site on a regular basis. If you see redness and swelling, feel unusual warmth at the site, hear the patient complain of tenderness or pain, or note that the site feels like a firm rope or that the cannula is no longer in a vein, notify your supervisor immediately. The supervisor may ask you to stop the IV infusion quickly, although do not remove the IV line without permission.

Complications of IV therapy include bleeding, infection, phlebitis, infiltration, catheter dislodgment, occlusion, vein irritation, severed catheter, hematoma, venous spasm, thrombosis, thrombophlebitis, circulatory overload, nerve, tendon, or ligament damage, systemic infection, air embolism, allergic reaction, incompatibility of medications, and irreversible medication error. The most common complications include the following.

■ **Infiltration** occurs when the IV catheter becomes displaced and allows IV fluids and medications to leak into the tissue surrounding the vein. This complication can cause a varying degree of injury, from discomfort to permanent damage to the tissue, depending on how quickly the problem is discovered and how caustic the medication is to the tissue.

■ **Thrombus** (blood clot) or **phlebitis** (vein inflammation) can result from extremes in solution pH, needle or catheter trauma, particulate material, irritating drugs, or selection of a vein too small for the volume of solution infused. Check the vein for signs of inflammation (e.g., redness, swelling, and warmth to the touch) or pain.

■ Air **emboli** (bubbles released into the bloodstream) can occur if air enters the vein. Small amounts of air in veins are not usually harmful, but rapidly injecting air into the vein can be fatal. Be careful to purge all air from the IV tubing before securing the line in the patient. Assess the patient's respiratory status, and report and document any changes.

■ Particulate material (small particles) can cause vein irritation. Small pieces of glass can chip away from the vial or bottle. For this reason, many pieces of IV tubing contain a final filter in the line. Swelling and redness at the site can signify that particulate matter has infiltrated the vein.

●●● SUMMARY

■ Parenteral medications include all medications that are not ingested or introduced into the gastrointestinal system.

■ Parenteral administration includes topical, ophthalmic, otic, nasal, inhalation, and injection.

■ Parenteral medications come in different forms and compositions, some ready to administer and others that need to be prepared before use.

■ Topical medications are applied directly to the skin as a patch, ointment, cream, lotion, plaster, or gel.

- Ophthalmic medications are placed directly in the eye as drops or ointments.
- Otic medications are placed directly into the ear canal.
- Vaginal medications are available in several forms: foams, gels, jellies, suppositories, and lotions.
- Nasal medications can be in the form of a spray, inhaler, or instillation.
- Inhalation medications are administered with cannulas, masks, continuous positive airway pressure (CPAP) machines, inhalers, and nebulizers.
- Injection administration includes intramuscular (IM), subcutaneous (SC), intradermal (ID), and intravenous (IV).
- A constant among all medications is that the medication and equipment must be kept sterile prior to administration.
- The seven "rights of safe medication administration" are important when administering every medication:
  - The right patient
  - The right drug
  - The right dose
  - The right time
  - The right route
  - The right documentation
  - The right technique
- Learning who is legally allowed to administer medications via which route in the organization and state in which you are working is very important.

Activities

To make sure that you have learned the key points covered in this chapter, complete the following activities.

True or False

Write true if the statement is true. Beside the false statements, write false and correct the statement to make it true.

1. Signs and symptoms of infection are redness, heat, swelling, and pain. _____

   _____

2. IV tubing is clamped off with a filter. _____

   _____

3. IM injections are given at a 90° angle. _____

   _____

4. An ampule is usually broken open to remove the solution. _____

   _____

5. Vials come only in single-dose units. _____

   _____

6. A 27-gauge needle is larger than a 20-gauge needle. _____

   _____

7. IM injections usually use 3/8-inch needles. _____

   _____

8. Drug viscosity determines needle length. _____

   _____

9. Tuberculin syringes are used to give insulin. _____

   _____

10. A U-100 insulin syringe holds 200 mL. _____

    _____

11. Cartridge holders are disposed of with the prefilled cartridge. _____

    _____

12. Otic medications go in the eye. _____

    _____

13. Always wash an ear dropper with soap and water after use. _____

    _____

14. Place used needles in biohazard sharps containers after use. _____

_____

15. Otic and ophthalmic solutions are interchangeable. _____

_____

Multiple Choice
Choose the best answer for each question.

1. By which route is insulin usually given?

    A. ID

    B. SC

    C. IM

    D. Z-track

2. At which angle is a TB test given?

    A. 10° to 15°

    B. 45°

    C. 90°

    D. 100°

3. An IM injection in an infant should be injected into which muscle?

    A. Deltoid

    B. Ventrogluteal

    C. Vastus lateralis

    D. Dorsogluteal

4. Which of the following is NOT true about Z-track injections?

    A. Insert the needle at a 90° angle.

    B. Inject medication slowly and completely.

    C. Release the skin before removing the needle.

    D. Do not massage the site after injecting.

5. Allergy testing is done via which route?

    A. IV

    B. ID

    C. IM

    D. SC

6. Childhood vaccinations are administered via which route?

    A. IV

    B. ID

    C. IM

    D. SC

7. A 90° angle is used with which of the following injections?
   A. IV
   B. ID
   C. IM
   D. SC

8. Minute amounts of medication such as 0.1 mL are usually administered via which route?
   A. IV
   B. ID
   C. Inhalation
   D. IM

9. Which of the following routes allows medication to reach the bloodstream the fastest?
   A. SC
   B. IV
   C. ID
   D. Transdermal

10. Ophthalmic medications are given in the _____.
    A. Buttock
    B. Eye
    C. Ear
    D. Arm

11. A suppository is a type of medication that can be given via what route?
    A. Rectal
    B. Vaginal
    C. Otic
    D. Both A and B

12. An IV solution can include all of the following EXCEPT _____.
    A. Lactated Ringer's
    B. D250NS
    C. Normal saline
    D. D5W

13. Dialysis is a procedure involving IV fluids for which of the following conditions?
    A. Kidney failure
    B. Hepatitis
    C. Cirrhosis
    D. Cystic fibrosis

14. An IV catheter should be discontinued during which circumstance?

    A. Phlebitis

    B. Infiltration

    C. Signs of infection

    D. All of the above

15. A Y-tubing setup is used to administer:

    A. Blood products

    B. Hyperalimentation

    C. Lipids

    D. None of the above

Short Answer Questions

1. Which syringe would be used for each of the following procedures?

    A. Insulin administration _____

    B. Allergy testing _____

    C. Flu shots _____

    D. TB testing _____

    E. IM injections _____

2. What length needles would you use for each of these procedures?

    A. Insulin administration _____

    B. Allergy testing _____

    C. Flu shots _____

    D. TB testing _____

    E. IM injections _____

Application Exercises

1. The physician orders you to give ID, IM, and SC injections. Which supplies would you assemble (remember gauge and needle length) for each type?

    A. ID _____

    B. IM _____

    C. SC _____

2. A patient needs an IV infusion with lactated Ringer's solution. You have been asked to obtain the necessary supplies. What do you obtain? _____

_____

_____

3. Dr. Mangrum asks you to obtain D2.5W/0.45NSS from the drug cabinet. What is it? _____

_____

_____

4. You are monitoring a patient who is receiving a blood transfusion, and he suddenly complains of chills and begins to have trouble breathing. What do you do? _____
_____
_____

5. You break an ampule, and get glass in your finger. What do you do? What could you have done to prevent this accident? _____
_____
_____

Medication Review

Fill in the following table with regard to the medication and routes you have learned in this chapter. "Subcutaneous" has been filled in for you.

Route	When Used	Example (May Vary)
Subcutaneous	Slow absorption	Insulin
Inhalation		
Intradermal		
Intramuscular		
Intravenous		
Vaginal		

Charting Activity

For all injections, it is important to document the name of the medication, dosage, site, and patient response. Practice documentation by completing the following exercises.

1. Document that you gave 1 mL of Depo-Provera in the left deltoid of a patient. _____
_____
_____

2. Document that you gave 0.1 mL of tuberculin in the right anterior forearm of a patient.
_____
_____

3. Document that you injected 7 units of insulin to the upper right of the umbilicus.
_____
_____

4. How would you document that you observed a patient after giving an ID injection?
_____
_____

5. If that patient experienced a rash after a TB test, how would you document it?

_____

_____

Internet Research

1. Go to www.osha.gov, and research the Occupational Safety and Health Administration regulation for needle safety. Be prepared to discuss the consequences to the employer of not following these regulations.

2. Use the keyword "safety needles" to research a minimum of two medical suppliers, and investigate the various safety devices offered for needles. Decide which two you think would be most effective in the workplace, and defend your answers.

Classifications of Drugs

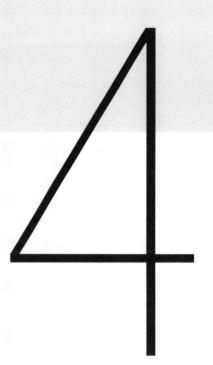

Chapters 11 to 21 discuss common medication classifications relative to body system. See Appendix A at the back of this text for a list of drug classifications and their general effects. Your knowledge of physiology will assist your understanding of how drugs work and how to administer them safely. Each chapter explores subcategories under the main classification of medications. For example, in Chapter 11, the main classification is integumentary system medications. This category is subdivided into many different medications, such as those that combat bacteria, viruses, parasites, injuries, autoimmune disorders, and others. A Master the Essentials table included in each systems chapter identifies key examples of medication side effects, contraindications, precautions, and interactions. Drug Spotlight boxes focus on one or more drugs important to each system.

Integumentary System Medications

*T*he skin is the major defense organ of the body. Any injury, infection, or disease that alters the skin's physiology can compromise the health of the individual. Skin infections are caused by bacteria, parasites, viruses, and fungi. Inflammatory conditions such as burns, atopic dermatitis, and psoriasis can cause pain, itching, and self-consciousness about body image, and some conditions can be life-threatening. Each of these skin conditions requires a specific type of medication for successful treatment. In addition, skin cancer can range from the common basal cell carcinoma to the much more serious squamous cell carcinoma and malignant melanoma. Skin cancer has a good prognosis if found at an early stage. Therefore, thorough skin assessment can detect problems early on, and an understanding of treatments and available medications is essential for true patient advocacy.

LEARNING OUTCOMES

At the end of this chapter, you should be able to:

11.1 Define all key terms.

11.2 Differentiate between two primary routes of medication administration in the integumentary system, and determine when each route would be chosen.

11.3 Recall at least seven conditions affecting the integumentary system and the medications used to treat them.

KEY TERMS

Acne	Keratinization	Nodule
Comedones	Metastasize	Psoriasis
Eczema	Nevus (nevi)	Rosacea
Impetigo	Nits	Thrush

■ INTEGUMENTARY SYSTEM: VULNERABLE BARRIER

The integumentary system consists of the skin, hair, and nails. The skin is the largest organ of the human body and is made of multiple layers, each providing different functions and levels of protection to the body (Fig. 11-1). These layers are the epidermis, dermis, and hypodermis. The skin is one of the most important keys to a healthy body because intact skin provides the greatest defense to invasion by disease-causing microorganisms. Skin has only a few openings, such as the eyes, ears, and nose. The skin is the only barrier our bodies have to the outside world, and it is particularly vulnerable to external injury. Injuries such as abrasions, blisters, calluses, cracks, cuts, irritated areas, inflamed areas, lesions, scrapes, sores, rashes, and sunburn can damage the skin and provide an opening for infection for bacteria, fungi, parasites, or viruses.

Some patients are more susceptible to skin irritations and/or tumors because of a genetic predisposition: their skin may be more delicate. People who have fair skin that has repeated exposure to the sun are more vulnerable to skin damage. Other environmental hazards may be responsible for causing the following skin conditions:

- ■ Skin discoloration
- ■ Alopecia (hair loss)
- ■ Seborrhea (oily skin lesions)
- ■ Psoriasis (scaly patches)
- ■ Verrucae (warts caused by viruses)
- ■ Nevi (moles)
- ■ Tumors

Skin disorders are classified as infectious, inflammatory, or cancerous. The medications used are based on the diagnosis in that classification. These medications are given either topically or systemically, depending on the severity of the skin disorder (see the Master the Essentials table for descriptions of the most common integumentary system drugs).

■ SKIN INFECTIONS AND MEDICATIONS

As mentioned earlier, bacteria, parasites, viruses, and fungi can invade the body through a skin injury. Different types of medications treat skin infections either topically or systemically, depending on the

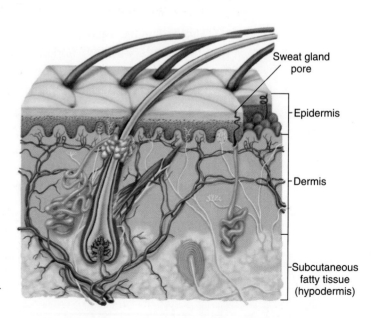

FIGURE 11-1: Layers and structures of the skin.

ailment. Generally, antibiotics fight bacteria, whereas antifungal medications treat fungi, antiviral medications fight viruses, and pediculicides and scabicides fight parasites.

Bacteria

Several bacterial infections can wreak havoc on the skin, the most common example being acne. **Acne** is an inflammatory disorder that affects the sebaceous glands. Acne occurs most commonly in adolescents due to an increase in androgens (male hormones present in both men and women). Bacteria can also cause acne, which affects adolescents and adults. Hormonal changes that occur during puberty cause **seborrhea,** a condition caused by an overproduction of skin oils. Abnormal **keratinization,** or hardening of the epithelial tissue, also occurs. A bacterium, *Propionibacterium acnes,* grows inside the sebaceous glands and makes an irritating, acidic substance. The skin produces inflamed bumps, called pustules, in response to this irritation.

Open **comedones,** or blackheads, are oil glands plugged with melanin granules. Closed comedones, or whiteheads, are white rather than black because they are produced just below the skin and lack melanin. Deeper lumps called **nodules** involve inflammation deep below the skin. Severe inflammation and pus can cause pain, deformity, and eventual scarring.

Rosacea is a type of skin irritation without pus. Small bumps, or papules, redden the skin. Even though these papules do not contain pus, they may produce pain because of the thickening and swelling. The patient with rosacea appears flushed, especially on the nose and cheek. Sunlight, stress, and hot temperatures can aggravate rosacea, as can alcohol, spicy foods, and hot beverages.

Medications used to treat acne and rosacea can be applied topically to the irritated areas, frequently the face, back, and neck. The active ingredient in these medications may be vitamin A, an acid, or an antibiotic. Over-the-counter (OTC) medications, such as a cream, gel, or lotion, usually contain benzoyl peroxide. Benzoyl peroxide is bacteriostatic (inhibits bacterial growth).

Retinoids contain vitamin A, which increases the body's resistance to infection by reducing the oil production that clogs the pores. Retinoids reduce both the function of the sebaceous glands and keratinization. Because of serious associated side effects (birth defects, emotional problems), oral retinoids are reserved for patients with severe acne who do not respond to other topical agents. For severe acne, salicylic acid, sulfur, or resorcinol may be used topically to remove the infected skin through shedding. Systemic antibiotics such as tetracyclines are sometimes necessary in extreme cases.

Oral contraceptives have also been effective in decreasing the symptoms of acne and are sometimes prescribed for this purpose. The hormones in some oral contraceptives can help stop acne from forming by reducing androgen production.

Another bacterial infection is **impetigo,** which most commonly occurs in children. A common example is a child with an upper respiratory infection who is constantly wiping his or her nose until the skin breaks down and allows entry of bacteria. This condition is treated with topical antibiotics, topical corticosteroids, and, if the infection is severe, systemic antibiotics.

 CRITICAL THINKING

> Think of ways to inhibit the growth of skin infections. (What conditions enhance growth of microorganisms?) List at least two ways (not including medications) that will slow down or stop the growth of these microorganisms.

 Fast Tip 11.1 Applying Skin Medications

When applying skin medications, teach the patient to wash the affected area with a clean damp cloth to remove any old medication and/or microorganisms, and apply medication in a very thin layer to the clean skin. Make sure the patient understands the importance of only using a clean cloth each time to prevent recontamination of the skin with the dirty cloth.

Parasites

Scabies is a parasitic infection caused by human itch mites that burrow into the skin and lay their eggs. This condition usually occurs in the webbing of the fingers and toes as well as the neck, axillae, and groin. Lice, which cause pediculosis (infestation of head, body, or pubic lice), live in hair and feed on blood. Scabicides and pediculicides are used to treat itch mite and lice infestations, respectively. These drugs are applied directly to the area of infestation.

Lice lay eggs called **nits.** After applying a pediculicide, the hair where the nits live should be combed with a special fine-toothed comb and the site inspected for at least 1 week to be sure all the nits are dead. Because bedding and clothing may hold eggs, they must be thoroughly cleaned daily for 1 week. Pediculicides are neurotoxins and may cause neurological side effects; therefore, they should be used only as prescribed.

Viruses

Viruses are the smallest of microorganisms, and because they depend on a host cell for survival, eradicating them can be difficult without killing the host cell. Some examples of viruses that affect the skin are the human papillomavirus (HPV), herpes simplex virus type 1 (HSV-1), and herpes simplex virus type 2 (HSV-2). HPV causes venereal warts and most of the cervical cancer in women, and it can become problematic and difficult to eliminate. Warts on the genitals are called condylomas; otherwise, warts are called verrucae. HPV can lie dormant in the system and flare up if it is not completely treated. The goal of wart treatment is to destroy affected skin superficially at the site of growth. Cryosurgery with liquid nitrogen or topical products containing salicylic acid may be necessary to remove persistent or prolific warts.

HSV-1 typically causes cold sores, or fever blisters, on the mouth and lips. HSV-2 is a sexually transmitted virus and usually affects the genital mucosa. Both HSV-1 and HSV-2 are treated with oral antivirals. Herpes zoster, or shingles, is a reactivation of the varicella-zoster virus that causes chickenpox. This is also treated with oral antiviral medications, which are covered in Chapter 17, Immunological System Medications.

Fungi

Fungal infections that affect the integumentary system include tinea and candidiasis. In tinea infections, dermatophytes invade keratin and can infect the hair, nails, and skin. Topical antifungals, such as

Drug Spotlight 11-1 *Silvadene (silver sulfadiazine topical)*

Classification	Antimicrobial
Availability	Topical cream, prescription
Indications	Used to treat or prevent serious infections on areas of the skin with second- or third-degree burns
Dosage/ Implementation	Burn area should be covered with Silvadene at all times. Should be applied once or twice a day to 1/16 of an inch thickness. Depending on doctor's orders, the burns may be cleaned and debrided prior to application.
Action	Kills bacteria by breaking down the cell membrane and cell wall.
Adverse Reactions/ Side Effects	Skin irritations (including rash, blistering, peeling or discoloration of skin or mucous membranes) or upset stomach.
Contraindications/ Precautions	Hypersensitivity to silver sulfadiazine. Do not use if pregnant patient is approaching or at term, or on newborn infants younger than 2 months of age.

clotrimazole (Lotrimin) or terbinafine (Lamisil), may be used when the infection is present on the trunk, extremities, groin, or feet. If the infection is on the scalp, oral agents may be needed.

Candidal infections, also known as yeast infections, are caused by *Candida albicans.* This infection is associated with a pruritic red rash that may be painful. When it occurs in the mouth, this infection is commonly known as **thrush;** white plaques are usually present on the oral mucosa. Topical antifungals such as nystatin may be ordered.

INFLAMMATORY CONDITIONS AND MEDICATIONS

Inflammatory conditions of the skin include burns, atopic dermatitis, and psoriasis. The most common treatments for burns are anesthetics and antibiotics. Atopic dermatitis is treated with corticosteroids, immunomodulators, and antihistamines. Antipsoriatic agents and ultraviolet (UV) therapy are used to treat psoriasis.

Burns

Burns damage the skin by removing water from it, by causing it to blister, or by removing it entirely. Burns are classified as first-, second-, or third-degree according to the level of tissue damage (Fig. 11-2).

First-degree burns involve only the epidermis. The skin becomes red and painful to touch. The most common first-degree burn is sunburn. People with few melanocytes (darkening cells), and thus fair skin, are especially vulnerable to sunburn.

Nonpharmacological treatment for sunburn includes application of cool water for 20 minutes and of an herb called aloe vera. An old home remedy of applying butter or lard to sunburn causes more damage and should not be used. Pharmacological treatment of sunburn includes lidocaine-containing medications such as Solarcaine.

A burn is classified as second degree if a blister forms over the burn due to tissue damage that extends into the dermis, and the burn turns yellow. Cover second-degree burns with a sterile dressing, and administer an antibiotic such as silver sulfadiazine (Silvadene) to the burn as prescribed. The dressing can help absorb exudate if the blister should break. Silvadene helps to prevent infection that could result because the natural barrier against microorganisms has been severely damaged.

A third-degree burn is the most severe and affects all layers of skin, subcutaneous tissue, and possibly even muscle and bone. The patient with such a burn has lost much skin integrity and is at great risk for infection and fluid loss. Immediate treatment includes maintaining the patient's airway (if burns are around the face and neck) and administering oxygen and intravenous fluids as needed. Collagenase (Santyl), which débrides (or removes) tissue, is sometimes prescribed to eliminate the dead tissue. However, it also removes healthy tissue and must be applied only to the wound as ordered. An antimicrobial nonstick dressing may be ordered. Other drugs may be ordered to absorb exudates (DuoDERM) or to stimulate formation of healthy new granulation tissue (e.g., becaplermin [Regranex]). Systemic medications may include analgesics, anti-inflammatory agents, and antibiotics. The patient may or may not complain of pain because the nerves have been destroyed in this area. Usually, if pain is present, it is caused by a mixture of second- and third-degree burns.

Atopic Dermatitis

Atopic dermatitis is also called **eczema.** It is an allergic disorder usually associated with other atopic diseases, such as asthma or allergic rhinitis. It causes cutaneous inflammation that is evidenced by extremely dry patches of itchy skin. Initial methods of treatment include avoiding allergens, removing irritants, and maintaining hydration. Agents that may be needed include topical corticosteroids, such as hydrocortisone acetate 1% (Cortef), or topical immunomodulators, such as tacrolimus (Protopic) or pimecrolimus (Elidel). Corticosteroids decrease inflammation to reduce the damage it causes. Immunomodulators (immune response modifiers) used for atopic dermatitis are topical preparations that temporarily modify the skin's immune reaction. They do not affect the immune system of the entire body. Oral antihistamines such as diphenhydramine (Benadryl) may relieve itching but can cause mood changes, bone defects, or hematological problems if they are used for prolonged periods.

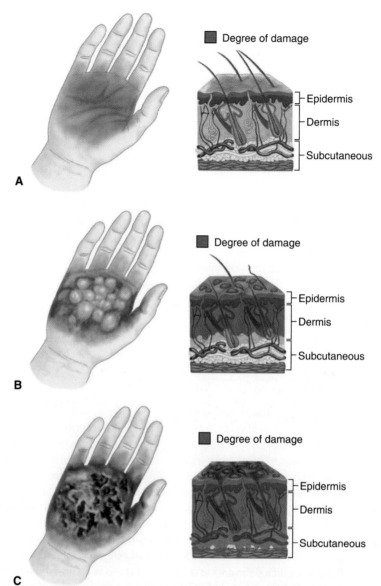

FIGURE 11-2: Burn degrees. (A) Burning of the top layer of skin is called a first-degree burn; it commonly causes red skin and swelling. (B) A burn that causes a blister is a second-degree burn; the blisters may open and ooze a clear fluid. This burn is often very painful. (C) A burn that removes the skin and tissue beyond it is a third-degree burn; the area looks brown, even charred.

Psoriasis

Psoriasis is a chronic inflammatory skin disease in which, for unknown reasons, the life cycle of skin cells is shortened (Fig. 11-3). Some investigators believe that the disease has a genetic factor, and others believe that environmental triggers exist. The normal life span of the skin cell is somewhere between 30 and 50 days. With psoriasis, the skin cell matures in 3 to 4 days. The dead skin cells in both healthy and psoriatic skin rise to the surface to be shed. Dead cells in this instance cannot be shed quickly enough, thus causing a buildup of skin cells on the surface. The dead cells take on a flaky white appearance atop a reddened (erythematous) plaque. Treatment of psoriasis may include topical

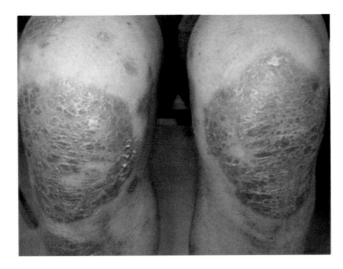

FIGURE 11-3: Psoriasis. *(Reprinted from Barankin, B, and Freiman, A: Derm Notes: Clinical Dermatology Pocket Guide. F.A. Davis, Philadelphia, 2006; p 133.)*

corticosteroids, low-dose antihistamines, salicylic acid, or phototherapy. Specific antipsoriatic agents include the cream anthralin (Psoriatec) and calcipotriene (Dovonex, Calcitrene), which is available as both a cream and an ointment. Oral or injectable methotrexate is used for severe disease unresponsive to other therapy.

Many countries, including Argentina, France, and Iceland, have spas that claim to have healing hot springs containing varying combinations of algae, thermal mud, mineral- and salt-rich water, and other natural substances that cure both psoriasis and dermatitis. Use of UV light has also shown some promise of improvement in psoriatic symptoms.

■ SKIN CANCER AND MEDICATIONS

Skin cancer can occur when the skin's tissue is damaged. The three major types of skin cancer are basal cell carcinoma, squamous cell carcinoma, and malignant melanoma. Basal cell carcinoma is the most common form of skin cancer and rarely **metastasizes** (spreads) (Fig. 11-4). Treatment may require surgical excision, but topical preparations for superficial basal cell carcinomas such as fluorouracil, which affects the rapidly dividing cancer cells, or imiquimod (a topical immunomodulator that stimulates the immune system) may be used. Liquid nitrogen cryotherapy is also an option.

Squamous cell carcinoma arises from malignant keratinocytes (the most common type of skin cells that produce keratin) (Fig. 11-5). This form of skin cancer can metastasize. Surgical removal is the treatment of choice, and radiation therapy may be needed. The third type of skin cancer is malignant melanoma, and its incidence is quickly rising (Fig. 11-6). This unpredictable cancer spreads through the lymphatic system and blood.

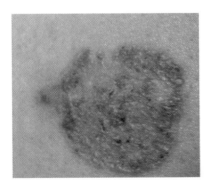

FIGURE 11-4: Basal cell carcinoma. *(Reprinted from Barankin, B, and Freiman, A: Derm Notes: Clinical Dermatology Pocket Guide. F.A. Davis, Philadelphia, 2006; p 70.)*

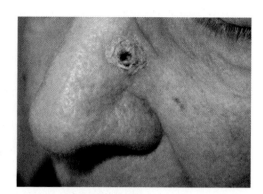

FIGURE 11-5: Squamous cell carcinoma. *(Reprinted from Barankin, B, and Freiman, A: Derm Notes: Clinical Dermatology Pocket Guide. F.A. Davis, Philadelphia, 2006; p 150.)*

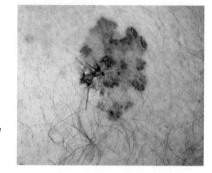

FIGURE 11-6: Melanoma. *(Reprinted from Barankin, B, and Freiman, A: Derm Notes: Clinical Dermatology Pocket Guide. F.A. Davis, Philadelphia, 2006; p 116.)*

Patients should be instructed to notify their physician if a **nevus** (mole) or discolored skin area changes in color, grows, or develops irregular borders, because this could be a sign of cancer, and a biopsy might be ordered. Treatment includes surgery, radiation, and chemotherapy. The medications used in treatment of these more invasive types of cancer are covered in Chapter 17, Immunological System Medications.

● ● ● SUMMARY

- ■ The integumentary system consists of the skin, hair, and nails.
- ■ The skin is the major defense organ of the body and consists of the epidermis, dermis, and hypodermis.
- ■ Skin disorders are classified as infectious, inflammatory, or cancerous.
- ■ Integumentary medications are given either topically or systemically based on the diagnosis.
- ■ Skin infections are caused by bacteria, parasites, viruses, and fungi. Medications include antibiotics, antifungals, antivirals, pediculicides, scabicides, and retinoids.
- ■ Inflammatory conditions include burns, atopic dermatitis, and psoriasis. Medications include anesthetics and antibiotics for burns; corticosteroids, immunomodulators, and antihistamines for atopic dermatitis; and antipsoriatic agents and ultraviolet (UV) therapy for psoriasis.
- ■ Types of skin cancer include the common basal cell carcinoma, squamous cell carcinoma, and malignant melanoma.
- ■ Thorough skin assessment can detect problems early on, and an understanding of treatments and available medications is essential for true patient advocacy.

Master the Essentials: Dermatologic Medications

This table shows the various dermatologic medications and key side effects, contraindications and precautions, interactions, and examples of each classification.

Class	Use	Side Effects	Contraindications and Precautions	Interactions	Examples
Benzoyl peroxide	Treatment of acne	Peeling, erythema, edema	Hypersensitivity	Tretinoin	Benzoyl peroxide (Clearskin, PanOxyl, many other brands)
Retinoids	Tretinoin: Treatment of severe acne; reduction in appearance of fine wrinkles Tazarotene: reduction in appearance of fine wrinkles	Photosensitivity, local reactions (topical); depression, suicidal ideation, pseudo-tumor cerebri, pancreatitis, visual changes, hepatotoxicity, hypertriglyceridemia (oral)	Hypersensitivity, pregnancy	Other topical products, photosensitizers	Tretinoin (Retin-A, Renova, Avita), tazarotene (Tazorac)
Scabicides and pediculicides	Infection with lice or scabies (parasites that lay eggs or live on hair or skin)	Eczema, rash, redness, itching, burning, headache	Hypersensitivity	Oils, pentobarbital, diazepam	Lindane, permethrin (Nix)
Keratolytics	Acne, dandruff, seborrhea, or psoriasis Removal of warts, corns, and calluses	Burning, irritation, tinnitus, dizziness, ototoxicity, headaches (oral)	Hypersensitivity, prolonged use, irritated skin, moles, birthmarks, or warts with hair growth, mucous membranes	Usually none with topical use	Salicylic acid (Compound W, Clearasil, Stridex), ammonium lactate (Lac-Hydrin lotion)
Topical antifungals	Fungal infection of the skin (ringworm, athlete's foot, jock itch, vaginal yeast infections, and diaper rash)	Burning, stinging, pruritus, erythema	Hypersensitivity	None reported	Clotrimazole (Mycelex, Lotrimin, Gyne-Lotrimin), ketoconazole (Nizoral), nystatin (Mycostatin)
Topical corticosteroids	Inflammation and rashes caused by allergic reactions, psoriasis, or eczema	Burning, itching, irritation	Hypersensitivity (use on the face, groin, or axillae), pregnancy	None reported	Hydrocortisone (Westcort, Cortaid), dexamethasone (Decadron)
Topical Immunomodulators	Severe atopic dermatitis	Burning, pruritus	Hypersensitivity, pregnancy, breastfeeding	Formal studies not performed	Pimecrolimus (Elidel), tacrolimus (Protopic)
Antipsoriatic agents	Dandruff, psoriasis, psoriatic arthritis, rheumatoid arthritis, skin cancer	Irritation to surrounding skin; discoloration of skin, hair, or fabrics	Hypersensitivity, use on the face, renal disease, pregnancy, breastfeeding, hypercalcemia (calcipotriene)	Topical corticosteroids	Coal tar (T/Gel, Neutrogena), anthralin (Dritho-Scalp, Psoriatec), cyclosporine (Gengraf, Neoral), etanercept (Enbrel), methotrexate (Trexall)
Topical fluorouracil	Scaly skin, superficial basal cell carcinoma	Erythema, burning, vesicle formation, insomnia, photosensitivity, malaise	Hypersensitivity, pregnancy	None reported	Fluorouracil (Efudex, Fluoroplex, Carac)

Activities

To make sure that you have learned the key points covered in this chapter, complete the following activities.

True or False

Write true if the statement is true. Beside the false statements, write false, and correct the statement to make it true.

1. Antifungals are used to treat impetigo. _____

   _____

2. Pediculicides kill nits and lice. _____

   _____

3. Vitamin A is used to treat acne. _____

   _____

4. Thrush is a bacterial infection. _____

   _____

5. Oral contraceptive drugs can treat acne. _____

   _____

6. Malignant melanoma is easily treatable with topical creams. _____

   _____

7. The topical antibiotic used for burns is called Silvadene. _____

   _____

8. A nevus is a mole. _____

   _____

9. Rosacea is a type of skin cancer. _____

   _____

10. Psoriasis occurs when a shortened life cycle of skin occurs. _____

    _____

Multiple Choice

Choose the best answer for each question.

1. HPV is an example of a _____.
   A. Bacterial infection
   B. Viral infection
   C. Parasitic infection
   D. Fungal infection

2. **A comedo is _____.**
   A. A louse egg
   B. A nodule
   C. A form of acne
   D. Earwax

3. **Rosacea includes skin irritations called _____.**
   A. Comedones
   B. Papules
   C. Verruca
   D. Nevus

4. **An example of a pediculicide is _____.**
   A. Compound W
   B. Nystatin
   C. Rid-X
   D. Decadron

5. **Thrush is caused by _____.**
   A. HSV-1
   B. HSV-2
   C. *Candida albicans*
   D. *Sarcoptes scabiei*

6. **Thrush is treated with what medication?**
   A. Nystatin
   B. Ampicillin
   C. Acyclovir
   D. Any of the above

7. **Which of the following is NOT a type of skin cancer?**
   A. Basal cell carcinoma
   B. Squamous cell carcinoma
   C. Small cell barceloma
   D. Melanoma

8. **Atopic dermatitis is also called _____.**
   A. Eczema
   B. Psoriasis
   C. Basal cell carcinoma
   D. None of the above

9. The layer of skin involved in a second-degree burn is the _____.
   A. Dermis
   B. Epidermis
   C. Hypodermis
   D. A and B
   E. All of the above
   F. None of the above

10. Scabies is caused by this parasite.
   A. Itch mite
   B. Body lice
   C. Head lice
   D. Pubic lice

Application Exercises

Respond to the following situations.

1. Harold has been told that his cold sores are caused by herpes. He is very upset and states that he is not promiscuous. What would you say to him? _____

   _____

   _____

2. Harold is given Abreva for cold sore treatment. What would you teach him about its use?

   _____

   _____

   _____

3. Cheryl suffers from psoriasis and is given topical corticosteroids. She is very upset and scared to use steroids. How would you explain what steroids are and why she is being

   asked to use them for her condition? _____

   _____

   _____

4. Bill has acne. He asks why he is being placed on an oral antibiotic when it is a skin problem. How would you answer his question? _____

   _____

   _____

5. Brenda has sustained a second-degree burn to her hands. She asks why she has to have her hands scrubbed as part of her treatment because it hurts so badly. What would you say?

   _____

   _____

   _____

Essentials Review

For further study and practice with drug classifications learned in this chapter, complete the following table to the best of your ability. Use resources such as the *PDR,* the Internet, or printed drug guides for help.

Medication	Classification	Purpose	Side Effects	Contraindications and Precautions	Examples	Patient Education
Lindane						
Resorcinol						
Topicort						
Elidel						

Internet Research

Using your favorite search engine, go to your local health department or similar website. Use the information there to create a patient teaching aid on lice infestation removal, and bring it to class to share.

12

Musculoskeletal System Medications

*T*he musculoskeletal system comprises muscles, bones, and joints. The skeleton provides the scaffolding for the body, and the muscles hold the bones in place and allow the body to move and interact with the environment. When the musculoskeletal system or any part of it malfunctions, it affects the ability to move. This chapter addresses the medications used to treat conditions that affect muscles, joints, and bones. Medications are used to prevent or treat disease or to decrease symptoms associated with disease that cannot be prevented or cured.

LEARNING OUTCOMES

At the end of this chapter, you should be able to:

12.1 Define all key terms.

12.2 Identify the key features of the musculoskeletal system.

12.3 Discuss the importance of healthy endocrine and nervous systems to proper musculoskeletal functioning.

12.4 Recall at least five muscular system disorders and one appropriate treatment for each.

12.5 Discuss at least four bone or joint disorders and one appropriate treatment for each.

KEY TERMS

Antispasmodic
Bisphosphonates
Calcitonin
Disease-modifying antirheumatic
   drugs (DMARDs)

Dystonia
Gout
Hypocalcemia
Osteoarthritis
Osteomalacia

Osteoporosis
Rheumatoid arthritis

THE MUSCULOSKELETAL SYSTEM

The musculoskeletal system consists of muscles, tendons, and ligaments that attach to the bones and joints (Fig. 12-1), and that rely on the nervous and endocrine systems to function properly. Coordinated and strong movement require healthy nerve signals, healthy muscle tissue, and adequate endocrine function. The nervous system provides the signals that make the muscles contract or relax and thus allow the body to perform tasks such as picking up a spoon and bringing it to the mouth. Even if the signals occur at the appropriate time, a muscle that is not healthy cannot perform its functions. The human skeleton is composed of 206 bones. The skeleton not only gives the body structure, it also stores minerals that help muscles move. Calcium is needed for nerves, bones, and muscles to function properly. If not enough calcium is stored in bones, the bones can break. If too much calcium is stored, not enough is available for the bloodstream to deliver to the muscles.

The endocrine system must be healthy to control the deposit of these minerals. The thyroid gland produces **calcitonin,** which allows calcium to remain in the bone and not move into the blood (Fig. 12-2).

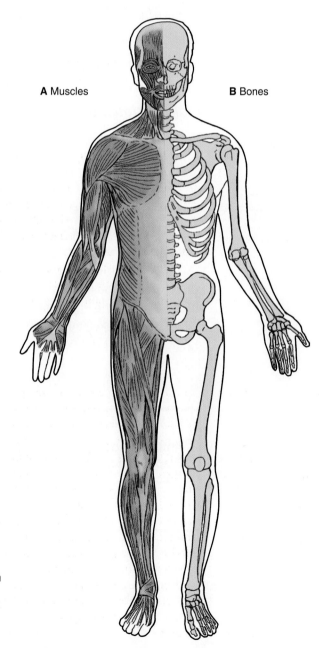

A Muscles   **B** Bones

FIGURE 12-1: The musculoskeletal system is made up of (A) muscles and (B) bones that form the skeleton. The musculoskeletal system gives the body its structure and is the force behind movement.

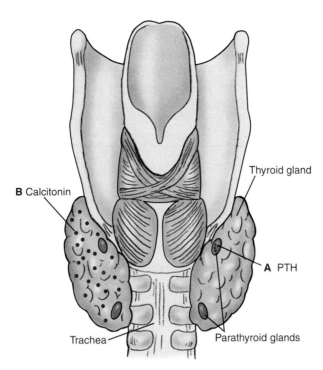

FIGURE 12-2: Thyroid and parathyroid glands. Parathyroid hormone (PTH) and calcitonin help keep calcium in the body in balance. (A) The parathyroid glands secrete PTH, which pulls calcium from the bones into the bloodstream. (B) The thyroid gland secretes calcitonin, which puts calcium into the bones.

Conversely, the parathyroid gland secretes parathyroid hormone, which increases the amount of calcium in the blood and leads to a loss of calcium in the bones. Both glands work together to keep calcium levels in balance. If these glands do not function appropriately, abnormal calcium levels may lead to bone abnormalities. Calcium also assists in muscle contraction and nerve impulses, so abnormalities can lead to altered muscle functioning. Other minerals (magnesium and potassium) stored in the bones also affect musculoskeletal functioning (see the Master the Essentials table for descriptions of the most common musculoskeletal system drugs).

Medications used for musculoskeletal disorders can be placed into two categories: those to treat muscular disorders and those to treat bone disorders. Disorders include conditions causing impaired movement, pain, and damage to muscles, bones, and/or joints.

MEDICATIONS USED TO TREAT MUSCULAR DISORDERS

Muscle disorders comprise a range of ailments. Some originate in the brain (e.g., cerebral palsy, stroke, and multiple sclerosis), and some arise in the muscle tissue itself. Muscle spasms can develop from these disorders or from the use of psychotropic drugs. Certain conditions (e.g., injury to a muscle in the back, muscular dystrophy) cause the patient's muscles to move in uncoordinated, or spastic, ways. Other patients have **dystonia,** which is abnormal tension in one area of the body, such as the limbs, neck, face, eyes, or spine. Medications used to treat some of the muscular problems found in these disorders include muscle relaxants such as Flexeril (cyclobenzaprine) and **antispasmodics** such as Skelaxin (metaxalone); these dugs relax muscles and relieve muscle spasms. Both types of medications work with the central nervous system (CNS) to inhibit the neurological activity that causes the spasms or rigidity. Sometimes the antispasmodics or muscle relaxants are classified as benzodiazepines (Valium [diazepam]) or have CNS effects to maximize effectiveness. One of the newer drugs on the market, Cymbalta (duloxetine), which is used for chronic low back pain, is an antidepressant. This drug may decrease the stress felt with chronic pain and help patients live more productive, mobile lives.

Other antispasmodics focus on the muscle itself. Botulinum toxin type A (Botox and Botox Cosmetic [onabotulinumtoxin A]) is a toxic substance derived from the bacterium *Clostridium botulinum,* which, in high doses, causes food poisoning (botulism). However, researchers have found that in lower doses it acts as an effective muscle relaxant by blocking acetylcholine release and thus paralyzing the muscle. The most common use of Botox Cosmetic is to reduce wrinkles associated with aging. Botox is used to treat chronic migraines, limb spasticity, abnormal head position and neck pain (cervical dystonia), severe underarm sweating, and certain eye muscle problems. In some situations, once the muscle is paralyzed, the patient can perform strengthening exercises to promote strength in other muscles to correct, for example, abnormal head position. This treatment reaches maximum effectiveness within 6 weeks and must be repeated every 3 to 6 months. Because botulinum toxin causes pain, it is usually administered with a local anesthetic.

Other muscle disorders that require medication include myasthenia gravis and fibromyalgia. Myasthenia gravis is a progressive, autoimmune disease of skeletal muscle fatigue and weakness that is caused by loss of acetylcholine receptors, basically a breakdown in communication between the nerves and the muscles. It can be debilitating. One type of medication for this disease consists of cholinesterase inhibitors, such as neostigmine, which block cholinesterase and therefore facilitate acetylcholine accumulation. Although the disease has no cure, treatment can help reduce symptoms to allow the individual to function more independently.

Fibromyalgia is a disorder of chronic pain in muscles and the soft tissue surrounding joints. This rheumatological illness is difficult to manage. Treatment includes decreasing the contributory factors (e.g., lack of exercise, poor coping response to stress), physical therapy, antidepressants, anti-inflammatory medications, trigger point injections, and narcotic analgesics.

■ MEDICATIONS USED TO TREAT ABNORMAL CALCIUM LEVELS

When calcium levels are low, supplements may be needed to correct the imbalance. Calcium supplements are prescribed for **hypocalcemia,** or low blood calcium. Vitamin D may be added to facilitate calcium usage. Vitamin D assists in the absorption of calcium from the stomach and helps to maintain adequate serum calcium levels for proper bone development. Risk factors for hypocalcemia include smoking, lack of exercise, high alcohol consumption, anorexia nervosa, estrogen or testosterone deficiency, poor nutrition, and obesity. Patients with hypocalcemia may be given calcitonin (Miacalcin), which is available as a nasal spray or in an injectable form. Calcitonin is naturally produced by the thyroid gland to deposit calcium into bones. Calcitonin can come from humans or fish such as salmon.

When there is a lack of calcium, the bones can become soft, brittle, and deformed. This condition is known as **osteomalacia** in adults or rickets in children. **Osteoporosis** is a common bone disease that also results from a lack of calcium in the body; this disease creates holes in the bones and gives bone a spongelike appearance. In all cases, the bones are not firm, and they break easily, even under little

Drug Spotlight 12-1 *Lyrica (pregabalin)*

Classification	Analgesics, anticonvulsants
Availability	Capsules, oral solution
Indications	Used for the treatment of fibromyalgia, shingles pain, and diabetic neuropathy pain
Action	Interrupts pain signals from the brain
Adverse Reactions/ Side Effects	May cause suicidal thoughts in a few patients. Risk for hypersensitivity reaction in patients taking ACE inhibitors. May cause edema of hands, feet, and legs; dizziness or sleepiness
Contraindications/ Precautions	Avoid abruptly stopping the medication unless discussed with the pre-scriber because symptoms may worsen

stress or pressure. Sometimes calcium and vitamin D are used to prevent bone breaks, as is the case with osteoporosis.

Some medications, such as estrogen (or hormone) replacement therapy (ERT), inhibit bone resorption of calcium and can reduce the extent of osteoporosis. However, this type of treatment has side effects, such as breast and uterine cancer and blood clots. For this reason, these drugs are used with caution. If a patient prefers not to take ERT, she may choose to take a **bisphosphonate,** which is a similar medication without the side effects. These drugs are similar to bisphosphate salts, which are found naturally in the body. An example of a bisphosphonate is alendronate sodium (Fosamax).

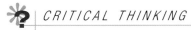

CRITICAL THINKING

Why would a woman choose to take ERT? Why would she choose not to take it?

Although too little bone calcium can cause fractures, too much bone calcium is a problem as well. Paget's disease is a chronic disease that debilitates patients by enlarging the bone. A patient with Paget's disease resorbs bone excessively, but the new bone is weak and fragile. The bones are deformed (e.g., bowing of the lower legs), leading to pain and fractures. Paget's disease can be diagnosed by a blood test. X-ray studies show irregular bones. Treatment for Paget's disease consists of calcitonin and bisphosphonates, which encourage strong bone formation; supplemental calcium and vitamin D may also be taken as needed.

MEDICATIONS FOR BONE AND JOINT INFLAMMATION

Arthritis and gout can cause inflammation of the bones and joints. Arthritis, as indicated in Table 12-1, can be one of two types: osteoarthritis or rheumatoid. In **osteoarthritis,** erosion of bone occurs where the bones meet at the joint. Those affected are mainly middle-age or older persons and also those who are either extremely sedentary or extremely active.

Rheumatoid arthritis is slightly different in that it is an autoimmune condition, in which the joints are affected by inflammation caused by a negative reaction from the immune system. Rheumatoid arthritis usually affects women 30 to 50 years of age or children. Nonsteroidal anti-inflammatory drugs (NSAIDs), such as Advil, Motrin (ibuprofen), and Aleve (naproxen), are the most common type of medications used to treat osteoarthritis and rheumatoid arthritis.

Gout is a form of arthritis characterized by a sudden, severe attack of pain, redness, and joint tenderness, most commonly at the joint of the big toe and foot. Before middle age, gout primarily affects men, but after women reach menopause, the numbers of men and women affected by gout start to equalize. Risk factors include excessive alcohol use, hypertension, diabetes, hyperlipidemia, and arteriosclerosis. In addition, certain medications and family history are risk factors. Gout is caused by a buildup of uric acid in the joints. Uric acid is a natural by-product of food metabolism

TABLE 12.1   Types of Arthritis

Type	Cause	Age Affected
Osteoarthritis	Degeneration (erosion) of bones where they meet, or articulate, at the joints	Strikes middle-age or older persons; extremely sedentary and extremely active persons are at increased risk
Rheumatoid arthritis	Autoimmune reaction: the body's immune system attacks the joints and causes inflammation	Can affect children, but mostly affects women 30 to 50 years of age at symptom onset

and is excreted via the kidneys. In this instance, too much uric acid is produced, or not enough is excreted by the kidneys. Medications used for treating gout are often not administered until the acute attack is over. If medications are given during a gout attack, uric acid may migrate to additional joints. Symptoms of a gout attack are treated first with NSAIDs. High doses may be prescribed to halt an acute attack, and lower doses may be used to prevent future attacks. For patients unable to take NSAIDs, Colcrys (colchicine) is used to relieve the pain. In addition, patients may be given glucocorticoids to control pain and inflammation. When the acute attack has ended, patients start taking antigout medication such as Zyloprim (allopurinol) or Uloric (febuxostat) to lower the uric acid level in the body.

NSAIDs

NSAIDs reduce inflammation, which is helpful to the patient with gout, osteoarthritis, or rheumatoid arthritis. Some of the concerns regarding NSAIDs are increased gastrointestinal bleeding and renal and cardiac damage caused by long-term use. Thus, these medications should be taken only as ordered, and long-term use should be monitored closely. Aspirin and other analgesics are used for pain. Topical medications containing medication such as menthol, salicylate, and trolamine are usually creams or gels that are rubbed into muscles and joints. Examples are Absorbine, Bengay, Icy Hot, and capsaicin. Stronger pain relief can be obtained by combining analgesics and antidepressants.

Cyclooxygenase-2 Inhibitors

Cyclooxygenase-2 (COX-2) inhibitors (celecoxib [Celebrex]), which technically belong to the larger group of NSAIDs, decrease the production of prostaglandins that cause pain and inflammation. Generally, NSAIDs block the production of both COX-1 and COX-2 enzymes. COX-2 inhibitors block only the production of the COX-2 enzyme and allow the COX-1 enzyme to continue to be produced. COX-1 enzymes are present in many tissues in the body, such as the stomach, where they provide protection to the stomach and intestines. By allowing this enzyme to continue production, the risk for ulceration and bleeding with prolonged use is reduced. COX-2 inhibitors cannot be used by patients who are allergic to sulfa drugs. These medications can also increase the risk for heart problems in certain patients.

Disease-Modifying Antirheumatic Drugs (DMARDs)

If anti-inflammatory drugs do not reduce the inflammation adequately, **disease-modifying antirheumatic drugs (DMARDs)** may be used in patients with rheumatoid arthritis. These medications suppress the

---

Drug Spotlight 12-2 *Capsaicin*

Classification	Analgesic
Availability	Topical cream, gel, lotion, and transdermal patch.
Indications	Used for pain relief from disorders such as diabetic neuropathy, cluster headaches, osteoarthritis, rheumatoid arthritis, shingles, and psoriasis
Action	Effective by activating the nerve signals and then decreasing them; patient may have initial increase in pain, followed by relief. Active ingredient comes from the substances that make hot peppers hot, such as chili
Dosage	Topical: May be used up to four times a day Transdermal: Apply up to 4 patches for 60 minutes.
Adverse Reactions/Side Effects	Side effects: Hypersensitivity reaction
Contraindications/Precautions	Education: Wash hands well after use to avoid transference to eyes, mouth, or other mucous membranes; do not apply to areas of broken skin

autoimmune response, but in doing so they suppress immunity systemically. Although not able to cure the disease, these drugs may be able to slow the continual joint destruction. The goal of treatment is not cure but continued joint mobility. Examples of DMARDs include Rheumatrex (methotrexate), Neoral (cyclosporine), and Azulfidine (sulfasalazine). One interesting example is Solganal (gold aurothioglucose). Given by injection or sometimes orally, it prevents joint damage and disability. Gold tends to work best in the early stages of rheumatoid arthritis, although it may also help with other types. Gold is used infrequently because the other DMARDs listed are more effective.

Corticosteroids

Glucocorticosteroids such as Decadron (dexamethasone) and Medrol (methylprednisolone) are medications manufactured to mimic cortisol, which is a hormone produced in the adrenal gland. Corticosteroids reduce inflammation by suppressing the production of materials that trigger allergic and inflammatory responses, but they do not cure inflammatory diseases such as arthritis and gout. Because corticosteroids reduce the body's ability to fight infection, they are used only for short-term therapy during acute symptomatic episodes.

■ MEDICATIONS TO TREAT PHANTOM LIMB PAIN

Patients who have had a limb amputated often experience pain in the missing limb. The pain impulse originating in the brain and spinal cord does not recognize that the limb is no longer there. Although some patients report that the pain fades over time, others experience a lifetime of pain management issues. One type of medication that may be effective in managing this chronic pain consists of tricyclic antidepressants such as Elavil (amitriptyline) and Pamelor (nortriptyline). Tricyclic antidepressants alter the chemical messengers that relay pain signals, and they also benefit by helping the patient with sleep. Anticonvulsants and narcotics are two other classifications of drugs that may help. Anticonvulsants such as Tegretol (carbamazepine) quiet damaged nerves to prevent or slow pain signals. Narcotics such as Roxanol (morphine) work by dulling the pain perception center of the brain.

 CRITICAL THINKING

Why is it important to know why a patient is taking a medication?

●●● S U M M A R Y

- ■ The musculoskeletal system consists of muscles, tendons, and ligaments that attach to the bones and joints.
- ■ The system relies on the nervous and the endocrine systems to function properly.
- ■ The thyroid and parathyroid glands work together to keep calcium levels in balance.
- ■ Bones can weaken from a lack of calcium (hypocalcemia osteomalacia, osteoporosis) or an excess of calcium (Paget's disease).
- ■ Examples of muscle disorders that originate in the brain include cerebral palsy, stroke, and multiple sclerosis.
- ■ Examples of muscle disorders that originate in the muscle tissue include spasms and dystonia.
- ■ Other muscle disorders include myasthenia gravis and fibromyalgia.
- ■ Many drugs are available to help treat muscular disorders, including antispasmodics, muscle relaxants, nonsteroidal anti-inflammatory drugs (NSAIDs), antidepressants, cholinesterase inhibitors, and narcotic analgesics.
- ■ Medications for the muscular system act in the brain or in muscle, depending on where the problem is located.
- ■ Osteoarthritis is caused by the erosion of bones at the joints.
- ■ Rheumatoid arthritis is an autoimmune condition that causes inflammation of the joints.

■ NSAIDs and corticosteroids are used to treat the inflammation in osteoarthritis and rheumatoid arthritis. Aspirin and topical analgesics are used for pain. Cyclooxygenase-2 (COX-2) inhibitors work to reduce pain and inflammation while decreasing the risk for ulceration and bleeding. Disease-modifying antirheumatic drugs (DMARDs) can be used for patients with rheumatoid arthritis.

■ Assisting the patient to maintain independent functioning should be one of the goals of every health-care worker. With independence, patients have dignity and a feeling of well-being.

Master the Essentials: Musculoskeletal Medications

This table shows the various classes of musculoskeletal medications and uses, key side effects, contraindications and precautions, interactions, and examples of each class.

Class	Use	Side Effects	Contraindications and Precautions	Interactions	Examples
Antigout drugs	Gout or kidney stones	Acute gouty attacks, headache, GI symptoms	Hypersensitivity, uric acid kidney stones, blood dyscrasias, active peptic ulcer	Antibiotics, antineoplastics, warfarin, salicylates, oral antidiabetics	Allopurinol (Zyloprim), colchicine (Colcrys)
Anti-inflammatory drugs (NSAIDs)	Swelling, fever, pain; to prevent heart attack, stroke or chest pain	Albuminuria, hematuria, bronchospasm, constipation, dizziness, epigastric pain, increased bleeding time, hypersensitivity reactions, GERD, GI ulcers and bleeding, headache, tinnitus and hearing loss, vision disturbances	Anemia, asthma, children with viral infections (aspirin), clotting disorders, disorders of the CV and GI systems, GERD, breastfeeding, liver and kidney failure, pregnancy, sulfonamide hypersensitivity, thyroid disorders	Alcohol, anticoagulants, corticosteroids and other steroids, oral hypoglycemics	Aspirin (Ecotrin, Bayer, Bufferin), diclofenac with misoprostol (Voltaren, Cataflam), ibuprofen (Motrin, Advil), naproxen (Naprosyn, Aleve)
Bisphosphonates	Osteoporosis with a high risk for bone fracture	Headache, abdominal pain, bone pain	Hypersensitivity, hypocalcemia, esophageal stricture or achalasia	Calcium supplements, antacids, ranitidine, aspirin	Teriparatide acetate (Forteo)
Calcitonin	Osteoporosis in postmenopausal women	Rhinitis, nasal irritation (nasal spray); hypertension, dizziness, injection site reaction, nausea, vomiting	Clinical allergy to drug, pregnancy, breastfeeding	None reported	Calcium carbonate (Tums, Os-Cal-D), calcitonin salmon (Miacalcin)

Master the Essentials: Musculoskeletal Medications—cont'd

Class	Use	Side Effects	Contraindications and Precautions	Interactions	Examples
Cholinesterase inhibitors	Myasthenia gravis	Bradycardia, hypotension, convulsions, rash, increased salivation, weakness, muscle cramps	Hypersensitivity, peritonitis, mechanical intestinal or urinary obstruction	Succinylcholine, aminoglycosides, anesthetics, antiarrhythmics, corticosteroids, magnesium	Neostigmine (Prostigmin)
COX-2 inhibitors	Pain or swelling caused by arthritis, ankylosing spondylitis, and menstrual pain	Headache, insomnia, rash, abdominal pain, diarrhea, dyspepsia, upper respiratory infection	Hypersensitivity to sulfonamides	Fluconazole, rifampin, theophylline, ACE inhibitors	Celecoxib (Celebrex)
DMARDs	Rheumatoid arthritis	Hepatotoxicity, bone marrow suppression, GI disturbances, blood dyscrasias, pruritus, rashes	Hepatic or renal impairment, pregnancy, breastfeeding, active infection, immunosuppression, known hypersensitivity, lupus, pulmonary fibrosis	Vaccines, NSAIDs, probenecid, corticosteroids	Auranofin (Ridaura), azathioprine (Imuran), gold sodium thiomalate (Mycochrysine), methotrexate (Rheumatrex)
Muscle relaxants and antispasmodics	Muscle spasms, pain, and stiffness	Anxiety, ataxia, blurred vision, confusion, decreased blood pressure and respirations, diarrhea, dizziness, drowsiness, dry mouth, headache, slurred speech, tremor, urinary incontinence, weakness	Asthma, breastfeeding, muscular dystrophy, myasthenia gravis, pregnancy	Alcohol, analgesics, antihistamines, psychotropics	Baclofen (Lioresal), cyclobenzaprine (Flexeril), dantrolene (Dantrium), metaxalone (Skelaxin)

ACE, angiotensin-converting enzyme; COX, cyclooxygenase; CV, cardiovascular; DMARDs, disease-modifying antirheumatic drugs; GERD, gastroesophageal reflux disorder; GI, gastrointestinal; NSAIDs, nonsteroidal anti-inflammatory drugs

Activities

To make sure that you have learned the key points covered in this chapter, complete the following activities.

True or False

Write true if the statement is true. Beside the false statements, write false, and correct the statement to make it true.

1. Gout is a disease caused by the buildup of calcium in the joints. _____
_____

2. Myasthenia gravis is a progressive autoimmune disease affecting the muscles. _____
_____

3. Capsaicin is a drug made from hot peppers. _____
_____

4. NSAIDs are used for phantom limb pain. _____
_____

5. Osteoporosis can lead to increased risk for fractures. _____
_____

6. Fibromyalgia is an acute disorder of the bones. _____
_____

7. Lyrica is a drug used to treat osteoarthritis. _____
_____

8. The endocrine system is very important in maintaining proper levels of calcium in the
bones. _____
_____

9. Side effects of estrogen replacement therapy (ERT) can include breast and uterine cancer.
_____
_____

10. Examples of topical NSAIDs for gout, osteoarthritis, and rheumatoid arthritis include
Icy Hot, Bengay, capsaicin, and Absorbine. _____
_____

Multiple Choice

Choose the best answer for each question.

1. Osteomalacia is a _____.
   A. Rheumatologic disease
   B. Gout
   C. Joint degeneration
   D. Calcium disorder

2. **Which is a buildup of uric acid in the joints?**

   A. Fibromyalgia

   B. Gout

   C. Paget's disease

   D. Myasthenia gravis

3. **Which is used to treat dystonia?**

   A. Muscle relaxant

   B. Antispasmodic

   C. Calcitonin

   D. Parathyroid hormone

   E. A and B

4. **Which disorder is characterized by chronic pain in muscles and soft tissue surrounding joints?**

   A. Paget's disease

   B. Myasthenia gravis

   C. Gout

   D. Fibromyalgia

5. **Examples of corticosteroids include _____.**

   A. Decadron

   B. Rheumatrex

   C. Celebrex

   D. Morphine

6. **Examples of DMARDs include _____.**

   A. Decadron

   B. Rheumatrex

   C. Celebrex

   D. Morphine

7. **Examples of narcotics include _____.**

   A. Decadron

   B. Rheumatrex

   C. Celebrex

   D. Morphine

8. **Examples of COX-2 inhibitors include _____.**

   A. Decadron

   B. Rheumatrex

   C. Celebrex

   D. Morphine

9. Which endocrine gland produces calcitonin?

   A. Parathyroid gland

   B. Thyroid gland

   C. Adrenal gland

   D. Pancreas

Application Exercises

Respond to the following situations.

1. Shelly is an army veteran who lost one of her legs in the Iraq War. She asks how she can feel pain in a foot that is no longer there. What would you say? _____

   _____

   _____

2. Harold has been diagnosed with Paget's disease. He does not understand why he is being told to make sure he eats enough calcium when his bones are already big. What would you tell him? _____

   _____

   _____

3. Joette is entering menopause. Why would she refuse estrogen replacement therapy? _____

   _____

   _____

4. Ruth has rheumatoid arthritis. She wants to know why the medications she is taking are not making the disease go away. What would you tell her about the goals of treatment for arthritis? _____

   _____

   _____

5. Vicki is taking NSAIDs for osteoarthritis. She has developed stomach pains. Should she be told to stop taking this medication? Why or why not? _____

   _____

   _____

Essentials Review

For further study and practice with drug classifications learned in this chapter, complete the following table to the best of your ability. Use resources such as the *PDR*, the Internet, or printed drug guides for help.

Example	Generic Name	Classification	Purpose	Side Effects	Contraindications and Precautions	Examples	Patient Education
Flexeril							
Capsaicin							
Azulfidine							
Elavil							

Internet Research

1. Using the Internet, locate information to create a patient education plan for someone with chronic back pain. Search for "patient education plan for chronic back pain."

2. Using the Internet, find information about Celebrex published within the last 2 years, and write a report about the safety of this drug.

Nervous System Medications

*T*he most complex system in the body is the nervous system. This system starts with the brain, which houses billions of neurons and innumerable internal connections. The brain is attached to the central nervous and peripheral nervous systems. The nervous system processes all incoming information before acting on it; it controls everything we do from breathing to walking. Nervous system medications, as described in this chapter, are used to treat pain, anxiety, depression, mania, insomnia, convulsions, and schizophrenia.

LEARNING OUTCOMES

At the end of this chapter, you should be able to:

13.1   Define all key terms.

13.2   Identify the two major branches of the nervous system.

13.3   Recall the five categories of nervous system medications.

13.4   Identify four categories of medications used to treat pain and fever.

13.5   Recall at least one category of medication used to treat anxiety, insomnia, sedation, and seizures.

13.6   Identify at least one category of medication used to treat behavioral, emotional, or mood disorders.

13.7   Discuss medications used to treat psychosis, and identify other disorders for which these medications may be prescribed.

13.8   Recall at least one category of drug used to treat dementia and two categories of drugs used to treat Parkinson's disease.

13.9   Compare and contrast the actions of local and general anesthetics.

13.10 Discuss how alcohol can influence medication use and its effect on the body.

KEY TERMS

Adrenergic (sympa-
   thomimetic)
Analgesic
Anxiolytic
Aura
Autonomic nervous
   system
Blood-brain barrier
Central nervous system
   (CNS)
Cholinergic (parasym-
   pathomimetic)

Drug holiday
Gamma-aminobutyric
   acid (GABA)
Hydantoins
Monoamine oxidase
   inhibitors (MAOIs)
Narcotic
Neuroleptic
Neurotransmitters
Parasympathetic
Peripheral nervous
   system (PNS)

Psychotropic
Selective serotonin
   reuptake inhibitors
   (SSRIs)
Somatic nervous system
Status epilepticus
Sympathetic nervous
   system
Synapse

■ THE NERVOUS SYSTEM

The nervous system is divided into the **central nervous system (CNS)** and the peripheral nervous system (PNS), which also includes the autonomic nervous system. The CNS includes the brain and spinal cord, which contain billions of neurons. Neurons make up nerves, which make communication and interaction possible between the brain and every part of the body. The brain processes both internal and external information and tells the body how to respond. For example, if the brain receives a signal via nerves that you are cold, it signals your body via nerves to shiver to raise its temperature. Additionally, if your body is not receiving enough glucose because you skipped lunch, nerves send a signal to the brain to stimulate a headache and remind you to eat.

Nervous system medications are used to treat pain, anxiety, depression, mania, insomnia, convulsions, and schizophrenia. Any medication that affects the mind, emotions, or behaviors is known as a **psychotropic.** Nervous system medications act on the CNS and the PNS (discussed in the next section) (Fig. 13-1). Because the PNS extends throughout the body, these drugs can affect other body systems. For example, a drug meant to ease uterine pain may also relieve leg pain.

Most of these drugs act at the **synapse** (gap) between nerves and can adjust the transmission of messages by **neurotransmitters,** which are chemicals that facilitate the movement of messages across the synapses. Medications work by either exciting the CNS or depressing it. Because these drugs are powerful enough to cross the **blood-brain barrier,** which is the barrier in the brain that prevents toxic substances and some medications from entering the brain, they frequently have serious side effects (see the Master the Essentials table for descriptions of the most common nervous system drugs).

The Peripheral Nervous System

The **peripheral nervous system** consists of the **somatic** (voluntary) and **autonomic** (involuntary) nervous systems. The somatic nervous system consists of those muscles over which we have conscious control (e.g., for lifting your arm to scratch your nose). The autonomic nervous system, conversely, controls our internal organs. For example, if you are watching a scary movie, and a monster jumps out from behind a door, your heart begins to race, your stomach may hurt, your pupils dilate, and/or your mouth gets dry, but you do not voluntarily cause these changes; they occur involuntarily based on a stimulus sent to your brain. Medications described in this section include those that affect the autonomic nervous system.

The Autonomic Nervous System

The **autonomic nervous system** is broken down further and consists of two parts: the **sympathetic nervous system,** which controls the body's "fight-or-flight" response, and the **parasympathetic** nervous system, which helps the body to rest and relax (see Fig. 13-1). Acetylcholine and norepinephrine are the two main neurotransmitters that affect the autonomic nervous system. A nerve cell that releases acetylcholine is referred to as **cholinergic,** which relaxes the body. One that releases epinephrine or norepinephrine is

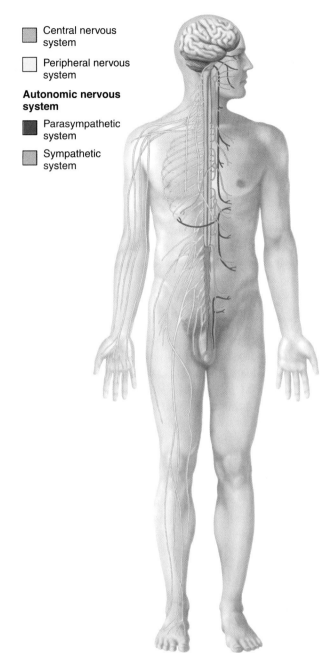

Central nervous system

Peripheral nervous system

Autonomic nervous system

Parasympathetic system

Sympathetic system

FIGURE 13-1: Central and peripheral nervous systems. The brain and the spinal cord make up the central nervous system. The PNS contains nerves outside the brain and spinal cord that lead to the arms, legs, hands, and feet. The autonomic nervous system is part of the PNS.

considered **adrenergic,** which excites the body. These cholinergic and adrenergic substances are naturally occurring in the body, but the substances must be provided artificially when the body's reaction is not appropriate to counteract disease states. The next section describes in more detail when cholinergic and adrenergic drugs are used and why.

THE AUTONOMIC NERVOUS SYSTEM AND MEDICATIONS

Autonomic drugs stimulate the sympathetic nervous system when the body needs to be excited. These drugs are also called **sympathomimetics** or adrenergic agonists. Drugs that stimulate the parasympathetic nervous system calm the nervous system. They are also called **parasympathomimetics** or **cholinergic agonists.**

Sympathomimetics (Adrenergic)

Adrenergic drugs are called sympathomimetics because they mimic the sympathetic nervous system and stimulate the fight-or-flight impulse. They work to stimulate the heart, increase blood flow to the skeletal muscles, and constrict peripheral blood vessels, which then dilate certain parts of the body, such as the bronchi for patients with asthma and pupils for patients who may be having an eye procedure. They are also used to restore heart rhythm during cardiac arrest and to increase blood pressure with drugs such as Levophed (norepinephrine) in cases of shock. They constrict capillaries if the patient is bleeding, such as during a nosebleed. The major contraindication for adrenergic drugs is hypersensitivity to the drug. These drugs should be used cautiously in patients with hypertension, myocardial infarction, atrial fibrillation, or hypovolemia, in children, and in women who are pregnant or breastfeeding.

Adrenergic Blockers

As the name suggests, adrenergic blockers block the action of adrenergics (naturally occurring substances in the body that stimulate the sympathetic nervous system) and thus have a parasympathetic effect. As discussed earlier, the parasympathetic effect calms the nervous system. Adrenergic blockers are useful for treating cardiac arrhythmias (heart rhythm problems), high blood pressure, migraine headaches, and chest pain because they slow the heart rate, relax the blood vessels, and allow blood to flow more freely, thus decreasing the workload on the heart.

Adrenergic blockers are broken down into two groups, based on the muscles they affect. Alpha blockers such as alfuzosin (Uroxatral), doxazosin (Cardura), prazosin (Minipress), tamsulosin (Flomax), and terazosin (Hytrin) affect vascular smooth muscle and are used to alleviate hypertension and benign prostatic hypertrophy (this condition, which affects the male reproductive and urinary systems, is discussed in Chapter 20). Beta blockers work by blocking the effects of the hormone epinephrine. This action affects the heart and blood vessels and causes the heart to beat more slowly and with less force, thereby reducing blood pressure. Beta blockers such as acebutolol (Sectral), atenolol (Tenormin), bisoprolol (Zebeta), metoprolol (Lopressor), nadolol (Corgard), nebivolol (Bystolic), and propranolol (Inderal LA) are used for hypertension, migraine headaches, and glaucoma.

Parasympathomimetics (Cholinergics)

Parasympathomimetics (cholinergics) are so named because they mimic the action of the parasympathetic nervous system; cholinergics release acetylcholine, which relaxes the body's fight-or-flight mechanism. Cholinergics are rarely used because they severely slow body system activity (including heart rate) and constrict respiratory passages. Nerve gases are an example of this class. One of the few cholinergic drugs still used is pilocarpine (Pilopine) for the treatment of open-angle glaucoma. This drug increases the drainage of fluid (aqueous humor) out of the eye to reduce ocular pressure. The drug must be stopped several weeks before surgical procedures because of an increased risk for intraoperative breathing problems.

Anticholinergics or Cholinergic Blockers

Anticholinergics or cholinergic blockers inhibit the parasympathetic branch of the autonomic nervous system and thus promote fight-or-flight symptoms. These drugs dry secretions, including those in the respiratory tract, and are used for asthma and motion sickness. They are also used for preoperative relaxation, for neuromuscular blocking of spasms, as antidotes to insect stings, and in cholinergic crises. A cholinergic crisis manifests with extreme muscular weakness and respiratory depression caused by surplus acetylcholine. This crisis is most commonly seen in patients with myasthenia gravis who are overmedicated with anticholinesterase drugs. In an emergency, atropine (Atropen) can be used to treat a slow heart rate, heart block, or bronchospasm.

◼ MEDICATIONS TO CONTROL PAIN AND FEVER

Pain is an unpleasant sensory and emotional experience arising from actual or potential tissue damage. The perception of pain varies greatly among patients, but it is important to treat each person's pain based on his or her description of it. Pain management is based on a thorough patient assessment that includes the location and intensity of pain.

Analgesics reduce pain without eliminating feeling or sensation, as occurs with anesthetics. Choices include salicylates, acetaminophen, nonsteroidal anti-inflammatory drugs (NSAIDs), and narcotics. Some of these drugs are also antipyretic, which means they reduce fever.

Salicylates

Salicylates, such as aspirin (acetylsalicylic acid), relieve mild to moderate pain and reduce inflammation and fever. Salicylates are also used to decrease inflammation in blood vessels, to improve cardiovascular flow. Aspirin has the disadvantage of causing gastrointestinal (GI) distress, and it should not be used in children with viral infections because of the danger of Reye's syndrome.

Methylsalicylate is a topical anti-inflammatory medication used to irritate the surface of the skin. This irritation increases blood flow to the area where it was applied and thus decreases pain. An example of this class is Bengay.

 CRITICAL THINKING

Based on what you learned in previous chapters and your understanding of how different routes of medication administration affect absorption, why would aspirin in a powder form that you place on your tongue work more rapidly than aspirin tablets?

Acetaminophen

Acetaminophen (Tylenol) decreases pain and fever, but it has no anti-inflammatory effect. Acetaminophen is often an ingredient in combination products used to relieve pain or in products used for cold and flu symptoms such as Alka-Seltzer Plus cold medications. Because it typically does not produce severe side effects, acetaminophen is frequently combined with narcotics, such as oxycodone with acetaminophen (Percocet), to treat moderate to severe pain. Additional acetaminophen should not be ingested with these combination pain medicines as excessive acetaminophen can lead to liver damage.

Nonsteroidal Anti-Inflammatory Drugs (NSAIDs)

NSAIDs, in the context of pain and fever relief, refer to medications such as ibuprofen (Motrin or Advil). These drugs reduce pain and swelling caused by inflammation. Fever is also reduced using this type of drug. As with acetaminophen, NSAIDs can be combined with narcotics to relieve moderate to severe pain. An example is oxycodone with ibuprofen (Combunox). Additional ibuprofen should not be used in combination with these pain medications as too much ibuprofen can lead to kidney damage.

Opioid Analgesics

Opioid analgesics are strong painkillers that suppress the CNS. They are an excellent choice when pain cannot be relieved by milder drugs. The active ingredient in most narcotics is opium, which is extracted from the poppy plant. Other opioid analgesics are obtained from synthetic or semisynthetic sources.

Patients taking narcotic medications to relieve pain must be closely monitored because of the possibility of severe side effects, particularly in large doses. An excess amount of a narcotic medication can slow respirations to dangerous levels. In this instance, the drug Narcan (naloxone) can be given to reverse opioid analgesic effects. It can also decrease blood pressure significantly as a result of peripheral vasodilation. Further drops in blood pressure occurring with changes in position lead to the risk for falls. Patients must use caution with certain activities, such as driving.

Opioid analgesics such as morphine, meperidine (Demoral), and fentanyl are the strongest. They are not routinely prescribed because of their addiction potential. Because narcotics produce euphoria, or happy feelings, they can cause physiological or psychological dependence (A Closer Look 13.1). In addition, limited amounts of medications are ordered, to force close supervision and reassessment of these patients. However, if a patient has pain that does not respond to other medications, he or she should not be denied adequate pain relief out of concern for addiction or dependence. Opioid analgesics are rarely addictive in patients who take them for relief of acute pain for a short period. Opioid analgesics can also be used for general anesthesia during surgery. As discussed in Chapter 4, opioid analgesics are classified as levels I to V controlled substances based on accepted use and addictive qualities.

Sometimes combining analgesics with alternative methods of pain relief, such as meditation, can reduce pain effectively.

A CLOSER LOOK 13.1: Opioid Analgesic Addiction Epidemic

The number of people addicted to opioid analgesics such as dilaudid, methadone, morphine, and oral prescription opioid analgesics such as oxycodone and hydrocodone is becoming an epidemic. This is a serious global problem, and it is estimated that 33 million users abuse opiates and prescription opiates worldwide.[1] Unintentional overdose deaths have quadrupled in the United States since 1999. According to the Centers for Disease Control and Prevention, more than 15,000 people died from prescription opioid overdoses in 2015 (one-half of all U.S. opioid overdose deaths).[2] Babies are being born daily to mothers who abused these drugs during pregnancy and who now are equally addicted. The withdrawal process on these infants is difficult for all involved. This epidemic is placing a huge financial and social burden on society to provide care for the addicts as well as the families of these addicts.

[1] Centers for Disease Control and Prevention, Prescription Opioid Overdose Data. https://www.cdc.gov/drugoverdose/data/overdose.html. Accessed 24 May, 2017.
[2] United Nations Office on Drugs and Crime. World Drug Report 2016. http://www.unodc.org/doc/wdr2016/WORLD_DRUG_REPORT_2016_web.pdf. Accessed 24 May, 2017.

CRITICAL THINKING

What other nondrug methods, aside from meditation, can be used to decrease pain?

MEDICATIONS TO TREAT ANXIETY, INSOMNIA, SEDATION, AND SEIZURES

The limbic system of the brain is integral to such emotions as love, fear, and anger, as well as being important to our memory and level of alertness. The connections in this part of the brain allow the limbic system to control and mediate these emotions. If the structures in this system are not operating optimally, difficulty with anxiety, sleeplessness, alertness, or seizures may occur. Medications help to relieve anxiety, promote sleep, increase alertness, or help stop seizures.

Anxiolytic Medications

Anxiety may be an uneasy feeling of discomfort or tension, or it may be an apprehension that originates from anticipating danger. Anxiety disorders are characterized by the recurrences of such reactions to the extent they interfere with a person's ability to function. Types of anxiety disorders include generalized anxiety disorder, panic disorder, posttraumatic stress disorder, obsessive-compulsive disorder, phobias, and many more. With anxiety disorders, the source of discomfort or danger is often unknown or unrecognized. Phobias are exaggerations of normal anxieties (heights, animals), and others are based on previous experiences (e.g., being trapped in an elevator).

Anxiolytic medications reduce the intensity of these fears, dangers, and/or tension that a patient may be experiencing. They can be taken routinely or only when the patient feels increasing anxiety. These drugs work in the limbic system of the brain by depressing the subcortical levels of the CNS and have a calming effect. This effect can range from mild sedation to coma, depending on the medication and dose used. CNS depressants comprise a type of anxiolytic used to treat anxiety and restlessness. The two main categories of CNS depressants are benzodiazepines and barbiturates. Benzodiazepines include lorazepam (Ativan), diazepam (Valium), and alprazolam (Xanax), and are used for anxiety, seizures, alcohol withdrawal symptoms, and muscle relaxation. They can also be used to reduce anxiety before general anesthesia. Barbiturates are an older type of medication including phenobarbital, which are not often used due to high levels of addiction and a very narrow window of effectiveness before serious problems occur. Barbiturates may still occasionally be used to control seizures. Other categories of medications used as anxiolytics include selective serotonin reuptake inhibitors (SSRIs) such as celexa (Citalopram), fluoxetine (Prozac), and sertraline (Zoloft); serotonin-norepinephrine reuptake inhibitors (SNRIs) such as venlafaxine (Effexor XR); and tricyclic antidepressants such as amitriptyline (Elavil). Although these drugs may not work as quickly as CNS depressants, they have very little dependence issues.

Insomnia and Medications

Insomnia (trouble sleeping) is a common complaint from patients. Sometimes barbiturates are used to induce sleep by depressing the CNS (slowing heart rate, respirations). They are also used to help the patient relax before a minor procedure or general surgery. Other newer non-narcotic benzodiazepine hypnotics such as zolpidem (Ambien) and eszopiclone (Lunesta) help to promote sleep with fewer side effects. Both types of medications target the same portion of the brain, but the newer non-narcotic medications are able to target just the areas promoting sleep without depressing the entire CNS. These medications are therefore becoming the preferred sleep aids, but they continue to pose a possible addiction risk. Therefore, they should be used on a limited basis.

Barbiturates and Antiseizure Medications

Barbiturates are also used to control seizures (A Closer Look 13.2). Barbiturates that are **hydantoins,** such as phenytoin (Dilantin), delay sodium from crossing the neural membranes. This effect decreases the potential for too much electrical activity and calms the cell. Hydantoins are the drug of choice for tonic-clonic (grand mal) and partial seizures. Other barbiturates such as phenobarbital (Luminal) are used for tonic-clonic and febrile seizures in children. Succinimides such as ethosuximide (Zarontin) comprise a class of antiseizure drugs that delay the movement of calcium over the neurons. Like hydantoins, they relax nerve cells. The succinimides are the drugs of choice for absence (petit mal) seizures.

The reason that traditional antiseizure medications decrease seizure activity has long been poorly understood. Researchers eventually discovered, however, that the naturally occurring **gamma-aminobutyric acid (GABA)** is a neurotransmitter inhibitor. In other words, GABA inhibits abnormal electrical activity in the brain, and an increased presence of this amino acid decreases seizure activity (Fig. 13-2). The discovery led researchers to look for agents that could affect GABA activity. An example of this category of drug is vigabatrin (Sabril). Benzodiazepines such as diazepam (Valium) can also intensify the effect of GABA transmitters in the brain and allow more GABA to reach the receptors in the brain to trigger the actions needed to suppress abnormal electrical activity. Other medications that work as anticonvulsants are lamotrigine (Lamictal), tiagabine (Gabitril), topiramate (Topamax), and carbamazepine (Tegretol).

A CLOSER LOOK 13.2: Seizures

Abnormal electrical activity in the brain can cause seizures. A patient may have a diagnostic test called electroencephalography (EEG) to detect seizure activity. Seizures may be mild (petit mal) or severe (grand mal). The most severe seizure is called **status epilepticus.** In this instance, the patient is having a tonic-clonic (grand mal) seizure that lasts for longer than 30 minutes and cannot regain consciousness. Because the patient is not breathing during this episode, there is a high risk for brain damage and death without immediate medical intervention, usually with IV benzodiazepines such as Valium.

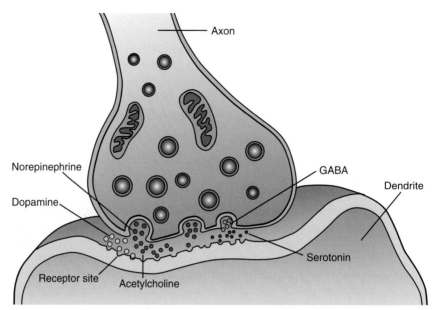

FIGURE 13-2: Nerve synapse. The gap between the axon and the dendrite of a nerve is called the synapse. Neurotransmitters such as gamma-aminobutyric acid (GABA), serotonin, dopamine, norepinephrine, and acetylcholine help transmit the electrical impulse from the axon to the dendrite. The neurotransmitters fit into receptors on the dendrites. Some psychotropic drugs act by inhibiting the work of the neurotransmitters, thereby slowing the electrical impulses; others act by stimulating neurotransmitters, thereby promoting electrical impulses.

■ MEDICATIONS TO TREAT BEHAVIORAL, EMOTIONAL, AND MOOD DISORDERS

Behavioral and emotional disorders are becoming more common in the United States. Behavioral and emotional disorders is a broad term used to include a wide variety of mental health diagnoses in which the individual may have difficulty initiating and maintaining relationships with peers and others. This includes diagnoses such as ODD (oppositional-defiant disorder), OCD (obsessive-compulsive disorder), anxiety disorders, schizophrenia, and autism. Mood disorders are typically characterized by the elevation or depression of one's mood. For example, a person with bipolar disorder experiences periods of mania, very elevated emotions, to very low emotions such as depression. Several categories of drugs, including antidepressants, mood stabilizer drugs, and antipsychotics, can be used to help patients with behavioral, emotional, and mood disorders.

Central Nervous System Stimulants

CNS stimulants are used to treat ADD, ADHD, obesity, and sleep disorders such as narcolepsy. Attention deficit disorder (ADD) and attention deficit–hyperactivity disorder (ADHD) are common in both children and adults. In the past, these were considered behavioral disorders, but today there is much debate as to whether they should be included in this category. These disorders stem from the ineffectiveness of the impulse control center of the frontal cortex of the brain.

It may seem counterintuitive to give a distracted, unfocused, overactive patient a stimulant, but CNS stimulants such as amphetamine/dextroamphetamine (Adderall), pemoline (Cylert), and methylphenidate (Ritalin) have the opposite effect in these patients in that they calm them and increase their ability to focus. An alternate way to view this disorder is to understand that the patient is being bombarded by a multitude of stimuli and is unable to focus on any one of them. The CNS stimulants help these patients to focus on only a few of the stimuli and not be distracted by the others and therefore allow patients to become more successful in their daily activities. People who do not have ADD or ADHD but who take the medication anyway find that it acts as a CNS stimulant.

Sometimes an amphetamine, a type of CNS stimulant, such as phentermine (Zantryl), is prescribed for obesity. Usually, it is given 30 to 60 minutes before meals to increase metabolism, but only for short periods. Diet and exercise regimens should be used concurrently with amphetamine use for weight loss.

The primary treatment in patients with narcolepsy is CNS stimulant drugs such as modafinil (Provigil) or armodafinil (Nuvigil) to help them to stay awake and alert.

 CRITICAL THINKING

Why should amphetamines not be prescribed routinely for obese patients who are trying to lose weight?

Antidepressants

Clinical depression is characterized by excesses of sleeping and eating, an inability to concentrate, avoidance of the companionship of other people, decreased interest in sex and activities one usually enjoys, and feelings of despair. Depression is usually a combination of genetic and environmental causes, which lead to a change in the brain's biochemistry, and can be devastating to the patient. When neurotransmitters are depleted, the patient does not think as clearly as usual, and mood becomes depressed. Antidepressants preserve neurotransmitters at the synapse.

Many medication options for depression exist, and most patients find that the first medication they try is a good fit. Other patients must try numerous medications before they find an antidepressant that works for them and has tolerable side effects. Four categories of antidepressant agents are monoamine oxidase (MAO) inhibitors (MAOIs), tricyclic antidepressants (TCAs), selective serotonin reuptake inhibitors (SSRIs) and serotonin-norepinephrine reuptake inhibitors (SNRIs).

Monoamine Oxidase Inhibitors (MAOIs)

MAOIs inhibit MAO, an enzyme that terminates the action of neurotransmitters at the synapse. Inhibiting or stopping MAO improves the retention of neurotransmitters at the site. An example of an MAOI is selegiline (Eldepryl). Unfortunately, this drug classification requires dietary exclusion of foods containing tyramine (Box 13-1). A patient who eats any of these foods while taking an MAOI can suffer critical hypertension. Because tyramine is common in many foods, these drugs are rarely prescribed today.

 CRITICAL THINKING

If a patient who is taking an MAOI went to a Super Bowl party, which typical party foods would he or she be unable to eat?

Tricyclic Antidepressants (TCAs)

TCAs are medications with a three-ring (tricyclic) chemical structure that keeps norepinephrine and serotonin at the nerve terminals and thereby helping electrical impulses cross the synapse (see Fig. 13-2). TCAs such as amitriptyline (Elavil) have been used for decades but have many more side effects than the more

---

BOX 13.1 Foods High in Tyramine	
Avocados	Papayas
Bananas	Paté, beef
Beer	Pepperoni
Bologna	Raisins
Chocolate	Salami
Dairy products, aged	Sausage
Fava beans	Soy sauce
Figs	Wine
Herring	Yeast
Hot dogs	

popular SSRIs. TCAs are still the drugs of choice for severe depression and inpatient treatment of depression. Patients suffering from insomnia are generally prescribed TCAs because of the sedative side effects of these drugs.

Selective Serotonin Reuptake Inhibitors (SSRIs)

SSRIs such as citalopram (Celexa), fluoxetine (Prozac), paroxetine (Paxil), and sertraline (Zoloft) prevent serotonin from being used up at the synapse. Serotonin is a chemical produced in the brain that acts as a neurotransmitter to help signals transfer from one part of the brain to another. Low serotonin levels have been implicated in depression, and keeping serotonin at the synapse improves mood. Because they have so few side effects compared with MAOIs and TCAs, SSRIs are frequently the first class of drug prescribed for depression. However, each drug within the classification can affect the patient differently. If one drug does not work well for the patient, the prescriber may change the dosage or change to another medication.

Serotonin-Norepinephrine Reuptake Inhibitors (SNRIs)

The newest category of medications to treat depression are the serotonin-norepinephrine reuptake inhibitors (SNRIs). These medications block the reuptake of both serotonin and norepinephrine. The increase in these levels are shown to elevate the mood. Examples of SNRIs are venlafaxine (Effexor XR), desvenlafaxine (Pritiz), and duloxetine (Cymbalta). Although these drugs are newer, the SSRIs have fewer side effects and therefore continue to be the most commonly prescribed for depression.

 CRITICAL THINKING

Why are antidepressants used to decrease pain?

Mood Stabilizers

Mood stabilizers (antimanic agents) stabilize the extreme mood shifts seen in patients with bipolar disorder and are also used in patients with schizophrenia. In a very short period, patients vacillate between severe depression and a manic state in which they make grandiose plans and possibly act on those plans because they feel invincible. Therapy can decrease the number and intensity of these manic episodes and the frequency of these shifts in mood.

A common drug used to treat bipolar disorder is lithium. Lithium is a salt, so it is important for patients who are taking lithium not to become dehydrated. These patients should avoid using table salt. Lithium has a small therapeutic range. Because lithium toxicity can be fatal, blood lithium assays (levels) must be performed regularly. Signs of toxicity include drowsiness, blurred vision, confusion, sensitivity to light, tremors, muscle weakness, cardiovascular collapse, seizures, and coma. Other mood stabilizing drugs include lamotrigine (Lamictal) and valproic acid (Depakene, Depakote).

Medications for Treating Psychoses

Psychoses comprise a class of disorders characterized by abnormal thoughts, disorganized communication, and lack of interaction with the environment. Delusions, hallucinations, paranoia, and bizarre thoughts and behaviors are frequent symptoms of psychoses and occur in schizophrenia.

Antipsychotic medications called **neuroleptics,** such as chlorpromazine (Thorazine), clozapine (Clopine), and thioridazine (Mellaril), treat the abnormal actions and behavior of psychoses such as talking and interacting with a situation that only patients can see and hear. Some antipsychotic medications are used for nausea and vomiting, dementia, agitation, and spasms, as well as for psychoses. Be sure you know why the neuroleptic was prescribed.

■ MEDICATIONS TO TREAT DEGENERATIVE DISORDERS

Degenerative disorders of the nervous system are characterized by a continuous decline in mental and/or physical functioning, and they have no cure. These disorders may be caused by genetics, environment, or injury to the nervous system, although the cause is often unknown. The goals of treatment are to relieve symptoms and to maintain independence for as long as possible. The following are two of the more common degenerative disorders affecting the nervous system.

Dementia

Dementia is a progressive, irreversible decline in mental function. Alzheimer's disease is the most frequent cause of dementia, but there are dozens of other less commonly known causes. Currently, few drugs are available to treat dementia, and the ones that do cause only a minor reduction in symptoms of confusion and decreased memory (Drug Spotlight 13.1). The goal of drug therapy is to prevent or slow further mental deterioration. Therefore, the best outcome is early diagnosis, so treatment can begin. Although it is unclear how they work, cholinesterase inhibitors are the drugs of choice in treating mild to moderate Alzheimer's disease. Research shows that this class of drugs prevents the breakdown of cholinesterase in the brain that is responsible for memory and thinking. Aricept (donepezil HCL) is an example of a cholinesterase inhibitor that shows some promise in slowing the progression of this disease.

CRITICAL THINKING

If a patient is diagnosed with dementia, what precautions may need to be taken in the home?

Parkinson's Disease

Parkinson's disease is a degenerative disorder of the CNS. When neurons that produce the neurotransmitter dopamine die, muscle movements become disorganized. The lack of dopamine and the increase in acetylcholine cause tremors, slow movement, rigid muscles, and balance problems. Antiparkinsonian drugs focus on keeping dopamine and acetylcholine at the nerve synapse and thereby promote the transmission of nerve signals. These drugs are classified as dopaminergic (replacing or increasing dopamine), such as selegiline (Eldepryl), bromocriptine (Parlodel), ropinirole (Requip), and carbidopa/levodopa (Sinemet), or cholinergic agents (those that inhibit the action of acetylcholine), such as biperiden (Akineton).

Because of the blood-brain barrier, it is difficult to ensure that a sufficient amount of dopamine reaches the brain to control the symptoms of this disease effectively. As a result, patients with Parkinson's

Drug Spotlight 13-1 *Namzaric (donepezil hydrochloride and memantine hydrochloride)*

Classification	Anti-Alzheimer's agents
Availability	Tablets
Indications	Treatment of moderate to severe dementia associated with Alzheimer's.
Dosage/Implementation	10 mg of donepezil hydrochloride once a day. May be taken with or without food, intact or opened, and sprinkled on a small amount of food.
Action	Improves the function of nerve cells in the brain by stopping the breakdown of acetylcholine.
Adverse Reactions/Side Effects	Most common is diarrhea, headache, and nausea. May include vomiting, anorexia, and ecchymoses.
Contraindications/Precautions	Hypersensitivity to memantine hydrochloride, donepezil hydrochloride, or piperidien derivatives. If patient is pregnant or plans to become pregnant or is breastfeeding, notify her physician.

disease are given a combination of drugs that allow smaller doses of medications to achieve the dopamine levels needed. These patients tend to become acclimatized or tolerant of their medication, and thus the doses must be increased to have the same effect. When the dose cannot be increased or the side effects become intolerable, the doctor will request a **drug holiday,** in which the patient stops taking antiparkinsonian medications for a week or so and then restarts them at a lower dose, to produce the desired effects.

LOCAL AND GENERAL ANESTHETIC MEDICATIONS

Anesthesia means loss of sensation. Anesthesia administered locally creates a lack of feeling without a loss of consciousness. For instance, lidocaine is used to numb the skin before stitches are placed to close a wound. General anesthesia causes patients to lose both feeling and consciousness, such as during a surgical procedure.

Local Anesthesia

Local anesthesia can be applied to a body surface to numb an area before a procedure. The local anesthetic blocks the entry of sodium ions into nerve fibers. Adequate amounts must be applied or injected to keep the area numb throughout the procedure. Local anesthetics come in a variety of forms: cream (lidocaine/prilocaine [EMLA]), aerosol spray (benzocaine/butamben/tetracaine [Exactacain]), otic (benzocaine [Americaine otic]) or ophthalmic drops (tetracaine [Tetcaine ophthalmic]), or an injectable solution such as lidocaine (Xylocaine). Local anesthetics are classified as esters or amides, depending on the structure of their molecules.

Amides, such as lidocaine and novocaine, tend to last longer, so they are more popular. Adverse effects and allergies are rare. The patient must be observed during the procedure to be sure that the anesthetic is still in effect and to monitor any negative reactions. Be sure to document your observations.

Esters, such as procaine and tetracaine, have the potential for severe allergic reactions such as anaphylactic shock because of the release of para-aminobenzoic acid (PABA), a known allergen, during the metabolism process. Because of this, the use of esters is limited to topical preparations, in which exposure to PABA is much less significant than in injections.

General Anesthesia

General anesthetics can be administered by intravenous (IV) infusion or inhalation. For longer procedures, an IV agent such as midazolam (Versed), propofol (Diprivan), or ketamine (Ketalar) may be used initially, followed by inhalation therapy with medications such as desflurane (Suprane), isoflurane (Forane), or sevoflurane (Ultane). Use of the IV agent allows smaller doses of inhalation therapy medications to be used and thus reduces the risk for severe side effects of these medications.

 CRITICAL THINKING

Why would an IV anesthetic be given before an inhaled gas is administered by mask?

Inhaled general anesthetics are volatile agents that can depress respiratory and cardiovascular function, so patients must be observed carefully during procedures in which these drugs are used. An example of an inhaled general anesthetic in ambulatory care is nitrous oxide, which is used for dental and brief surgical procedures.

Contraindications to inhalation anesthetics include any known hypersensitivity to specific anesthetic agents or respiratory system disease.

◼ ALCOHOL

Alcohol, which is a CNS depressant, is rarely prescribed as a medication. However, because it interacts with other medications and can have powerful effects on the body, it is included in this discussion. Alcohol added to medication can cause confusion, peripheral vasodilation, increased heart rate, electrolyte imbalances, decreased motor coordination, unsteady gait, and slurred speech. Prolonged use can permanently damage the CNS and liver.

Signs and symptoms of chronic alcoholism include irritability, tremors, GI disorders, frequent falling accidents, blackouts, memory loss, confusion, neural and muscular weakness, and conjunctivitis. Treatment includes disulfiram (Antabuse), behavior modification, vitamin B injections, and dietary changes (e.g., supplements to replace vitamins lost through poor nutrition).

Patients abusing alcohol should be assessed for respiratory problems, vomiting, convulsions, cerebral swelling, electrolyte imbalances, and tremors when they are withdrawing from alcohol.

●●○ SUMMARY

- ◼ The nervous system consists of the central nervous and the peripheral nervous systems.
- ◼ The central nervous system consists of the brain and spinal cord.
- ◼ The peripheral nervous system consists of the network of all nerve tissue outside of the brain and spinal cord.
- ◼ The peripheral nervous system is broken down into the somatic (voluntary) nervous system and the autonomic (involuntary) nervous system.
- ◼ The autonomic (involuntary) nervous system is further broken down into the sympathetic nervous system and the parasympathetic nervous system.
- ◼ Two main neurotransmitters affect the autonomic system: cholinergic nerve cells release acetylcholine, and adrenergic nerve cells release norepinephrine.
- ◼ The categories of nervous system medications include sympathomimetics (adrenergic), adrenergic blockers, parasympathomimetics (cholinergics), anticholinergics (cholinergic blockers), and analgesics.
- ◼ The categories of medications to treat pain and fever are salicylates, acetaminophen, nonsteroidal anti-inflammatory drugs (NSAIDs), and opioid analgesics.
- ◼ Medications to treat anxiety, insomnia, sedation, and seizures include anxiolytic medications and barbiturates and antiseizure medications.
- ◼ Medications to treat behavioral, emotional, and mood disorders include CNS stimulants, antidepressants, mood stabilizers, and antipsychotic medications (neuroleptics).
- ◼ Cholinesterase inhibitors can help treat dementia, and dopaminergic or cholinergic agents are used to treat Parkinson's disease.
- ◼ Local anesthetics produce a loss of feeling in a specific area of the body without a loss of consciousness. General anesthesia causes a loss of feeling and consciousness.
- ◼ Alcohol is a sedative/hypnotic and commonly increases the action of nervous system medications.

Master the Essentials: Nervous System Medications

This table shows the various classes of nervous system medications and key side effects, contraindications and precautions, and interactions for each class.

Class	Use	Side Effects	Contraindications and Precautions	Interactions	Example
Adrenergics	Extreme hypotension, severe wheezing, severe allergic reactions (anaphylactic shock)	Chest pain, fast heart rate, headache, increased blood glucose, nervousness, tissue death, tremors	Brain damage, CV and heart problems, glaucoma, hyperthyroidism	Adrenergic blockers, CNS drugs	Norepinephrine (Levophed), epinephrine
Adrenergic blockers	BPH, hypertension, cardiac arrhythmias, angina, prevention of heart attack, migraine headache	Confusion, decreased blood pressure, blood glucose, energy, heart rate	Asthma, atrioventricular block (heart block), chronic heart failure, diabetes, low blood pressure	Alcohol, digitalis, epinephrine, insulin, MAOIs, theophylline, TCAs	Alfuzosin (Uroxatral), doxazosin (Cardura), prazosin (Minipress) tamsulosin (Flomax), terazosin (Hytrin), acebutolol (Sectral), atenolol (Tenormin), bisoprolol (Zebeta), metoprolol (Lopressor), nadolol (Corgard), nebivolol (Bystolic), propranolol (Inderal LA)
Cholinergics	Glaucoma or other ocular hypertension, dementia associated with Alzheimer's disease	Bronchospasm; decreased heart rate, respirations, blood pressure; increased salivation, tears, and sweating; muscle cramps and weakness	Asthma, benign prostatic hypertrophy, cardiac disease, GI disorders, hyperthyroidism	Quinidine, procainamide	Pilocarpine (Pilopine), donepezil (Aricept)
Anticholinergics	Bladder, stomach, or intestinal spasms, poisoning	Blurred vision, confusion, decreased GI motility, dilation of pupils, drying of secretions, fever, flushing, headache, increased heart rate	Asthma, cardiac arrhythmias, COPD, GI or GU obstruction, glaucoma, hypertension	Digoxin, nitroglycerin, TCAs	Atropine (Atropen)
Salicylates	Pain, fever, inflammation. Heart attack, stroke, or angina prevention	Coma, depression, dizziness, headache, drowsiness, increased bleeding time, bruising, GI bleeding, liver and kidney disorders, tinnitus, rash	Asthma, bleeding disorders, lactation, pregnancy, vitamin K deficiency	Alcohol, antacids, anticoagulants, heparin, NSAIDs, insulin	Salicylic acid (aspirin)

Master the Essentials: Nervous System Medications—cont'd

Class	Use	Side Effects	Contraindications and Precautions	Interactions	Example
Acetaminophen	Pain, fever	Rash, urticaria (high dosages can cause liver failure)	Alcohol abuse, hypersensitivity, liver disease, malnutrition	Alcohol, oral contraceptives, phenytoin, loop diuretics	Acetaminophen (Tylenol)
NSAIDs	Pain, fever, inflammation	Blurred vision, constipation, dizziness, drowsiness, dyspepsia, edema, GI bleeding, headache, hepatitis, irregular heart rate, kidney disorders, prolonged bleeding, psychic disturbances, rash, tinnitus	Active GI bleeding, CV disease, hypersensitivity, liver disease, pregnancy, renal disease, ulcer	Corticosteroids, salicylates, cyclosporine, anticoagulants, beta blockers, digoxin	Ibuprofen (Advil, Motrin)
Opioid analgesics	Moderate to severe pain	Decreased blood pressure, heart rate, and respirations; agitation, blurred vision, confusion, constipation, flushing, headache, oversedation, rash, restlessness, seizures, urinary retention	Lactation and pregnancy, patients with head injury, CNS depression, COPD, hypothyroidism, liver or kidney disease; used with caution in addicted patients, children, elderly patients, hypersensitive patients, suicidal patients	Alcohol, antiemetics, antihistamines, antihypertensives, antiarrhythmics, muscle relaxers, psychotropics, sedative-hypnotics	Morphine, meperidine (Demerol), hydromorphone (Dilaudid), fentanyl (Sublimaze)
Non-narcotic benzodiazepine hypnotics	Insomnia	Outgoing or aggressive behavior, confusion, agitation, hallucinations, worsening of depression, suicidal thoughts or actions, memory loss, anxiety, sleep activity	Hypersensitivity to ingredients, pregnancy, lactation, children	Alcohol, paroxetine, lorazepam, olanzapine	Zolpidem (Ambien), eszopiclone (Lunesta)

Continued

Master the Essentials: Nervous System Medications—cont'd

Class	Use	Side Effects	Contraindications and Precautions	Interactions	Example
Antiseizure medications	Epilepsy (seizures), nerve pain, anxiety disorders, muscle spasms, alcohol withdrawal	Multiple side effects different for each medication	Dilantin: hypersensitivity, caution in pregnancy, impaired liver function; Luminal: blood disorder porphyria, patients taking GHB; Zarontin: hypersensitivity to succinimides; Sabril: none; Lamictal: hypersensitivity; Gabitril: hypersensitivity; Topamax: hypersensitivity, glaucoma; Tegretol: history of bone marrow depression, hypersensitivity; Valium: hypersensitivity, children younger than 6 months of age, myasthenia gravis, severe respiratory or hepatic insufficiency, sleep apnea, acute narrow-angle glaucoma	Alcohol, salicylates, succinimides, sulfonamides, valproic acid, oral contraceptives, rifampin, and many more than possible to list	Phenytoin (Dilantin), phenobarbital (Luminal), ethosuximide (Zarontin), vigabatrin (Sabril), lamotrigine (Lamictal), levetiracetam (Keppra), tiagabine (Gabitril), topiramate (Topamax), carbamazepine (Tegretol), diazepam (Valium), pentobarbital (Nembutal)
Anxiolytics	Anxiety disorders, panic disorders, alcohol withdrawal, muscle spasms	Agitation, amnesia, bizarre behaviors, confusion, decreased white blood cell count, depression, drowsiness, hallucinations, headache, lack of coordination, lethargy, oversedation, sensitivity to light, tremors	Not used in children, decreased vital signs, depression, lactation, pregnancy, suicidal ideation; observe for addiction and for evidence that the patient is considering suicide	Alcohol, antiemetics, antihistamines, analgesics, CNS depressants, digoxin, grapefruit juice, muscle relaxants, phenytoin, psychotropics	Alprazolam (Xanax), diazepam (Valium), lorazepam (Ativan)

Master the Essentials: Nervous System Medications—cont'd

Class	Use	Side Effects	Contraindications and Precautions	Interactions	Example
Barbiturates	Insomnia, preoperative sedative, seizures	Lethargy, dizziness, irritability, constipation, vessel swelling, confusion, decreased respirations and heart rate, bone softening, coma, fatal overdose, unsteady balance, liver inflammation, bone marrow suppression, vision disorders, anorexia, inflammation of the gums	Pregnancy, hypersensitivity, hepatitis, cardiac and renal disease, hemolytic disorders, decreased heart rate	Alcohol, analgesics, antacids, antineoplastics, CNS depressants, corticosteroids, folic acid, grapefruit juice, MAOIs, oral anticoagulants, oral contraceptives, theophylline, sedatives	Secobarbital (Seconal), pentobarbital (Nembutal)
CNS stimulants	ADD, ADHD, narcolepsy, obesity	Nervousness, insomnia, irritability, seizures or psychosis; increased heart rate, blood pressure, and irregularity of heart rhythm; dizziness, headache, blurred vision, GI disorders, dependence	Nervousness, insomnia, irritability, seizures, or psychosis; increased heart rate, blood pressure, and irregularity of heart rhythm; dizziness, headache, blurred vision, GI disorders, dependence	Antacids, anticoagulants, anticonvulsants, clonidine, TCAs	Methylphenidate (Ritalin), amphetamine/ dextroamphetamine (Adderall), phentermine (Zantryl)
MAOIs	Parkinson's disease	Nervousness, headache, stiff neck, increased heart rate and blood pressure, diarrhea, blurred vision	Known hypersensitivity, heart disease, hepatic or renal impairment, headaches, cerebrovascular disease, pregnancy, lactation, foods containing tyramine	Adrenergics, diuretics, antidepressants, CNS depressants, insulin, levodopa, foods containing tyramine, herbs such as St. John's wort	Selegiline (Eldepryl)

Continued

Master the Essentials: Nervous System Medications—cont'd

Class	Use	Side Effects	Contraindications and Precautions	Interactions	Example
TCAs (tricyclic antidepressants)	Depression	Dry mouth, increased appetite, weight gain, blurred vision, drowsiness, dizziness, constipation, urinary retention, postural hypotension, irregular heart rhythms, headache	Pregnancy and lactation; cardiac, kidney, liver, and GI disorders; glaucoma; obesity; seizures	Alcohol, CNS drugs, MAOIs	doxepin (Sinequan), imipramine (Tofranil), nortriptyline
SSRIs	Depression, panic disorders, OCD, bulimia, anxiety disorders, PTSD, PMDD	Sexual dysfunction, anorexia, diarrhea, sweating, insomnia, anxiety, nervousness, tremor, fatigue, dizziness, drowsiness, headache	Pregnancy and lactation; patients with thoughts of suicide, diabetes, bipolar disorders, eating disorders	CNS drugs, MAOIs, anticoagulants, beta blockers, antiarrhythmics	Fluoxetine (Prozac), sertraline (Zoloft), paroxetine (Paxil), citalopram (Celexa)
SNRIs	Depression	Nausea, constipation, dizziness, drowsiness, anorexia, excessive diaphoresis, dry mouth, weight gain	Patients using MAOIs or IV methylene blue, hypersensitivity to any ingredients of medication, may cause worsening of depression and suicidal ideation, may increase blood pressure, may increase risk for bleeding events	Alcohol, MAOIs, triptans, anticoagulants, antihistamines, Theophylline, ketoconazole	desvenlafaxine (Pristiq), duloxetine (Cymbalta), venlafaxine (Effexor)
Lithium	Bipolar disorder (manic-depressive disorder)	GI distress, hypotension, cardiac irregularities, polyuria, tremors, thyroid problems	Seizure disorders; Parkinson's disease; CV, kidney, and thyroid diseases; dehydration, pregnancy, lactation	NSAIDs, diuretics, ACE inhibitors, sodium salts	Lithium citrate
Antipsychotics	Schizophrenia, bipolar disorder, severe behavioral and conduct disorders in children, nausea and vomiting, severe hiccups	ECG changes, hypotension, agitation, dizziness, sedation, drowsiness, dystonia, headache, constipation, dry mouth, photosensitivity, nausea	Known hypersensitivity, cardiac arrhythmias, seizure disorder, thyroid disease, renal or hepatic impairment	Anticholinergics, CNS depressants, alcohol, beta blockers, caffeine, antidepressants, lithium	Clozapine (Clopine), phenothiazine (Mellaril), chlorpromazine (Thorazine)

Master the Essentials: Nervous System Medications—cont'd

Class	Use	Side Effects	Contraindications and Precautions	Interactions	Example
Antiparkinsonian drugs	Parkinson's disease, acromegaly	Involuntary movements, loss of appetite, anxiety, confusion, depression, psychosis, decreased blood pressure, dizziness, fainting	Pregnancy and lactation, asthma and emphysema, cardiac disease, decreased blood pressure, peptic ulcer, diabetes, glaucoma	Benzodiazepines, pyridoxine, phenothiazines, haloperidol, antihypertensives, phenytoin, vitamin B_6, MAOIs	Ropinirole (Requip), selegiline (Eldepryl), bromocriptine (Parlodel), benztropine (Cogentin), carbidopa/levodopa (Sinemet), biperiden (Akineton)
Local anesthetics	Minor surgery/procedure preparation, pain and/or itch relief	Heart block, hypotension, bradycardia, arrhythmias, restlessness, anxiety, dizziness, headache, nausea, vomiting	Known hypersensitivity, severe hypertension, shock, hematologic disorders, psychosis	Sedatives, sulfonamides	Lidocaine/prilocaine (EMLA cream), benzocaine/butamben/tetracaine (Exactacain), benzocaine (Americaine otic), lidocaine (Xylocaine), tetracaine (Tetcaine ophthalmic)
General anesthetics	Sedation of patient prior to minor or major surgery, or procedure	Cardiopulmonary depression, confusion, sedation, nausea, vomiting, hypothermia, malignant hyperthermia	Known hypersensitivity, hepatic disorder, malignant hyperthermia, pregnancy, lactation	CNS depressants, neuromuscular blockers, catecholamines	Midazolam (Versed), propofol (Diprivan), ketamine (Ketalar), desflurane (Suprane), isoflurane, sevoflurane (Ultane), nitrous oxide

ACE, angiotensin-converting enzyme; ADD, attention deficit disorder; ADHD, attention deficit–hyperactivity disorder; BPH, benign prostatic hypertrophy; CNS, central nervous system; COPD, chronic obstructive pulmonary disease; CV, cardiovascular; ECG, electrocardiogram; GI, gastrointestinal; GU, genitourinary; MAOI, monoamine oxidase inhibitor; NSAID, nonsteroidal anti-inflammatory drug; OCD, obsessive-compulsive disorder; PMDD, premenstrual dysphoric disorder; PTSD, post-traumatic stress disorder; SSRI, selective serotonin reuptake inhibitor; TCA, tricyclic antidepressant.

Activities

To make sure that you have learned the key points covered in this chapter, complete the following activities.

True or False

Write true if the statement is true. Beside the false statements, write false, and correct the statement to make it true.

1. Parasympathomimetics have many therapeutic uses because of relatively few side effects.

_____

_____

2. Some antipsychotic drugs are used to manage alcohol withdrawal. _____

_____

3. Benzodiazepines are a type of local anesthesia. _____

_____

4. Salicylates have the side effect of prolonging bleeding time. _____

_____

5. Barbiturates are used for insomnia. _____

_____

6. The nervous system is divided into three sections: the central, peripheral, and lateral nervous systems. _____

_____

7. The somatic nervous system controls voluntary movement such as lifting your hand. _____

_____

8. The somatic nervous system controls involuntary movements such as the constriction of pupils. _____

_____

9. The blood-brain barrier restricts very few substances from entering the brain. _____

_____

10. Hydantoins are used to control seizures. _____

_____

Multiple Choice

Choose the best answer for each question.

1. The classification of drugs used to treat depression is _____.
   A. Benzodiazepines
   B. Antidepressants
   C. CNS stimulants
   D. Narcotic analgesics

2. The classification of drugs usually used for surgical procedures is _____.

   A. Benzodiazepines

   B. Anesthetics

   C. Barbiturates

   D. Beta blockers

3. The disease most commonly associated with a drug holiday is _____.

   A. Parkinson's disease

   B. Alzheimer's disease

   C. Myasthenia gravis

   D. Fibromyalgia

4. The classification of drugs usually used for treating psychosis is _____.

   A. SSRIs

   B. EEGs

   C. Benzodiazepines

   D. Neuroleptics

5. Which type of anesthesia has a high risk for allergic reaction?

   A. Amides

   B. Esters

   C. Both A and B

   D. None of the above

6. Which is the site of drug action?

   A. Neurotransmitter

   B. Blood-brain barrier

   C. Synapse

   D. Neural tube

7. Which part of the autonomic nervous system controls the body's fight-or-flight response?

   A. Sympathetic

   B. Parasympathetic

   C. MAO

   D. SSRI

8. Which part of the autonomic nervous system controls the body's rest and relaxation responses?

   A. Sympathetic

   B. Parasympathetic

   C. MAO

   D. SSRI

9. Which of the following is a side effect of cholinergic drugs?

A. Increased heart rate

B. Hypertension

C. Decreased heart rate

D. Decreased salivation

10. Which is NOT a side effect of tricyclic lithium?

A. GI distress

B. Hypotension

C. Polyuria

D. Hyperglycemia

Application Exercises

Respond to the following situations.

1. Harry is taking an MAOI. He is very skeptical about the food interactions that occur with this drug and indicates that he will not be following the recommended diet. What would

   you do? _____

   _____

   _____

2. Sandy is taking an SSRI, but at a lower dose than her sister. She wants to know why the same dose is not used and whether she should take as much as her sister. What would you

   tell her? _____

   _____

   _____

3. Harold is in the office with his wife. She is diagnosed with Alzheimer's disease, and he is wondering when the prescribed medications will begin to reverse her symptoms. What

   education would you provide for this couple? _____

   _____

   _____

4. Sheldon has been taking medication for Parkinson's disease for 2 years. The doctor has prescribed a drug holiday for him, and he is very upset because he feels he needs these medications to function. Explain to him why it will help him to take a break from his

   medicine for a little while. _____

   _____

   _____

Essentials Review

For further study and practice with drug classifications learned in this chapter, complete the following table to the best of your ability. Use resources such as the *PDR,* the Internet, or printed drug guides for help.

Example	Generic Name	Classification	Purpose	Side Effects	Contraindications and Precautions	Examples	Patient Education
Pilopine							
Motrin							
Morphine							
Eldepryl							
Thorazine							

Internet Research

1. Search the Internet to find the following, and write a paragraph on each and turn in for credit:

   ▪ The latest research on new medications to treat Alzheimer's disease.

   ▪ Local support groups for families and patients with Alzheimer's disease.

   ▪ The latest research on new medications to treat Parkinson's disease.

   ▪ Local support groups for families and patients with Parkinson's disease.

2. The following is a list of phobias (fears). Use a medical dictionary or Internet research site to define them on a separate sheet.

   ▪ Acrophobia   ▪ Claustrophobia

   ▪ Agoraphobia   ▪ Mysophobia

   ▪ Ailurophobia   ▪ Xenophobia

   ▪ Arachnophobia   ▪ Zoophobia

14

Eye and Ear Medications

*T*he eyes and ears gather sensory data from the environment and send it to the brain. When any of these organs do not work properly, information may be blocked or distorted, leading to pain, anxiety, and the inability to react properly to the environment. For example, someone who has poor eyesight may fall because he or she cannot clearly see stairs. Patients should be encouraged to be alert to changes in their vision and hearing. They should also have a thorough assessment of these organs regularly because some diseases, such as glaucoma, can be symptom free until quite advanced. Early detection and treatment may save the individual's eyesight or hearing for many years to come. Fortunately, several medications are available for conditions of the eyes and ears. These medications must be given carefully to have optimal effect.

LEARNING OUTCOMES

At the end of this chapter, you should be able to:

14.1 Define all key terms.
14.2 List five parts of the eye and the function of each structure.
14.3 Recall three conditions related to the eye that require treatment with medication and an example of an appropriate medication.
14.4 Classify parts of the ear as belonging to the external ear, middle ear, or inner ear, and discuss the function of each part.
14.5 Recall three conditions related to the ear that require treatment with medication and an example of an appropriate medication.

KEY TERMS

Aqueous humor	Ototoxicity	Tonometer
Cerumen	Schlemm canal	Vertigo
Intraocular pressure (IOP)	Tinnitus	Vitreous humor

THE EYE

It is important to review the anatomy of the eye (Fig. 14-1). The eyes are protected by their placement in the orbits of the skull. Eyelids, eyelashes, and eyebrows protect the eye from irritants and infectious microbes. A hard sclera protects the outer eye. The sclera contains a layer called the choroid, which consists of a network of blood vessels that nourish the majority of the eye with oxygen and nutrients. The iris regulates the amount of light that enters the eye by dilating and constricting the pupil. The pupil is basically a hole in the iris. The outer eye is bathed with tears. The anterior chamber contains a watery **aqueous humor** (fluid). The clear structure that covers the iris, the pupil, and the anterior chamber is the cornea. The cornea is provided with oxygen and nutrients through tears, not blood vessels; thus, it is clear. The dark cavern of the posterior chamber contains a viscous (thick) **vitreous humor.**

Images are projected through the pupil and lens onto the rods (black and white) and cones (color) of the retina. The retina is the light-sensitive tissue located at the back of the eyeball. The inverted images are then sent to the brain via the optic nerve for interpretation.

EYE MEDICATIONS

The eye is vulnerable to several disorders, irritations, and infections, such as glaucoma, conjunctivitis, macular degeneration, keratitis, chalazion, and cataracts, all of which require medication as part of

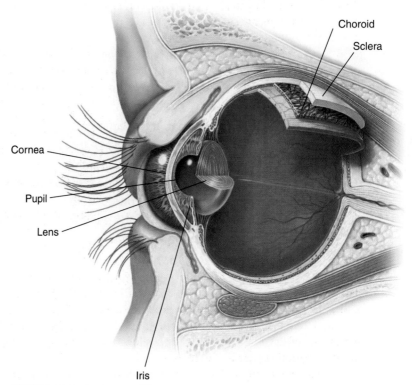

FIGURE 14-1: Anatomy of the eye.

a treatment plan. Some medications, such as atropine, are also used to facilitate eye examinations (see the Master the Essentials table for descriptions of the most common medications for disorders of the eye).

A CLOSER LOOK: Eye Health

Good eye health requires that patients have their eyes assessed annually. Family practitioners should encourage their patients, particularly older patients, to see an ophthalmologist or optometrist annually. These specialists use a **tonometer** to measure pressure in the eye. If pressure builds in the eye, it is usually because the aqueous humor is not flowing out of the eye correctly. This causes intraocular pressure (IOP) to increase. Pressure on the optic nerve eventually can lead to blindness.

Medications for Glaucoma

Glaucoma is a leading cause of blindness. In this disease, an increase in pressure in the eye damages the optic nerve and thus impairs its ability to transmit visual information from the eye to the brain. Glaucoma is actually a group of diseases. Primary open-angle glaucoma, the most common form, occurs when the eye's **Schlemm canal** (drainage tube for aqueous humor) becomes obstructed, thus leading to a gradual increase in pressure. This disease traditionally has no symptoms, and if not diagnosed, it can cause loss of vision. Primary open-angle glaucoma is routinely treated effectively with medications, especially when it is diagnosed early.

Another type of glaucoma is angle-closure, also known as acute or narrow-angle, glaucoma. This type is rarer, and it differs from open-angle glaucoma in that eye pressure usually increases very rapidly. Angle-closure glaucoma occurs when drainage is obstructed, but at a different place in the eye. The iris is usually too small, and it covers up the drainage canals. Symptoms of this type of glaucoma include headache, eye pain, nausea, multicolored halos around lights at night, and blurred vision. Angle-closure must be corrected surgically.

A third type of glaucoma is called normal-tension glaucoma. As the name implies, the optic nerve is damaged even though the pressure in the eye is not elevated enough to indicate this likelihood. The patient has no symptoms, and diagnosis is made only by examining the optic nerve for damage. Because the cause of this type of glaucoma is still a mystery to physicians, treatment consists of lowering the pressure in the eye as much as possible through medications or surgery.

A few other types of glaucoma fall into an "other" category. These include congenital glaucoma, in which an infant is diagnosed early with increased pressure resulting from a hereditary congenital malformation or abnormal fetal development. Secondary glaucoma is secondary to another disease that causes or contributes to increased eye pressure or is a result of injury or certain medications. Some medications, such as glucocorticoids, antihypertensives, antihistamines, and antidepressants, can predispose a patient to increased **intraocular pressure (IOP)** because of a decrease in aqueous humor flow in the eye. In many cases, this is temporary and subsides with discontinuation of the medication. In a few rare instances, it is permanent. Pigmentary glaucoma results when the pigment granules giving the eye its color break off and lodge in the drainage system.

Miotic and prostaglandin medications treat glaucoma by increasing the flow of aqueous humor. Miotics include drugs such as pilocarpine HCl (Isopto Carpine, Pilocarpine HCl Ophthalmic Solution USP), carbachol (Isopto Carbachol), and pilocarpine HCl gel 4% (Pilopine HS Gel). They also constrict the pupil. Some of these drugs activate cholinergic receptors, which decrease the IOP. They dilate the meshwork of the Schlemm canals, and allow increased output of aqueous humor. As more aqueous humor is absorbed, the IOP decreases.

Prostaglandins such as bimatoprost (Lumigan), latanoprost (Xalatan), and travoprost (Travatan Z) do not affect pupil diameter but rather dilate the meshwork in the anterior chambers of the Schlemm canals. However, one side effect of prostaglandins is that they change the pigmentation of the iris and thus the color of the eye.

Other medications decrease IOP by reducing the flow of aqueous humor. These agents include alpha and beta blockers, carbonic anhydrase inhibitors, and osmotic diuretics.

■ *Alpha blockers.* Alpha blockers such as apraclonidine HCl (Iopidine) and brimonidine tartrate (Alphagan P) dilate blood vessels in the eye and have a mild effect on the cardiovascular and respiratory systems. They treat glaucoma by decreasing the production of and increasing the drainage of aqueous humor.

■ *Beta blockers.* Beta blockers such as betaxolol HCl (Betoptic S) and timolol maleate (Istalol) also work by decreasing the production of intraocular fluid. In low dosages, beta blockers affect the eye but do not have a systemic effect. If they do enter the cardiovascular system, these drugs can constrict the bronchi, slow the heart rate, and cause hypotension. These systemic effects can be minimized by closing the eyes following application to prevent the drops from entering the tear drainage duct.

■ *Carbonic anhydrase inhibitors.* Medications such as acetazolamide (Diamox and Sequels) decrease IOP by reducing the production of intraocular fluid. They can be administered topically or systemically, although systemic use is reserved for patients who do not respond to the topical medications.

■ *Osmotic diuretics.* This class of medications, which include glycerin (Osmoglyn, Ophthalgan Solution), are used for eye surgery to decrease the amount of aqueous humor rapidly.

Although the cause is not clear, glaucoma is more prevalent among patients with hypertension, diabetes, migraines, nearsightedness, farsightedness, and patients of advanced age.

Medications for Eye Irritations and Infections

Minor eye injury and irritation can be treated with local anesthetics, antimicrobials, nonsteroidal anti-inflammatory drugs (NSAIDs), and glucocorticoids. The local anesthetics include tetracaine (Pontocaine 0.5% solution) and proparacaine (Ophthaine, Ophthetic 0.5% solution). The antimicrobials typically used are gentamicin, tobramycin, and erythromycin. The NSAIDs are ketorolac tromethamine 0.5% solution (Acular) and nepafenac 0.1% suspension (Nevanac). The glucocorticoids include dexamethasone (Maxidex suspension, Decadron solution and ointment) and hydrocortisone acetate (Hydrocortone). All of these medications can be administered as drops or salves or by injection. For milder irritations and injuries, the medications, such as eye lubricants, simply soothe the outer eye. For more serious irritations and injuries such as keratitis (an inflammation of the cornea caused by irritation or microbial infection), the medications must penetrate beyond the surface. Ophthalmic glucocorticoids should not be used for long-term treatment because they can suppress the immune response.

Anti-infectives are used for eye infections. Similar to infections elsewhere in the body, eye infections must be treated swiftly and completely. One of the most common infections of the eye is conjunctivitis (pinkeye), and it is treated with an antibiotic such as gentamicin ophthalmic ointment. Eye infections can spread to other parts of the body, especially if patients rub their eyes with their fingers and then touch another part of the body. Meticulous hand washing is important, and patients should be advised to not rub the infected eye. Another common eye infection is a stye. A stye is a bacterial infection in an oil gland in the eyelid that causes a painful red bump. Persistent or multiple styes are usually treated with topical ophthalmic antibiotics or oral antibiotics such as doxycycline (Vibramycin, Oracea, Adoxa).

 CRITICAL THINKING

How would you instruct the patient to administer eye medications to prevent the spread of infection?

Medications for Eye Examinations

Some drugs are used to make it easier for a health-care professional to examine the eyes. Cycloplegic mydriatics, for example, relax ciliary muscles and dilate the pupils so the examiner can peer into the eye.

Local ophthalmic anesthetic agents are used for removing foreign objects. The blink reflex is impaired, so it is important to inform the patient to wear darkened glasses when going outside until the effect of the medication wears off.

Staining agents are nontoxic, water-soluble dyes used to diagnose corneal epithelial defects caused by infection or injury. They can also be used to find foreign bodies or contact lenses in the eye. The stain colors the object green.

Miscellaneous Eye Medications

Immunomodulators such as Restasis work to treat a certain type of chronic dry eye by increasing tear production. The patient must understand that it will take time before the effects of this drug are felt and up to 6 months for maximum benefit. The liquid portion of the medication is castor oil, which provides some immediate moisturizing benefit. See Drug Spotlight 14.1 for a new medication (Xiidra) used to treat chronic dry eye.

Macular degeneration progression may be slowed with the used of ranibizumab (Lucentis) or aflibercept (Eylea). These medications are injected into the affected eye approximately once a month.

■ THE EAR

To understand ear disorders, you must understand the anatomy of the ear, which is divided into the outer, middle, and inner ear (Fig. 14-2). The outer ear consists of the pinna, which is the visible part of the ear, and the external auditory canal. The pinna protects the middle and inner ear, and it also collects sound and funnels it through the external auditory canal. The external auditory canal contains glands that secrete **cerumen** (earwax). The purpose of this wax is to protect the inner ear from damage and infections. Thus, a lack of wax can lead to an increased risk for ear infections. Too much earwax can cause a blockage leading to loss of hearing.

The middle ear is separated from the outer ear by the tympanic membrane (eardrum), and it includes the auditory ossicles (malleus, incus, stapes), the middle ear cavity (hollow area containing ossicles), and the eustachian tube. Once sound waves hit the tympanic membrane, three flexible bones called the ossicles convert that sound into mechanical vibrations. The eustachian tube connects the ear and the throat and functions to equalize pressure on both sides of the tympanic membrane.

The inner ear includes the oval window, round window, cochlea, and semicircular canals. The oval window is located directly behind the stapes and vibrates when that bone strikes it. This sets in motion the fluid-filled tubes, which generate nerve impulses that travel to the brain. The round window serves

Drug Spotlight 14-1 *Xiidra (lifitegrast ophthalmic)*

Classification	Artificial tears/Ocular lubricant
Availability	Ophthalmic solution
Indications	Used to treat symptoms of dry eye disease.
Dosage/Implementation	One drop in each eye every 12 hours.
Adverse Reactions/ Side Effects	Changes in vision, eye irritation or discomfort, blurred vision, redness of the white part of sclera.
Contraindications/ Precautions	No contraindications, use cautiously in elderly, pregnancy/lactation, and children younger than 17 years of age as there are insufficient studies at this time in these populations.

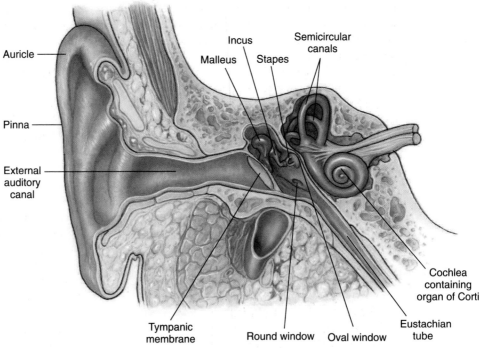

FIGURE 14-2: Anatomy of the ear.

as a pressure relief valve, bulging outward as pressure rises. The inner ear consists of fluid-filled tubes containing the actual hearing cells of the body. The front portion contains the following: the cochlea, which helps with hearing; the semicircular cells, which help maintain balance; and the vestibule, which also is responsible for balance. Thus, hearing and equilibrium are very closely intertwined in the anatomy of the ear.

■ EAR MEDICATIONS

Otic, or ear, medications can be used to treat inflammation, wax buildup, or infections. The most common disorders requiring ear medications are infections (Fast Tip 14.1). Other common conditions requiring medication are impaction of cerumen and motion sickness. See the Master the Essentials table for descriptions of the most common medications for disorders of the ear.

Medications for Ear Infections and Pain
Several types of medication are used to treat infections depending on their location. Swimmer's ear (otitis externa) is an infection of the outer ear, and otitis media is a middle ear infection. Antibiotics

---

● *Fast Tip 14.1*

Otic medications are usually deposited in the outer ear, or pinna, from where they flow through the auditory canal toward the eardrum. If the eardrum is intact, it provides a barrier that prevents infection from entering the inner ear. Otic medications are sterile so that if the eardrum is ruptured they will not transmit bacteria beyond the eardrum; however certain medications may be harmful, such as those used to loosen cerumen as they contain caustic ingredients. If you or the patient suspect a rupture, discuss this with the physician before instilling any otic medication.

such as acetic acid and aluminum acetate otic (Domeboro Otic), ofloxacin otic (Floxin), and acetic acid (Vosol) can be administered directly into the ear to fight infections. In the case of swimmer's ear, they may be combined with a glucocorticoid to reduce associated inflammation. Examples of these combination drops are as follows: ciprofloxacin and dexamethasone otic (Ciprodex); hydrocortisone, neomycin, and polymyxin B otic (Cortisporin); and hydrocortisone and acetic acid (Vosol HC). Systemic antibiotics, such as amoxicillin (Amoxil, Trimox), amoxicillin and clavulanate potassium (Augmentin), sulfamethoxazole and trimethoprim (Bactrim, Septra), cefaclor (Ceclor), and erythromycin and sulfisoxazole (Pediazole), are needed for middle or inner ear infections.

Pain medications such as antipyrine and benzocaine (A/B otic, Aurodex, and Auroguard) may also be prescribed for the pain that accompanies trauma or infection.

Medications for Cerumen and Motion Disorders

As discussed earlier, cerumen is a normal product of a healthy ear. Mineral oil, earwax softeners (cerumenolytics), and hydrogen peroxide can be used to decrease the amount of earwax if problems are occurring. Although earwax can protect the ear from infection, a buildup of earwax can decrease hearing, cause pain, and sometimes trap and promote growth of bacteria.

In addition to hearing, the ear is also responsible for balance. Motion sickness is caused by the ear's inability to determine the body's position relative to its motion. It can be treated with tablets or transdermal patches that are placed behind the ear. Medications such as Dramamine or Bonine should be taken 20 to 60 minutes before travel.

Drugs such as meclizine (Antivert), which is an anticholinergic, are given for dizziness, or **vertigo,** and the nausea that sometimes accompanies it.

■ MEDICATIONS AND OTOTOXICITY

As discussed in Chapter 2, many drugs can cause **ototoxicity** (damage to ears). Commonly, this occurs with certain antibiotics such as gentamicin. Symptoms of ear damage include **tinnitus** (ringing in the ears), hearing loss, and severe headache, ataxia, and balance disturbances.

 CRITICAL THINKING

A patient is taking Abreva, Ecotrin (aspirin), Xanax, and a multivitamin. What is the first medication you should suspect when the patient complains of tinnitus?

●●● SUMMARY

■ The eyes and ears provide critical sensory information to the brain.

■ The eye is made up of many interconnected structures working together to provide clear vision.

■ Conditions, disease, infections, and other irritants can disrupt sensory communication and cause pain and discomfort not only at the source but also systemically.

■ Glaucoma is a term for a group of diseases that cause increased pressure in the eye that, if untreated, will lead to blindness.

■ The basis of treatment for all types of glaucoma is the reduction of aqueous humor in the eye to decrease intraocular pressure (IOP).

■ Medications to reduce IOP include miotics, prostaglandins, alpha and beta blockers, carbonic anhydrase inhibitors, and osmotic diuretics.

■ Eye infections such as conjunctivitis and styes vary from minor to serious and must be treated with appropriate antibiotics.

■ The ear is made up of three major parts: the outer, inner, and middle ear. These parts work together to provide hearing and balance.

■ Otic medications include antibiotics, glucocorticoids, antivertigo drugs, cerumenolytics, and pain medications.

Master the Essentials: Eye and Ear Medications

This table shows the various classes of eye and ear medications, the key side effects, contraindications, precautions, interactions, and examples of each class.

Class	Indications for Use	Side Effects	Contraindications and Precautions	Interactions	Examples
Ophthalmic alpha blockers	Treatment of eye irritation	Hypertension, somnolence, oral dryness, ocular hyperemia, eye burning or stinging	Hypersensitivity	MAOIs, tricyclic antidepressants, beta blockers, antihypertensives, digoxin	Apraclonidine HCl (Iopidine), brimonidine tartrate (Alphagan P), dipivefrin (Propine), epinephrine (Epifrin, Glaucon)
Ophthalmic beta blockers	Treatment of open-angle glaucoma	Headache, depression, arrhythmia, syncope, nausea, keratitis, visual disturbances, bronchospasm	Bronchial asthma, COPD, sinus bradycardia, AV block, heart failure, hypersensitivity	Oral beta blockers calcium antagonists, digoxin, quinidine, phenothiazines	Betaxolol (Betoptic S), levobunolol HCl (Betagan), metipranolol (OptiPranolol), timolol hemihydrate (Betimol), timolol maleate (Timolol Maleate USP, Istalol), timolol maleate ophthalmic gel (Timoptic-XE)
Carbonic anhydrase inhibitors	Treatment of glaucoma	Ocular burning or sting, blurred vision, bitter taste	Hypersensitivity	Salicylates, amphetamines, quinidine, methamine	Acetazolamide (Diamox, Sequels), brinzolamide ophthalmic suspension (Azopt), dorzolamide HCl (Trusopt)
Cycloplegic mydriatics	Dilation of pupil in inflammatory conditions or for diagnostic or surgical procedures	Increased IOP, transient burning/ stinging, blurred vision, dry mouth, dry skin	Hypersensitivity, children with history of reaction to atropine, pregnancy	None reported	Pilocarpine (Isopto Carpine Solution), homatropine (Isopto Homatropine Solution 2%–5%), scopolamine (Scopace)
Immunomodulators	Used to increase tear production	Burning, itching, discharge, red eyes, blurred vision, overflow of tears	Active infections, hypersensitivity, contacts	None reported	Cyclosporine (Restasis 0.05% emulsion)
Miotics	Treatment of glaucoma	Corneal edema, clouding, stinging, burning, tearing, headache	Hypersensitivity, any condition in which pupillary constriction is undesirable	Topical NSAIDs	Carbachol (Isopto Carbachol), pilocarpine HCl (Isopto Carpine, Pilocarpine HCl

Master the Essentials: Eye and Ear Medications—cont'd

Class	Indications for Use	Side Effects	Contraindications and Precautions	Interactions	Examples
					Ophthalmic Solution USP), pilocarpine HCl gel (Pilopine HS Gel)
Ophthalmic antibiotics	Infection	Burning sensation in the eyes, conjunctivitis, hypersensitivity reactions, rash, urticaria	Allergy, fungal or viral diseases in the eye	Corticosteroids	Gentamicin ophthalmic (Garamycin ophthalmic, Genoptic, Gentasol), tobramycin (Tobrex, Tobralcon), ciprofloxacin (Ciloxan), azithromycin (AzaSite), erythromycin (Eyemycin, Ilotycin, Romycin), bacitracin/polymyxin B (Ocumycin, Polycin-B, Polysporin ophthalmic), neomycin/polymyxin B
Ophthalmic corticosteroids	Inflammation and pain resulting from injury or surgery	If used for prolonged period: immunosuppression	Immunosuppression, purulent drainage from infection	None reported	Dexamethasone (AK-Dex, Ocu-Dex), prednisolone ophthalmic (Econopred Plus, Omnipred, Pred Forte, Prednisol)
Ophthalmic local anesthetics	Anesthetic before surgery	Stinging, burning	Hypersensitivity, prolonged use	None reported	Tetracaine (Altacaine, Opticaine), proparacaine (Alcaine, Ophthetic)
Ophthalmic anti-inflammatories	Inflammation and pain in eye, chronic dry eye	Burning, stinging, irritation, corneal edema, risk for increased bleeding	Diabetes mellitus, children, infections, pregnancy, hypersensitivity, bleeding disorders	None reported	Diclofenac 0.1 % solution (Cambia, Voltaren), ketorolac tromethamine 0.5% solution (Acular), nepafenac 0.1% suspension (Nevanac), lifitegrast ophthalmic (Xiidra)

Continued

Master the Essentials: Eye and Ear Medications—cont'd

Class	Indications for Use	Side Effects	Contraindications and Precautions	Interactions	Examples
Osmotic diuretics	Treatment of glaucoma; decreases intra-ocular pressure	Dizziness, dry mouth, fluid and electrolyte imbalances, headache, tremors, nausea, vomiting, disorientation, confusion	Anuria, dehydration, pulmonary edema, hypersensitivity	Amphetamines, quinidine	Glycerin (Osmoglyn, Ophthalgan Solution)
Ophthalmic prostaglandin agonists	Treatment of open-angle glaucoma and ocular hypertension	Ocular hyperemia, decreased visual acuity, eye discomfort	Hypersensitivity, pregnancy	None reported	Bimatoprost (Lumigan), latanoprost (Xalatan Solution), travoprost (Travatan Z)
Antivertigo agents	Prevention and treatment of motion sickness	Blurred vision, confusion, extrapyramidal symptoms, restlessness, sedation, hypotension, rash, dry mouth	Benign prostatic hypertrophy, children, glaucoma, hypertension, lactation, pregnancy, seizures, hypersensitivity	Alcohol, CNS depressants, muscle relaxants	Meclizine (Anti-Vert, Bonine), diphenhydramine (Benadryl), dimenhydrinate (Dramamine), scopolamine (Transderm-Scōp Transdermal Patch)
Otic antibiotics	Treatment of ear infection	Irritation in the ear	Hypersensitivity, eardrum rupture, breastfeeding, pregnancy	Other ear drops	Acetic acid and aluminum acetate otic (Domeboro Otic), ofloxacin otic (Floxin), acetic acid (Vosol)
Otic combination drugs	Treatment of ear infection with inflammation	Unusual taste in the mouth	Hypersensitivity to antibiotics or steroids, eardrum rupture, pregnancy, breastfeeding	Other ear drops	Ciprofloxacin and dexamethasone otic (Ciprodex), hydrocortisone, neomycin and polymyxin B otic (Vosol HCl)
Cerumenolytics	Softening of earwax (cerumen)	None	Hypersensitivity, ear drainage or discharge, recent ear injury, surgery, dizziness, ruptured eardrum	None reported	Carbamide peroxide solution (Auro, Debrox)

AV, atrioventricular; CNS, central nervous system; COPD, chronic obstructive pulmonary disease; MAOI, monoamine oxidase inhibitor; NSAID, nonsteroidal anti-inflammatory drug.

Activities

To make sure that you have learned the key points covered in this chapter, complete the following activities.

True or False

Write true if the statement is true. Beside the false statements, write false, and correct the statement to make it true.

1. Half-angle is a type of glaucoma. _____

_____

2. Pinkeye is an injury occurring from surgery. _____

_____

3. Aqueous humor is located behind the eardrum. _____

_____

4. The Schlemm canal is located in the eye. _____

_____

5. Mydriatics are used to examine the inner eye. _____

_____

6. The stapes is located in the inner ear. _____

_____

7. Cerumen is another name for earwax. _____

_____

8. Glaucoma can occur suddenly or gradually over time. _____

_____

9. IOP stands for in other places. _____

_____

10. The pinna functions by funneling sound through the outer ear canal._____

_____

Multiple Choice

Choose the best answer for each question.

1. Which physician is an ear specialist?
   A. Audiologist
   B. Ophthalmologist
   C. Optician
   D. Dermatologist

2. **Which of the following are used to treat edema in the eye?**
   A. Cerumenolytics
   B. Glucocorticoids
   C. Mydriatics
   D. Miotics

3. **Which drug is used to treat glaucoma?**
   A. Cerumenolytics
   B. Glucocorticoids
   C. Mydriatics
   D. Miotics

4. **What class of drugs is used to treat pinkeye?**
   A. Miotics
   B. Antibiotics
   C. Diuretics
   D. Corticosteroids

5. **Scopolamine is given via which route?**
   A. Oral
   B. Injection
   C. Transdermal
   D. Rectal

6. **A stye is caused by _____.**
   A. Bacteria
   B. Fungus
   C. Parasite
   D. Virus

7. **The part of the eye covering the outer eye is called the _____.**
   A. Iris
   B. Cornea
   C. Eyelid
   D. Sclera

8. **Signs of ototoxicity include _____.**
   A. Tinnitus
   B. Severe headache
   C. Ataxia
   D. All of the above

9. The category of ophthalmic medication that may alter the color of the iris and change the patient's eye color is called _____.

   A. Glucocorticoids

   B. Prostaglandins

   C. Antibiotics

   D. Beta blockers

10. Oral motion sickness medication should be taken _____.

   A. 1 hour before travel

   B. 1 day before travel

   C. 20 to 60 minutes before travel

   D. At the time of travel

Application Exercises

Respond to the following situations.

1. Barry is having eye surgery for cataract removal next week. He is worried about postoperative pain management. How do you counsel him? _____

   _____

   _____

2. Adam is using corticosteroid eye drops and calls to inform you that he has new yellow discharge draining from his eyes. Should he continue the eye drops? What would you tell him and why? _____

   _____

   _____

3. Bruce was prescribed gentamicin for an infection. He calls your office and complains of tinnitus and ataxia. What is your response? _____

   _____

   _____

Essentials Review

For further study and practice with drug classifications learned in this chapter, complete the following table to the best of your ability. Use resources such as the *PDR,* the Internet, or printed drug guides for help.

Example	Generic Name	Classification	Purpose	Side Effects	Contraindications and Precautions	Examples	Patient Education
Transdermal Scopolamine							
Oxymetazoline							
Levobunolol							
Pilocarpine							
Glycerin							

15

Endocrine System Medications

*T*he endocrine system controls many of the body's functions; there-fore, disorders affecting this system can have profound implications for the health of the patient. The endocrine system helps the body maintain homeostasis by transferring messages in the form of hor-mones between systems and organs to keep both working efficiently. Extremely high or extremely low hormone levels can cause various illnesses, so it is important to be aware of the various types of hor-mones and their functions. The endocrine system also helps the body use energy, regulates temperature when the body sleeps, and assists the reproductive organs by allowing the right amount of hormones to be excreted for reproduction. Medications are most frequently used to suppress or replace hormones normally produced by the endocrine glands.

LEARNING OUTCOMES

At the end of this chapter, you should be able to:

15.1 Define all key terms.
15.2 Discuss six of the major endocrine glands and their functions.
15.3 Differentiate between hypothyroidism and hyperthyroidism, and identify the effects of each on the body and the medications used to treat each disorder.
15.4 Contrast hyperglycemia and hypoglycemia, and discuss the medications used to treat each one.
15.5 Explain the proper way to handle, store, and administer insulin.
15.6 Differentiate between adrenal gland insufficiency and oversecretion, and discuss the medications used to treat each one.

KEY TERMS

Addison's disease
Adrenocorticotropic
  hormone (ACTH)
Antidiuretic hormone
  (ADH)
Calcitonin
Cretinism
Cushing's disease
Diabetes mellitus
Goiter
Graves' disease

Hormone replacement
  therapy (HRT)
Hyperglycemia
Hypoglycemia
Insulin-dependent diabetes
  mellitus (IDDM)
Ketoacidosis
Melatonin
Myxedema
Negative feedback
  system

Non–insulin-dependent
  diabetes mellitus
  (NIDDM)
Parathormone
Thyroid-stimulating
  hormone (TSH)
Thyroid storm
Thyroxine (T_4)
Triiodothyronine (T_3)

■ THE ENDOCRINE SYSTEM

The endocrine system uses chemicals known as hormones, acting as messengers to various parts of the body, to trigger a reaction. Several components make up this system (Fig. 15-1), which is controlled by the hypothalamus. The hypothalamus gland, located in the brain, secretes chemicals called releasing factors that trigger the release of several hormones from the pituitary gland. The pituitary gland, also located in the brain, is known as the master gland because it secretes most of the body's hormones. The pituitary gland secretes follicle-stimulating hormone (FSH) and luteinizing hormone (LH), which are important to female reproduction, and **antidiuretic hormone (ADH),** which helps prevent loss of water by the kidneys. In addition, the pituitary gland secretes **thyroid-stimulating hormone (TSH),** which triggers thyroid gland function. Table 15-1 and Figure 15-2 provide a more in-depth look at all the hormones secreted by the pituitary gland. The hypothalamus is the body's coordinator—it tells the pituitary gland which hormones to send out to the body. When a hormone level becomes too high, the body tells the hypothalamus, which, in turn, tells the pituitary gland to stop producing the hormone. This is called a **negative feedback system.**

The gonads (sex organs) consist of the ovaries in females and the testes in males. These glands are responsible for secreting hormones in response to those released by the pituitary gland. The ovaries produce and release both estrogen and progesterone, and the testes produce and release androgens, which include testosterone. Chapter 20 covers the medications used to treat reproductive disorders.

The thyroid gland, which is located in the neck surrounding the esophagus, regulates metabolism, including temperature and body weight. The thyroid gland also regulates blood and bone calcium by secreting calcitonin. **Calcitonin** helps force calcium ions into bone. If the patient has insufficient calcitonin, the blood calcium level remains high and the bone calcium level remains low, thus leading to bone fractures. Replacement hormones help with both energy and calcium storage, but the prescriber may order only calcium supplements.

The four parathyroid glands are located on the surface of the thyroid gland and are responsible for the concentration of sodium and calcium in the blood and urine. The parathyroid glands, which are embedded in the thyroid gland, also help regulate calcium balance. They counter calcitonin with **parathormone,** which pulls calcium out of the bones into the bloodstream.

The pancreas, located in the abdominal cavity, has two major functions. First, it secretes digestive enzymes into the small intestine and thereby allows what we eat to be digested and used. The second function of the pancreas is achieved by secreting two hormones: insulin, which decreases blood glucose by moving it into the tissue, where it can be used; and glucagon, which increases blood glucose. The liver helps the pancreas determine blood glucose levels, so the liver and pancreas must be functioning properly to control blood glucose.

The adrenal glands are located above the kidneys. These glands are made up of the inner (adrenal medulla) and outer (adrenal cortex) portions. The secretion of **adrenocorticotropic hormone (ACTH)**

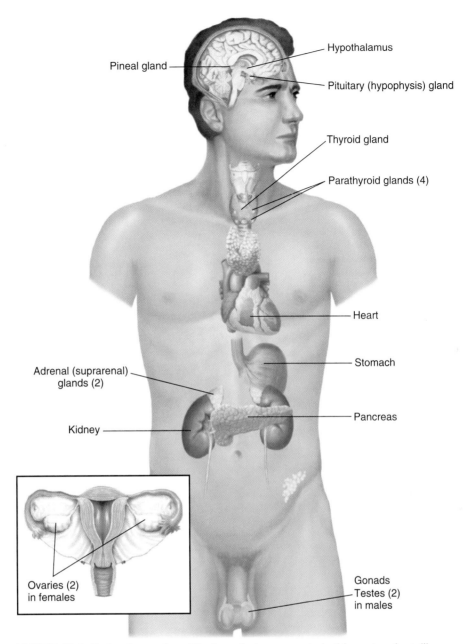

FIGURE 15-1: Endocrine system. The hypothalamus controls this system by telling the pituitary gland which hormones to secrete. Hormones have a wide range of effects on body organs, including the thyroid gland, pancreas, adrenal glands, and reproductive organs (testes and ovaries).

by the pituitary gland stimulates the adrenal medulla to release epinephrine and the adrenal cortex to release glucocorticoids.

Epinephrine, more commonly known as adrenaline, controls the fight-or-flight response, the physiological reaction to a perceived threat to survival or fright and other situations such as stress and anger. The epinephrine increases the body's heart rate; improves blood flow to major organs, skeletal muscles, and the brain; dilates airways to the lungs, and increases blood sugar. The adrenal medulla also secretes noradrenaline (norepinephrine) to constrict blood vessels, which increases blood pressure. These physical changes all help the body to exert maximum effort to meet or flee the situation.

The adrenal cortex secretes the glucocorticoids cortisol, cortisone, and corticosterone, which helps to regulate metabolism, provide resistance to stress, maintain blood pressure and cardiovascular

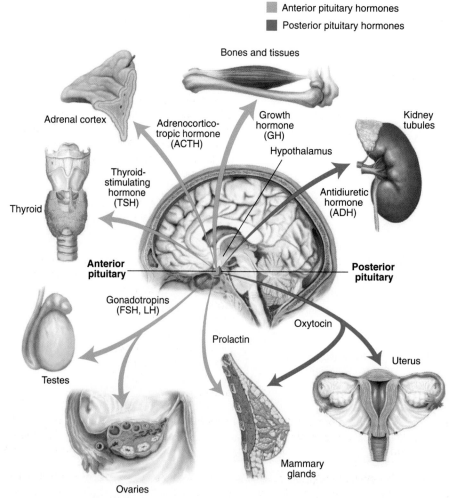

FIGURE 15-2: Pituitary hormones and target glands.

TABLE 15.1 Hormones Secreted by the Pituitary Gland

Hormone	Target Organs and Effect	Overproduction Causes...	Underproduction Causes...
Front or Anterior Pituitary Gland			
Adrenocorticotropic hormone (ACTH)	Regulates the release of epinephrine and glucocorticoids from the adrenal glands, which determines fight-or-flight responses of the autonomic nervous system	Cushing's disease	Addison's disease
Thyroid-stimulating hormone (TSH)	Regulates the release of hormones in the thyroid gland, which affects energy	Graves' disease	Myxedema in adults, cretinism in children

TABLE 15.1   Hormones Secreted by the Pituitary Gland—cont'd

Hormone	Target Organs and Effect	Overproduction Causes...	Underproduction Causes...
Front or Anterior Pituitary Gland			

Somatotropin, or growth hormone (GH)	Regulates the growth of bone, muscles, and other tissues by affecting the liver and adipose tissue	Gigantism (abnormally tall stature; patient becomes a "giant")
		    Acromegaly (growth of hands and feet after puberty when growth is supposed to stop)
		    Treatment of acromegaly: medications that suppress growth hormones
			Dwarfism (abnormally short stature)
			    Treatment: growth hormone

Prolactin	Stimulates milk production in the mammary gland	Overproduction of breast milk in women
		    Milk production in a nonlactating patient can be a sign of a pituitary tumor
		    Parlodel is used to suppress lactation in women who choose not to breast-feed, but a side effect is increased fertility
			Underproduction of milk in women; baby has difficulty nursing

Follicle-stimulating hormone (FSH)	Stimulates sperm production in men and egg production in women	Increased fertility	Men: sterility Women: irregular or absent menses
Luteinizing hormone (LH)	Stimulates the release of a ripened egg in women (ovulation); also helps in the production of female hormones (**estrogens** and **progestins**)	Multiple gestations (e.g., twins, triplets)	Infertility (woman cannot ovulate and therefore cannot conceive)
Interstitial cell–stimulating hormone (ICSH)	Stimulates the production of androgens (the male hormone testosterone)	Aggressiveness, excess hair	Feminine attributes in men (e.g., high voice, small muscles)
Back or Posterior Pituitary Gland			

Antidiuretic hormone (ADH)	Conserves fluids by changing the permeability of the kidneys	Syndrome of inappropriate antidiuretic hormone (SIADH): too much fluid is retained
		    Treatment: diuretics
			Diabetes insipidus; too much fluid is excreted by the kidneys, with resulting dehydration
			    Treatment: desmopressin (DDAVP)*

Oxytocin	Contracts the uterus and milk ducts in the breasts; contracts the prostate gland in men	The uterus or prostate can contract so much that it ruptures (rarely)	Labor may be slowed or milk expulsion constricted Treatment: Pitocin (oxytocin in synthetic form) may be given intramuscularly or intravenously to the laboring or postpartum patient to increase the force of contractions

*DDAVP is also used to help chronic bedwetters stop urinating at night and to stop bleeding in patients with hemophilia.

function, slow the immune response of the body, and maintain steady glucose levels. Ninety-five percent of the glucocorticoids are cortisone.

The pineal gland, which is in the brain, secretes **melatonin** in response to input from the eyes. The more light that enters, the less melatonin is released. Melatonin is what helps us to sleep; thus, in the darker hours of night and winter, we tend to feel sleepier. When the pineal gland fails, sleep is impaired, and melatonin or barbiturates (see Chapter 13) may be prescribed to correct this disorder. See the Master the Essentials table for descriptions of the most common endocrine system drug classifications.

■ ENDOCRINE SYSTEM MEDICATIONS

Medications used to treat disorders of the endocrine system can be separated into three categories: medications for thyroid and parathyroid disorders, medications for pancreatic disorders, and medications for adrenal disorders.

Medications for Thyroid and Parathyroid Disorders

The thyroid gland cues individual cells to work. It is an "on" switch for the body. The thyroid gland has an integral role in the body's metabolism. It produces two hormones, **triiodothyronine (T_3)** and **thyroxine (T_4),** which stimulate every tissue in the body to produce proteins and increase the amount of oxygen used by cells. Therefore, when the thyroid gland fails to work properly, the patient has less energy, and every cell in the body is affected. Decreased levels of these two hormones indicate hypothyroidism. Prolonged hypothyroidism can lead to a skin and tissue disorder called **myxedema,** which may be difficult to treat. A decrease of thyroid hormone secretion in utero and early infancy causes **cretinism** (slowed brain growth) in children. Rapid treatment can prevent both mental retardation and growth retardation.

To treat hypothyroidism, patients take oral doses of these hormones. These medications are prepared from natural sources, such as dried porcine thyroid gland, which include thyroid (Armour Thyroid, Bio-Throid) and liothyronine (Cytomel), or they are synthetically manufactured tablets such as levothyroxine (Synthroid, Levoxyl). This is known as **hormone replacement therapy (HRT).** Because a naturally occurring substance is being replaced, this medication is safe for use during pregnancy, although breastfeeding should be discussed with the physician. Caution should be used in elderly patients and those with heart problems or diabetes.

Hyperthyroidism results from an excess of thyroid hormone, leading to **Graves' disease,** characterized by bulging eyes, hyperactive metabolism, **goiter** (enlarged thyroid), and weight loss. **Thyroid storm,** which is a life-threatening condition and includes such symptoms as tachycardia, hyperthermia, chest pain, sweating, weakness, heart failure, anxiety, shortness of breath, and disorientation, can occur if hyperthyroidism is untreated. The thyroid gland can be inhibited from secreting T_3 and T_4 by thyroidectomy or with radioactive sodium iodide I-131 (Iodotope). The sodium iodide I-131 is taken by mouth; it is trapped within the thyroid gland and damages the thyroid's ability to function. Other oral antithyroid drugs, such as propylthiouracil or methimazole (Northyx, Tapazole), can also be used. These medications should be avoided in pregnancy and in breastfeeding mothers.

 CRITICAL THINKING

How does removal of the thyroid gland affect calcium in the body?

Medications to Treat Pancreatic Disorders

The pancreas functions properly when it secretes the correct amount of both insulin and glucagon. When this does not happen, the patient may develop one of two serious conditions: hyperglycemia or hypoglycemia. **Hyperglycemia** results from an excess of glucose in the blood. This condition can lead to problems with wound healing, high blood pressure, and nerve damage, among others. **Hypoglycemia** is caused by too little glucose in the blood and can lead to death. If the patient has low blood glucose, energy to fuel the cells is insufficient. Signs and symptoms of hypoglycemia are restlessness, shaky hands, lethargy, seizures, and coma (Fast Tip 15.1). Hypoglycemia is normally treated with a small dose of glucose such as hard candy, but patients may also choose to carry glucose preparations such as

Fast Tip 15.1 Emergency Treatment of Hypoglycemia

If an insulin dose is too high and low blood glucose results, immediately give juice, oral glucose gel, or hard candy if the patient is awake. A physician may also order dextrose IV or glucagon IM or IV to correct low blood glucose levels, especially if the patient is not conscious.

Insta-Glucose (gel) or BD Glucose (chewable tablet) that they take by mouth at the first sign of hypoglycemia. If patients cannot tolerate anything by mouth or are unconscious, they may be given injections such as glucagon (GlucaGen).

Diabetes mellitus is a disease characterized by hyperglycemia, or excessive blood glucose. Diabetes is categorized as type 1 or type 2. In type 1 diabetes or **insulin-dependent diabetes mellitus (IDDM),** destruction of the beta cells of the pancreas causes a decrease or lack of insulin secretion. Insulin in a healthy body serves to move glucose into the body tissues where it is needed, to assist in all functions at the cellular level. When the insulin is missing, glucose is elevated in the blood and unavailable to the tissues. When insulin is unavailable to remove accumulating glucose from the bloodstream, cells excrete water to flush out the vessels and send the glucose to the kidneys. For this reason, signs and symptoms of hyperglycemia include increased urination (from diuresis), increased thirst (the cells are dehydrated), and increased hunger (glucose is in the bloodstream but does not make it into the cells that desperately need it). Worsening damage occurs in the eyes, kidneys, heart, and nerves as long as glucose levels are elevated. Eventually, body organs can become severely affected. Vision worsens, wounds do not heal normally, fingers and toes may become numb, and kidney functions may be impaired. When blood glucose is very high, the patient may become lethargic and exhibit fruity-smelling breath and ketoacidosis (inefficient burning of fat). This can lead to seizures, coma, and death. Although type 1 diabetes is typically diagnosed in childhood or adolescence, it can occur at any age. Genetics, virus exposure, and pancreatic injuries are the contributing factors to the development of this chronic disease.

In type 2 diabetes or **non–insulin-dependent diabetes mellitus (NIDDM),** patients are insulin resistant; that is, their bodies produce adequate amounts of insulin but it does not lower the glucose levels as expected. The pancreas responds by increasing its production of insulin. Eventually, the pancreas cannot keep up with the body's need for insulin. Genetics, a sedentary lifestyle, and obesity are the main contributing factors for type 2 diabetes. Type 1 and type 2 diabetes are summarized in Table 15-2.

Patients with type 1 diabetes require insulin for treatment, whereas patients with type 2 diabetes may be managed with diet alone or with oral diabetic (antihyperglycemic) agents. Some antihyperglycemic drugs encourage the pancreas to release insulin, and others encourage the liver to trigger the

TABLE 15.2 Types of Diabetes

Diabetes Type	Contributing Factors	Insulin Production	Treatment
Type 1: insulin-dependent diabetes mellitus (IDDM)	Family history, pancreatic trauma	Pancreas makes little or no insulin	Insulin is destroyed in the stomach, so patients are dependent on subcutaneously injectable insulin; diet modification and exercise
Type 2: non–insulin-dependent diabetes mellitus (NIDDM)	Family history, obesity, poor diet	Pancreas does not secrete enough insulin, or body does not use insulin properly; if dietary fat intake is excessive, pancreas may not be able to keep up with demand	Diet modification and exercise may be enough; if not, oral antihyperglycemic agents; if these do not work, insulin

pancreas to release insulin. The choice of drug prescribed depends on the patient's individual problem. These medications are categorized as first- or second-generation, based on when they were released. First-generation sulfonylurea antihyperglycemic medications include acetohexamide (Dymelor), chlorpropamide (Diabinese), tolazamide (Tolinase), and tolbutamide (Orinase). The major drawback to the first-generation medications is that they can be dislodged from the proteins they bind to by other drugs, leading to very serious and prolonged hypoglycemia. The newer second-generation sulfonylurea antihyperglycemic medications are more potent and tend to be safer because they are not so easily dislodged. They include glimepiride (Amaryl), glipizide (Glucotrol), and glyburide (Diabeta, Micronase Glynase).

In addition, there are multiple other categories of antihyperglycemics. Sodium-glucose cotransporter 2 (SGLT-2) inhibitors such as empagliflozin (Jardiance), canagliflozin (Invokana), and dapagliflozin (Forxiga, Farxiga) inhibit the absorption of glucose by the kidneys. Dipeptidyl Peptidase-4 (DPP-4) inhibitors such as linagliptin (Tranjenta), sitagliptin (Januvia), and anagliptin (Suiny) inhibit DPP-4, an enzyme that inactivates incretion hormones GLP-1 and GIP (Drug Spotlight 15.1). Glucagon-like glucosidase peptide 1 (GLP-1) inhibitors such as liraglutide (Victoza) and dulaglutide (Trulicity) decrease blood glucose levels without causing hypoglycemia. Biguanides such as metformin improve peripheral glucose utilization. Thiazolidinediones (glitazones) such as rosiglitazone (Avandia) and pioglitazone (Actos) improve insulin sensitivity. Meglitinides such as nateglinide (Starlix) and repaglinide (Prandin, NovoNrom) stimulate insulin secretion from the pancreas, lowering glucose levels.

It is important to understand the types of insulin, its proper handling, and its proper injection to care safely for patients with diabetes mellitus.

CRITICAL THINKING

Why may too much glucose in the blood affect wound healing and nerve health?

CRITICAL THINKING

What would you do if a patient with diabetes mellitus came to your office and collapsed in the waiting room?

Types of Insulin

Insulin preparations are divided into five categories based on how quickly they start working and the length of action: rapid-acting, short-acting, intermediate-acting, long-acting, and premixed insulin preparations (Table 15-3). When a patient's blood glucose level is high, you may need to use short-acting insulin to lower it. Short-acting insulin is usually prescribed on a sliding scale, depending on the assessed blood glucose level. It may also be taken before meals so that it starts to work as food is being

Drug Spotlight 15-1 *Sitagliptin (Januvia)*

Availability	25-, 50-, and 100-mg tablets
Indications	Type 2 diabetes mellitus in combination with diet and exercise to improve control of glucose levels
Action	Helps to increase two hormones found in body that help control glucose levels (GLP-1 and GIP).
Adverse Reactions/ Side Effects	Body aches or pain, muscle aches, cough, loss of voice, rhinorrhea, stuffy nose, sneezing, ear congestion, fever, difficulty breathing, sore throat, abdominal pain, diarrhea
Contraindications	Hypersensitivity reaction to sitagliptin

TABLE 15.3   Types of Insulin

Type	Action	Onset of Action (Hours)	Duration of Action (Hours)
Insulin Lispro	Rapid	0.25–0.50	3–5
Insulin Aspart	Rapid	0.25	3–5
Insulin Glulisine	Rapid	0.25–0.50	1–1.5
Regular	Short	0.5–1	5–8
NPH	Intermediate	1–2	18–24
Lente	Intermediate	1–2.5	18–24
Levemir	Long	6–8	Up to 24
Lantus	Long	1–1.5	20–24
Ultralente	Long	0.5–3	20–36
Humulin 70/30	Premixed	0.5	2–4
Novolin 70/30	Premixed	0.5	2–12
NovoLog 70/30	Premixed	0.25	1–4
Humulin 50/50	Premixed	0.5	18–24
Humalog 75/25	Premixed	0.25	16–20

digested. If a patient is allowed nothing by mouth (NPO) for a test, insulin is not given because food is not given.

Intermediate-acting insulin is insulin mixed with a substance that makes the body absorb the insulin more slowly. This type of insulin looks cloudy in the bottle and must be mixed before injection.

Long-acting insulin can last up to one and a half days. It is usually taken in the morning or at bedtime.

If a patient's diabetes is fairly stable, different categories of insulin can be mixed to cover the next meal and beyond in one dose. For instance, a short- or immediate-acting insulin is used to treat the blood glucose increase that will occur with the meal the patient is eating or will soon eat. At the same time, the patient will receive a longer-acting insulin to help treat blood sugar increases that may occur in the hours following the meal, thus possibly preventing more injections throughout the day or night. This mixing is done by the patient or health-care worker, or a commercially prepared mixture can be used. The name of the insulin states the ratio of long-acting to short-acting insulin (e.g., 70/30). Commercially prepared insulin mixtures are available in a 10-mL vial (100 units per mL) or in an insulin pen. Insulin pens are ready to use with very little preparation. The patient screws on a sterile needle, dials in the desired dosage, and it is ready to inject (Fig. 15-3).

Patients with a history of hypoglycemia or poor control of blood glucose levels may receive insulin through a pump (discussed later in this chapter). The only category of insulin used with a pump is rapid- or short-acting insulin, and it is delivered at a base rate with programming available to provide extra insulin as needed.

Handling Insulin

Insulin should be refrigerated until the vial is opened because refrigeration extends the shelf life for 1 to 2 years (depending on manufacturer). Once the vial is opened, it may be kept at room temperature to avoid painful injections, but it must be discarded within 1 month. Insulin should never be kept at

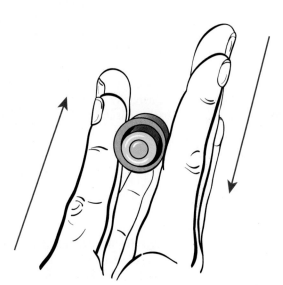

FIGURE 15-3: Insulin pens *(Credit: Ondrej83/Shutterstock)*

temperature extremes (freezing or very hot) because they will severely damage the insulin. Always label a container with the time and date that it was opened. After you have opened an insulin vial, gently roll it between your fingers (Fig. 15-4). Do not shake it.

Injecting Insulin

Rotate insulin injection sites on the patient's body. This is necessary for several reasons: (1) if a site is used too frequently, the body may develop scar tissue that thickens, thus preventing insulin absorption; (2) abscesses may form; and, most important, (3) rotating sites allows insulin to be evenly absorbed and thereby helps to maintain steady glucose levels and delay or minimize the complications of diabetes such as neuropathy, eye and kidney damage, and cardiovascular disease. If the patient is self-injecting, you may need to help the patient develop a chart of site rotation, such as that shown in Figure 15-5. A good rule of thumb to teach patients is that each site should only be used once a month, and each injection site should be 1 inch away from other sites.

The patient is spared discomfort and cost if you draw up regular and longer-acting insulin into one syringe before injection. Follow your agency protocol, but typically, the ordered amount of the clear, regular insulin is drawn up first, followed by the cloudy, longer-acting insulin. Following these directions ensures that you do not inadvertently put some of the cloudy, longer-acting insulin into the clear, regular insulin vial.

Another method of delivering insulin to patients with type 1 diabetes is the insulin pump (Fig. 15-6). This method uses a small needle, small-bore tubing, and a small pager-sized pump that delivers a steady dose of insulin to the patient 24 hours a day, 7 days a week. The pump also delivers a bolus (rapid injection) at mealtimes to help with the size of each meal eaten. In addition, some pumps monitor the blood

FIGURE 15-4: Proper insulin handling. Be sure to roll the insulin vial between your fingers before drawing up the injection; do not shake the vial.

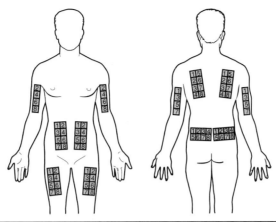

Sunday	Monday	Tuesday	Wednesday	Thursday	Friday	Saturday
Above navel	Below navel	Left thigh	Right thigh	Left of navel	Right of navel	Back of either arm

FIGURE 15-5: Site rotation for insulin injections. Use a chart to remind patients to rotate injection sites.

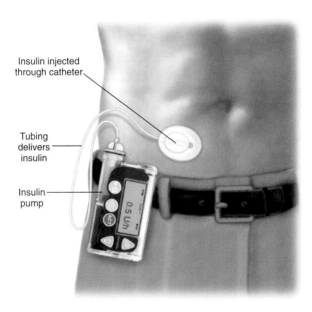

Insulin injected through catheter

Tubing delivers insulin

Insulin pump

0.5 U/h

FIGURE 15-6: Insulin pump. This provides continuous and steady administration of insulin to the patient with type 1 diabetes.

sugar level continuously and allow the patient to make needed adjustments. This method allows for injections to be reduced to once every few days instead of multiple times per day.

One other major function of the pancreas is the secretion of digestive enzymes. In patients with cystic fibrosis, the ducts in the pancreas become blocked with thick mucus and are unable to secrete these enzymes. For this reason, these patients must take replacement enzymes such as pancrelipase (Pancreaze, Ultresa, or Creon) for the rest of their lives every time they eat.

MEDICATIONS THAT TREAT ADRENAL DISORDERS

As with the thyroid gland, treatments for adrenal disorders are a response to the secretion of either too much or too little hormone. If the levels of naturally secreted hormones are too low, they must be replaced to help with symptoms such as weakness, hypoglycemia, and hypotension. If the adrenal gland is oversecreting hormones, the patient needs medication to inhibit cortisol to treat hypertension and hypertension symptoms.

Corticosteroid Medications

Glucocorticoid hormones available as medications are known as corticosteroids because their actions are identical to those of the naturally occurring hormones cortisone and cortisol. Chemically, these medications are steroids and are used as replacement therapy when these hormones are absent or diminished. Corticosteroid medications are used to treat Addison's disease, autoimmune diseases, inflammatory reactions, cerebral edema, dermatologic disorders, allergies, asthma, cancer, Crohn's disease, dermatitis, edema, rash, rheumatoid arthritis, rhinitis, shock, transplant rejection, and ulcerative colitis.

Addison's disease occurs when the adrenal cortex undersecretes glucocorticoid hormones. Patients with Addison's disease suffer from chronic fatigue that eventually worsens, muscle weakness, anorexia, nausea, vomiting, diarrhea, hypotension, hypoglycemia, sweating, irritability, and weight loss. The disease is treated with hydrocortisone USP tablets, a synthetic corticosteroid. If the level of aldosterone is also insufficient, it is replaced with oral doses of fludrocortisone acetate (Florinef).

In **Cushing's disease,** the adrenal cortex oversecretes the glucocorticoids mentioned earlier. Patients with Cushing's disease have symptoms similar to those of Addison's disease, except these patients suffer hypertension and hyperglycemia instead of hypotension and hypoglycemia. They also develop a fatty hump between their shoulders. Most patients have upper-body obesity and a rounded face, and women have excessive hair growth on their face, chest, abdomen, and thighs. Treatment is based on the cause of the excess production and may include surgery, irradiation, chemotherapy, and cortisol-inhibiting drugs such as metyrapone (Metopirone).

Anabolic Steroids

Anabolic steroids are mainly composed of male hormones called androgens, which change the natural balance between tissue breakdown and building. They can be used to prevent muscle wasting in patients with AIDS or to help patients with severe trauma to rebuild tissue. Examples of anabolic steroids are oxandrolone (Oxandrin) and nandrolone decanoate. Side effects of these medications include aggressive behavior, rage, atherosclerosis, sterility, and liver cancer. Because of these side effects and because anabolic steroids are frequently abused by athletes trying to build muscle mass, they are Schedule III controlled substances.

●●○ SUMMARY

- Components of the endocrine system produce hormones to control many of the body's functions.

- The endocrine system consists of the hypothalamus gland, pituitary gland, thyroid and parathyroid glands, pancreas, adrenal glands, pineal gland, and gonads.

- Disorders affecting this system can have profound implications for the health of the patient.

- Extremely high or extremely low hormone levels can cause various illnesses.

- Hormones from the thyroid and parathyroid glands regulate blood and bone calcium.

- Patients may need to take medications to suppress hormone secretion or hormone supplements to compensate for missing hormones.

- Hormone replacement therapy (HRT) to treat hypothyroidism consist of natural or synthetic hormones in oral doses.

- Medications to treat hyperthyroidism, which can lead to Graves' disease, include sodium iodide I-131 and other oral antithyroid drugs such as propylthiouracil or methimazole. Patients who do not respond to medication may need surgery (thyroidectomy).

- Pancreatic dysfunction causes two major problems that require medication. The first is the inability to digest food, and the second is the inability to regulate blood sugar.

■ In type 1 diabetes, destruction of the beta cells of the pancreas causes a decrease or lack of insulin secretion, which is needed to remove accumulating glucose from the bloodstream.

■ In type 2 diabetes, the pancreas produces adequate amounts of insulin, but the insulin does not lower the glucose levels, resulting in hyperglycemia.

■ Insulin or oral antihyperglycemic medications are required to lower blood glucose levels.

■ Insulin preparation types are divided into rapid-acting, short-acting, intermediate-acting, long-acting, and premixed insulin preparations.

■ The hormones of the adrenal glands help regulate metabolism, the immune response, blood pressure, and response to stress.

■ Corticosteroid medications are used to treat low or missing adrenal hormones to help with symptoms such as weakness, hypoglycemia, and hypotension.

■ Cortisol-inhibiting drugs such as metyrapone are used to reduce oversecretion of adrenal hormones to treat hypertension and hypertension symptoms.

■ Overall, patients need normally functioning endocrine glands. If this is not the case, the physician will use medication along with surgery and/or radiation to return hormones to levels as close to normal as possible, to maintain optimum health.

Master the Essentials: Endocrine Medications

This table shows the various classes of endocrine medications and key side effects, contraindications and precautions, interactions, and examples of each class.

Class	Indications for Use	Side Effects	Contraindications and Precautions	Examples	Interactions
Anabolic steroids	Weight gain following severe illness or injury, some anemias	Acne, hirsutism, depression, altered libido, edema, glucose tolerance, aggression, liver cancer, atherosclerosis	Breast cancer, prostate cancer, pregnancy, hypercalcemia, liver failure	Oral anticoagulants, oral hypoglycemic agents	Nandrolone decanoate, oxandrolone (Oxandrin)
Antithyroid medications	Hyperthyroidism	Paresthesia, headache, rash, agranulocytosis	Hypersensitivity, pregnancy, breastfeeding	Anticoagulants	Methimazole (Northyx, Tapazole), propylthiouracil I-131 (Iodotope)
Cortisol-inhibiting medications	Cushing's disease	Dizziness, drowsiness, headache, nausea, vomiting	Pregnancy, breastfeeding	Insulin, oral hypoglycemic agents, corticosteroids, estrogen, hydantoins, acetaminophen	Metyrapone (Metopirone)
Corticosteroids	Severe allergies, asthma, multiple sclerosis, arthritis, Addison's disease	Adrenocortical insufficiency, anxiety, cessation of menses, constipation, decreased wound healing, decreased growth in children, diarrhea, dizziness, fluid and electrolyte imbalances, GI upset, headache, hyperglycemia, increased eye pressure, increased infection, muscle pain and weakness, osteoporosis, psychosis, petechiae	Pregnancy, breastfeeding, children; history of clots, seizures, or immunosuppression; not used for long-term therapy; cautious use with infection, hypothyroidism, cirrhosis, increased blood pressure, congestive heart failure, emotional instability, diabetes, glaucoma, or GI upset; do not use in patients with a history of clots, seizures, or immunosuppression	Barbiturates, contraceptives, diuretics, NSAIDs, vaccines	Hydrocortisone USP, fludrocortisone acetate (Florinef)

Classification	Side Effects	Contraindications/Precautions	Drug Interactions	Generic (Trade) Names
Insulin	Headache, increased sweating, irritability, tingling, tremor, blurred or double vision, weakness, hypoglycemia, hypokalemia	Hypoglycemia, sensitivity, kidney impairment, liver impairment	Alcohol, MAOIs, salicylates, anabolic steroids	Lispro (Humalog, NovoLog), regular insulin (Iletin I, Iletin II, Humulin R, Novolin R), isophane (NPH) insulin (Humulin N, Novolin N), lente insulin (Humulin L, Novolin L), ultralente insulin (Humulin U, Ultralente), glargine insulin (Lantus)
Oral antidiabetic medications	Hypoglycemia; abdominal pain (alpha-glucosidase inhibitors); nausea, vomiting, metallic taste (metformin); aplastic anemia, rash, nausea (sulfonylureas); swelling, weight gain (thiazolidinediones)	Hypersensitivity, diabetic ketoacidosis, cirrhosis; inflammatory bowel disease (alpha-glucosidase inhibitors); kidney or liver dysfunction (metformin)	Alcohol, MAOIs, corticosteroids, salicylates, warfarin	**First-generation sulfonylureas** Acetohexamide (Dymelor), chlorpropamide (Diabinese), tolazamide (Tolinase), tolbutamide (Orinase) **Second-generation sulfonylureas** Glimepiride (Amaryl), glipizide (Glucotrol), glyburide (Diabeta, Micronase Glynase) **Biguanides** metformin (Glucophage, Fortamet) **Thiazolidinediones (Glitazones)** rosiglitazone (Avandia), pioglitazone (Actos) **Meglitinides** nateglinide (Starlix), repaglinide (Prandin, NovoNorm) **GLP-1 agonists** liraglutide (Victoza), dulaglutide (Trulicity) **DPP-4 inhibitors (gliptins)** anagliptin (Suiny), linagliptin (Trajenta), sitagliptin (Januvia) **SGLT-2 inhibitors** canagliflozin (Invokana), dapagliflozin (Forxiga, Farxiga), empagliflozin (Jardiance)
Pancreatic enzymes	Nausea, vomiting, stomach pain, diarrhea, constipation, greasy stools, gas	Allergy to pork, pregnancy or lactation	None known	Pancrelipase (Pancreaze, Ultresa, or Creon)
Thyroid medications	Palpitations, fast heart rate, irregular heartbeat, increased blood pressure nervousness, tremor, headache, insomnia, weight loss, diarrhea, abdominal cramps, intolerance of heat, fever, menstrual irregularities	Adrenal insufficiency, diabetes, cardiovascular disease	Adrenergics, insulin, oral anticoagulants, oral hypoglycemics	Levothyroxine (T_4) (Levothroid), desiccated thyroid (T_3, T_4) (Armour)

GI, gastrointestinal; MAOI, monoamine oxidase inhibitor; NSAID, nonsteroidal anti-inflammatory drug.

Activities

To make sure that you have learned the key points covered in this chapter, complete the following activities.

True or False

Write true if the statement is true. Beside the false statements, write false, and correct the statement to make it true.

1. Hypoglycemia is low blood sugar. _____

_____

2. Cushing's disease is caused by too much thyroid hormone. _____

_____

3. Lack of insulin causes hypoglycemia. _____

_____

4. A goiter may be a symptom of Graves' disease. _____

_____

5. Ketoacidosis is the inefficient burning of fat. _____

_____

6. Different categories of insulin cannot be mixed in one injection. _____

_____

7. Insulin pumps are used for 8 hours of every day. _____

_____

8. Regular short-acting insulin can be used on a sliding scale. _____

_____

9. Anabolic steroids are never legal to use. _____

_____

10. Addison's disease is caused by too little adrenal cortex hormone. _____

_____

Multiple Choice

Choose the best answer for each question.

1. Which of the following is a symptom or sign of Addison's disease?
   A. Tremor
   B. Dehydration
   C. Restlessness
   D. Weight loss

2. Which organ secretes insulin?

A. Pancreas

B. Renal

C. Adrenal

D. Thyroid

3. Which hormone triggers the release of hormones from the thyroid gland?

A. FSH

B. TSH

C. GH

D. ICSH

4. When should insulin be refrigerated?

A. Before opening (while storing)

B. After opening

C. Never

D. Always

5. Which is a common reason for an insulin pump to be prescribed?

A. Patient's aversion to shots

B. Good insurance

C. History of hyperglycemia

D. Poor control of blood sugar

Application Exercises

Respond to the following situations.

1. Barbara is a 10-year-old patient with newly diagnosed diabetes. Her mom wants to know why Barbara needs to have injections three to five times a day while her father just has to take pills. Explain the reason for this. _____

_____

_____

2. Steve was in a devastating car accident. He is taking anabolic steroids to help repair the body tissues injured in the accident. His wife is concerned about the serious side effects of these drugs. What are the side effects, and is she justified in being concerned? What would you say to her? _____

_____

_____

3. David has been recently diagnosed with IDDM. He is a traveling salesman and states that he leaves his insulin and injection supplies in the car for convenience. Explain to him the reason this is a bad idea, and give him some suggestions on better ways to handle his insulin needs. _____

_____

_____

4. Cindy is told that she has hyperparathyroidism. She has had two episodes of kidney stones. She is confused about how these two things are connected; what would you say to her? _____

_____

_____

Essentials Review

For further study and practice with drug classifications learned in this chapter, complete the following table to the best of your ability. Use resources such as the *PDR,* the Internet, or printed drug guides for help.

Example	Generic Name	Classification	Side Effects	Contraindications and Precautions	Examples	Patient Education
Oxandrin						
Solu-Medrol						
Iletin I						
Glucotrol XL						
Levothroid						

Internet Research

1. Using your favorite search engine, find out the latest information about inhaled insulin. Is it currently on the market? If so, is it widely used?

2. Go to the American Diabetes Association website (www.diabetes.org) to find information to help you to create a teaching aid for diabetic patients.

16

Cardiovascular System Medications

*T*his chapter discusses medications that affect the cardiovascular system. The heart is a vital organ, and cardiovascular disorders can cause serious conditions, such as chest pain or even death. Fortunately, cardiovascular disease has been well researched, and many medications exist to help patients. Medications that affect this system are prescribed for a variety of illnesses. This chapter covers medications used to prevent myocardial infarction, stroke, and clotting; to promote blood cell development; to lower blood pressure; to treat heart failure; to regulate heart rhythm; to treat shock; and to treat lipid disorders.

In addition, many other medications that patients take have implications for the cardiovascular system. Medications taken for migraine, for example, may cause severe hypotension, which puts the patient at risk for falls. Patients taking aspirin for chronic back pain are at increased risk for bleeding. Therefore, finding out what medications (both over-the-counter and prescription) your patients are taking is extremely important to providing the best care and education possible.

LEARNING OUTCOMES

At the end of this chapter, you should be able to:

16.1   Define all key terms.
16.2   Discuss how the cardiovascular system functions.
16.3   Describe 10 categories of cardiovascular medications and their uses and actions.

KEY TERMS

ACE inhibitors
Angina pectoris
Angiotensin receptor
  blockers (ARBs)
Anoxia
Atherosclerosis
Cerebrovascular
  accident (CVA)
Congestive heart
  failure (CHF)
Contractility

Cyanosis
Deep vein thrombosis
  (DVT)
Dysrhythmias
Embolus
Hemostasis
High-density lipoprotein
  (HDL)
Hypertension (HTN)
Hyperlipemia
Hypoxia

Infarction
Ischemia
Low-density lipoprotein
  (LDL)
Myocardial infarction (MI)
Pulmonary circulation
Shock
Thrombus
Very low-density
  lipoprotein (VLDL)

■ THE CARDIOVASCULAR SYSTEM

The cardiovascular system consists of the heart and blood vessels. The heart has four chambers, called the left and right atrium and the left and right ventricles, which are continuously contracting and relaxing in a coordinated rhythm (Fig. 16-1). This rhythmic pumping of the heart sends the blood out

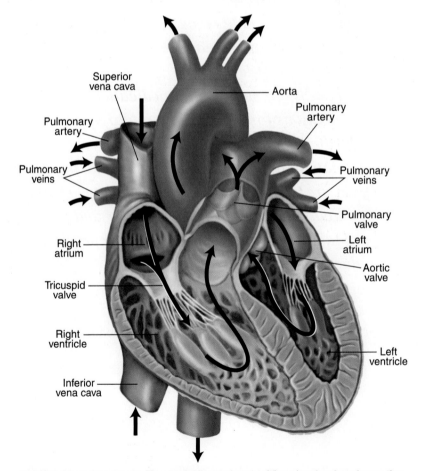

FIGURE 16-1: The heart. The heart is made up of four basic chambers: the left and right atrium and the left and right ventricle. In addition, the major blood vessels are attached to the heart to circulate blood from heart to the body and back again.

to the lungs via the pulmonary artery to obtain oxygen, which the heart and body tissues need to survive (Fig. 16-2). This oxygen-rich blood is then returned to the heart via the pulmonary veins. This sequence is known as the **pulmonary circulation.** The oxygenated blood is then sent out to the upper and lower parts of the body via the aorta, which subdivides into a system of arteries. Finally, the blood, which is now depleted of oxygen and rich in carbon dioxide, returns from the body to the heart via a network of veins, where it again is pumped to the lungs to exchange the carbon dioxide for more oxygen in a never-ending cycle.

The cardiovascular system plays two major roles in the human body. One is to deliver much-needed nutrients such as oxygen, hormones, and immune and clotting factors to every part of the body including the heart. The other role is to carry waste products such as carbon dioxide out of the cells. If any area of this system is damaged through accident or disease, the effects on health can be devastating.

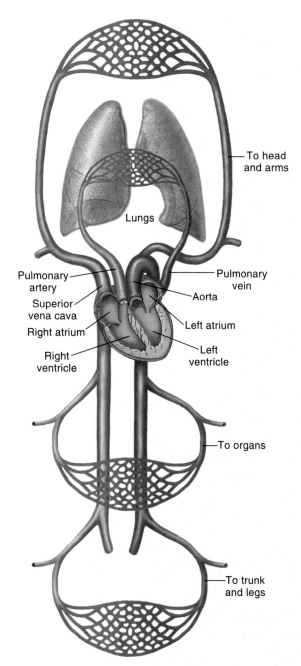

FIGURE 16-2: Cardiopulmonary circulation. The red blood vessels represent oxygen-rich blood, and the blue blood vessels represent oxygen-poor blood.

MYOCARDIAL INFARCTION, STROKE, AND CLOTTING

Myocardial infarction (MI) or heart attack, stroke, and clots all cause damage when blood flow is impeded to the chest, brain, or lungs. Chest pain can be a symptom of a total lack of oxygen, called **anoxia,** or significantly reduced oxygen, called **hypoxia,** in the heart muscle (myocardium). The lack or reduction of oxygen prevents the tissues of the heart from receiving enough nourishment, and this can lead to tissue injury or **ischemia** or even death, referred to as an **infarction.** The classic signs of MI are chest pain, sweating, pale skin, and **cyanosis** (a bluish tint to the skin), particularly around the mouth. Chest pain can also be caused by noncardiovascular conditions, including broken ribs, gastrointestinal (GI) disorders, anxiety, or injured skeletal muscles (A Closer Look 16.1).

A CLOSER LOOK 16.1: Heart Attacks and Women

Women tend to have atypical symptoms, such as upper back or shoulder pain, light-headedness, and unusual fatigue that lasts for several days. These atypical symptoms make rapid diagnosis more difficult. Health-care professionals and the public are becoming more educated about these atypical symptoms to help with quick diagnosis and treatment in women.

A stroke or **cerebrovascular accident (CVA)** occurs when the brain is deprived of oxygen and blood flow for several minutes. CVAs are a major cause of death and disability. MIs are caused by ischemia of heart muscle; CVAs are caused by ischemia of the brain. For this reason, medications that prevent ischemia can be prescribed to prevent stroke as well as MI.

CARDIOVASCULAR MEDICATIONS

Cardiovascular medications function in a few basic ways. Certain medications, such as atropine, increase the heart rate. Others, such as diltiazem (Cardizem) or verapamil (Calan), slow the heart rate. Drugs such as digoxin (Lanoxin) make the heart function more efficiently. Other medications, such as propafenone (Rythmol) and sotalol (Betapace), make it less irritable. In addition, drugs may be given to make the environment in which the heart functions less hostile. For example, if the heart is having a difficult time pumping, a backup of fluid may occur, leading to breathing problems. In this instance, administration of a diuretic such as furosemide (Lasix) decreases the amount of fluid that the heart must circulate through the body. This reduces the workload of the heart (see the Master the Essentials table for descriptions of the most common cardiovascular system drugs).

Antianginal Medications

Angina pectoris is chest pain caused by a lack of oxygen and nutrients in the heart tissue. As discussed earlier, ischemia (damage) occurs, and if continued, infarction, or the death of heart tissue, will ensue. Antianginal drugs decrease angina pectoris by dilating arteries and veins. An example is nitroglycerin (Nitrolingual, Nitroquick, Nitrostat, Nitro-Bid, Nitro-Dur), which can be administered via different routes such as sublingual, buccal, spray, or IV, depending on the patient's circumstances. The most common route is sublingual. The patient places a tablet or sprays the medication under the tongue at home when chest pain begins, with instructions to repeat the procedure every 5 minutes, for a maximum of three times. If pain continues, the patient should call emergency medical services (EMS) so that he or she can be evaluated for a possible MI.

A transdermal patch such as nitroglycerin topical (Nitro-Bid or Nitrol Appli-Kit) may also be used for prevention of angina pectoris. This patch is used daily as maintenance to prevent tissue ischemia and infarction. Angina can be treated with more than just medicine (Fast Tip 16.1). Nitroglycerin is also given in IV form by EMS or in the hospital setting for acute chest pain.

⬤ *Fast Tip 16.1* Nonpharmacological Treatment for Angina Pectoris

All the following strategies can help treat angina: decrease dietary fats, lower blood pressure, develop coping mechanisms for stress, exercise, decrease alcohol consumption, stop smoking, and decrease dietary sodium. If these changes do not improve heart function, nitrates may be prescribed.

If chest pain is caused by a skeletal muscle condition rather than by heart muscle problems, pain relievers such as nonsteroidal anti-inflammatory drugs (NSAIDs) may be effective. Be sure to teach patients to rule out heart problems (excluded as a diagnosis) before medicating chest pain with NSAIDs.

Anticoagulants, Antiplatelet, and Thrombolytic Medications

The clotting process is complex and has several stages that can be affected by different categories of medication. Anticoagulants interrupt the clotting process and ensure that blood flows smoothly through the vessels. Antiplatelet medications prevent platelets from clumping together to form clots. Thrombolytics dissolve clots that have already formed. Aggressive treatment of thrombolytic stroke with anticoagulants and thrombolytics (as well as antihypertensives, discussed later) can increase survival by increasing blood flow to the brain. Thrombolytics can also be used to prevent CVA and MI.

Anticoagulants and Antiplatelet Medications

Anticoagulants such as warfarin (Coumadin), heparin, and enoxaparin (Lovenox) prevent blood from clotting by interrupting the production of proteins called cofactors that work together in the clotting process. Vitamin K controls creation of these cofactors. Coumadin, which is taken orally, decreases the body's vitamin K levels and thus reduces clot formation. Heparin blocks the cofactors thrombin and fibrin from functioning to form clots. Exactly how Lovenox works is not clearly understood. It is believed that the drug attaches to one of the cofactors and neutralizes its effectiveness. Heparin and Lovenox are given by subcutaneous injection several times a day in patients at risk for developing **deep vein thrombosis (DVT)**. DVT is the formation of a blood clot in a vein that is located deep inside the body. Most commonly, this occurs in the lower extremities. However, portions of a clot can break off and travel to the brain, heart, or lungs and can cause serious injury or death. Patients at risk are those that are on bedrest and those with fractures to the pelvis, obesity, recent surgery, and a family history of blood clots.

After surgery, a patient may develop DVT because of inactivity. Physicians may prescribe not only anticoagulants to prevent clots but also tight stockings that cover most of the leg. These stockings compress the veins and aid the smooth return of blood to the heart, even if the veins in the leg are weakened. These antiembolic stockings are usually prescribed in addition to, not instead of, medications.

Patients taking anticoagulants must have their blood monitored for safety to ensure it has the desired ability to clot. Too little of the medication and the patient is at risk for blood clots and embolisms; too much of the medication and they are at risk for hemorrhage. If a patient taking anticoagulants has a break in the skin or mucosal integrity, profuse bleeding can occur because the clotting mechanism is disturbed (Fast Tip 16.2).

Antiplatelet medications such as aspirin, ticlopidine (Ticlid), clopidogrel (Plavix), abciximab (ReoPro), eptifibatide (Integrilin), and Tirofiban (Aggrastat) prevent platelets from clumping together to form clots. Because aspirin is an over-the-counter (OTC) medication, patients may not understand its potency relative to interfering with clotting. Always ask a patient whether OTC medications, including aspirin, are being taken. Aspirin is showing promise in the survival rates of heart attack victims when the drug is taken when initial symptoms occur and in prevention of subsequent heart attacks when it is taken routinely following an initial heart attack (Drug Spotlight 16.1).

Fast Tip 16.2 Patient Teaching About Anticoagulants

Patients taking an anticoagulant should be educated about the risks associated with this medication. If these patients are injured, clotting will likely be delayed. The following precautions should be taken to avoid injury and thus clotting delays.

- Use an electric razor to avoid injury.
- Reduce intake of green leafy vegetables, green tea, hummus, and other foods that are high in vitamin K, a vitamin necessary for coagulation. These foods include cabbage, cauliflower, spinach, cereals, and soybeans.
- Watch for signs of abnormal bleeding, such as frequent bruising, bleeding gums, and black, tarry stool.
- Keep appointments to have blood drawn to monitor the effect of anticoagulants.

Drug Spotlight 16-1 *Aspirin (Acetylsalicylic Acid)*

Classification	Analgesic
Definition and History	A substance used for pain relief and fever reduction in the form of a powder made from willow bark as far back as 400 to 500 B.C.; patented February 27, 1900, by a German company named Bayer; Bayer was forced to give up the patent as a result of the treaty of Versailles in 1919
Availability	Tablets
Indications	Used today for pain, inflammation, and fever reduction; taken in high doses for arthritis therapy; side effects must be monitored closely; also taken in low doses to decrease the risk for heart attack and stroke in older adults
Adverse Reactions/ Side Effects	Stomach upset, stomach ulcerations, increased bleeding time
Contraindications/ Precautions	Cited as a link in Reye's syndrome in children when taken after a viral infection; therefore, aspirin is not routinely given to children

Two other types of antiplatelet medications are adenosine diphosphate (ADP) receptor blockers and glycoprotein IIb/IIIa inhibitors. ADP receptor blockers interfere with the plasma membrane of platelets that prevents clots from forming. An example of this thrombus prevention drug is clopidogrel (Plavix). These medications provide long-term prevention against clot formation.

Glycoprotein IIb/IIIa inhibitors prevent the enzyme that aggregates platelets from working. They are sometimes given before cardiac procedures to prevent clots from forming during surgery or a procedure.

Patients taking antiplatelet medications should also learn the signs of bleeding and precautions. In addition, patients should be educated to avoid foods high in vitamin K because they interfere with anticoagulant therapy (see Fast Tip 16.2).

Thrombolytic Medications

If other medications fail to prevent clots from blocking blood vessels, thrombolytics can dissolve them. A clot in a vessel such as in DVT is known as a **thrombus.** A clot that breaks loose and travels is an **embolus.** A clot can form in the heart, lung, or brain or in the peripheral circulation. If a thrombus forms in a peripheral vein, as in DVT, the patient will complain of pain and swelling of the extremity. When this clot breaks loose, the embolus can travel and cause a heart attack (MI), a pulmonary embolus (blood clot in the lung), or a stroke (blood clot in the brain). In addition, a clot that lodges in the kidney, liver, or other organ may cause damage resulting from lack of blood flow to that organ.

A patient who can be diagnosed and treated within 60 minutes of onset of symptoms of a CVA can be given a treatment called tissue plasminogen activator (tPA). This thrombolytic medication is given by the IV route and is approved for use in acute stroke. If it is given within 60 minutes of onset of symptoms, the effects of the stroke are minimized. The treatment carries the risk for intracranial and/or systemic hemorrhage and angioedema; therefore, treatment protocol may require consent from the patient's next of kin for its use.

Thrombolytics can also be used to clear IV catheters and cannulas blocked with blood, but these medications must be used with extreme caution. If the blood has been in the cannula too long, injecting the drug can break off the clot rather than dissolve it.

Uncontrolled bleeding is just as dangerous as clotting. Clots must be dissolved quickly to prevent ischemia and infarction; however, a patient can die of uncontrolled bleeding as well. Therefore, frequent testing is necessary to ensure that the dose of anticoagulants, antiplatelets, or thrombolytics is therapeutic. The most common tests are prothrombin time (PT), activated partial thromboplastin time (aPTT), and international normalized ratio (INR). These tests are also used with anticoagulant, antiplatelet, and antithrombolytic therapy. PT is a blood test used to evaluate the ability of blood to clot and is often performed before surgical procedures. The aPTT blood test is usually used to evaluate the effectiveness of heparin therapy. An INR is a blood test used to determine how long it takes blood to clot and is performed primarily in patients taking Coumadin.

Antifibrinolytic Medications

Antifibrinolytic medications have an effect opposite to that of thrombolytics in that they help form clots when the patient is losing too much blood (hemorrhaging) and thereby provide **hemostasis** (stops the bleeding). This effect is useful, for example, in women with unusually heavy menstrual bleeding because it decreases the amount of blood lost each month. "Anti" means against, and "lytic" means to break down. These drugs prevent the destruction of fibrin and thus allow fibrin to form a clot. Examples include aminocaproic acid (Amicar) and tranexamic acid (Cyklokapron).

Blood loss can also be treated with other hemostatic drugs, such as vitamin K, protamine sulfate, and desmopressin acetate (DDAVP). They help regulate the clotting process. As described earlier, vitamin K is responsible for the formation of the cofactors responsible for clotting. Vitamin K is an antidote for anticoagulant overdose because it increases the production of those cofactors. Protamine sulfate is specifically administered by the IV route as an antidote to heparin overdose. DDAVP is an artificially made hormone that naturally occurs in the pituitary gland. This medication is used specifically in the treatment of hemophilia (bleeding disorders) in which the patient is lacking factor VIII and von Willebrand factor. DDAVP can raise the levels of these necessary clotting factors without the administration of blood products.

Medications that Promote Blood Cell Development (Hematopoietic Stimulants)

Some medications stimulate the growth of blood cells. Hematopoietic stimulant medications are used to treat anemias such as sickle cell and pernicious anemia (vitamin B_{12} deficiency). They are also used to treat patients with low blood iron levels, which decrease the ability of the red blood cells to carry oxygen. In addition, patients who are receiving chemotherapy often have lowered blood levels resulting from the bone marrow–suppressing effects of that treatment.

One example of a hematopoietic stimulant is ferrous sulfate (Feosol, Fer-in-Sol, Ferra-TD). This medication is taken by mouth and specifically treats iron-deficiency anemia. Another medication is cyanocobalamin (vitamin B_{12}) and is used in patients who cannot absorb vitamin B_{12} in the GI tract, such as those with pernicious anemia. Therefore, injectable vitamin B_{12} is usually administered to facilitate blood cell development for the remainder of their lifetime. This, in turn, promotes oxygen delivery to the cells and boosts the patient's energy. Medications such as filgrastim (Neupogen), pegfilgrastim (Neulasta), and sargramostim (Leukine) are given to stimulate blood cell development (see the Master the Essentials table for contraindications to and precautions for these medications).

Medications that Decrease Blood Pressure

Cardiac output, peripheral resistance, and blood volume interact to create blood pressure. Cardiac output is the product of the heart rate and the stroke volume (amount of blood that is pumped with each heartbeat). Peripheral resistance is determined by the size and flexibility of the arteries. Therefore, the force of the heart's contraction, the amount of blood that is pumped, and the resistance, or "give," of the blood vessels all influence blood pressure. The kidneys also play a key role by regulating circulating fluid volume (A Closer Look 16.2).

A CLOSER LOOK 16.2: Cardiac Output, Peripheral Vascular Resistance, Blood Volume, and Blood Pressure

Cardiac output (CO), peripheral resistance, and blood volume all interact to create blood pressure (BP). CO relates to the volume of blood that fills the heart, the force of the heart contraction, and the ability of the heart to relax. It is calculated by multiplying heart rate (HR) and stroke volume (SV), the amount of blood in the left ventricle.

$$CO = HR \times SV$$

The sympathetic and parasympathetic nervous systems control the HR, so medications that affect HR may also affect CO. BP is the product of CO and peripheral vascular resistance (PVR).

$$BP = CO \times PVR$$

PVR is the amount of force in the peripheral blood vessels. If the PVR is higher than normal, the heart has to work harder to maintain appropriate CO, which is the volume of blood the heart pumps each minute.

SV may be referred to as preload, and PVR is referred to as afterload. If a medication decreases the preload of the heart, the **contractility** (ability of the heart to contract) improves. If a medication decreases the afterload, the heart works more efficiently.

Poor heart action, **atherosclerosis** (fatty plaques in the arteries), kidney failure, narrowed peripheral blood vessels caused by diabetes mellitus, and chronic stress can cause hypertension.

Hypertension (HTN), or high blood pressure, is a major cause of death and disability. Chronic high blood pressure can reduce the kidney's ability to remove excess fluid and consequently puts a strain on circulatory organs.

Antihypertensives, which reduce blood pressure, include angiotensin-converting enzyme (ACE) inhibitors, autonomic nervous system agents, diuretics, and calcium channel blockers. Many of these drugs are also used to treat heart failure and are discussed later. To help you understand where in the process each class of medications works, please review A Closer Look 16.3 to refresh your understanding of blood pressure regulation.

A CLOSER LOOK 16.3: Blood Pressure Regulation

Blood pressure regulation is a complex process. The primary regulation is carried out by the medulla oblongata (the vasomotor center in the brain), chemoreceptors, and baroreceptors. Chemoreceptors recognize oxygen and carbon dioxide levels and pH in the blood. Baroreceptors sense pressure in the large blood vessels. Both types of receptors pass on their information to the medulla, which then tells the body how to respond.

A CLOSER LOOK 16.3: **Blood Pressure Regulation—cont'd**

The endocrine system also plays a role through the renin-angiotensin system, illustrated here. This system increases blood pressure through its effects on the blood vessels and the kidneys.

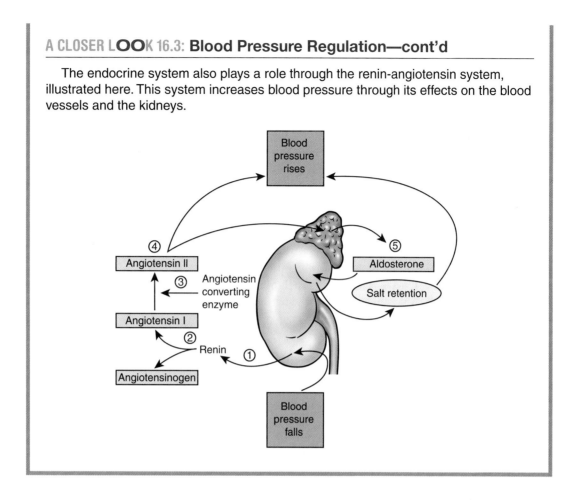

ACE inhibitors block the renin-angiotensin pathway from the kidneys to decrease blood pressure. They also help reduce the possibility of heart failure by blocking the action of the renin-angiotensin system. These drugs stop the enzyme that converts angiotensin I to angiotensin II. Angiotensin II is a polypeptide in the blood that causes constriction of the blood vessels that, in turn, increases blood pressure. If there is less angiotensin II, the blood vessels will not constrict, and the blood pressure will not increase. ACE inhibitors include benazepril (Lotensin), captopril (Capoten), enalapril (Vasotec), and fosinopril (Monopril). For further examples, see the Master the Essentials table.

Angiotensin receptor blockers (ARBs) block the action of angiotensin. These medications work similarly to ACE inhibitors. ARBs prevent angiotensin from attaching to receptors and thus prevent blood vessels from contracting and increasing blood pressure. These medications are sometimes used when patients are unable to tolerate the side effects of ACE inhibitors. Examples of ARBs include candesartan (Atacand), eprosartan (Teveten), irbesartan (Avapro), losartan (Cozaar), olmesartan (Benicar), telmisartan (Micardis), and valsartan (Diovan).

Autonomic nervous system agents, such as adrenergic blockers (see Chapter 13), relax the fight-or-flight stress response. They can act on alpha- and beta-adrenergic receptors. Beta-adrenergic blockers such as acebutolol (Sectral), atenolol (Tenormin), bisoprolol (Zebeta), metoprolol, nadolol (Corgard), nebivolol (Bystolic), and propranolol (Inderal LA) are autonomic nervous system agents that decrease the fight-or-flight response, which causes blood vessels to constrict and the heart to beat faster (see the Master the Essentials table for a full list of beta-blocker medications). These drugs are used to manage hypertension and angina pectoris, slow the heart rate, prevent MI, reduce congestion associated with heart failure, and treat glaucoma. Reducing the body's perception that it is in a threatening situation can improve cardiovascular function.

Diuretics clear excess fluid from the body and regulate blood pressure by encouraging the kidneys to excrete fluid. Less fluid in the body creates less blood volume and thus less pressure in the blood vessels (decreased peripheral vascular resistance). Diuretics are also used in the treatment of heart failure. The three major classifications of diuretics are thiazides, potassium-sparing diuretics, and loop diuretics. They are classified based on their site of action in the kidney.

■ Thiazide diuretics such as hydrochlorothiazide (HydroDIURIL, Aquazide H, Esidrix, Microzide) and chlorothiazide (Diuril, Diuril Sodium) are the most common classification of diuretic prescribed. Thiazide diuretics work by diminishing the amounts of sodium and chloride reabsorbed by the distal tubule of the kidneys. This effect increases fluid loss and thus decreases blood volume.

■ Potassium-sparing diuretics such as amiloride (Midamor), spironolactone (Aldactone), and triamterene (Dyrenium) produce diuresis by interrupting the sodium-potassium exchange in the distal tubule as do the thiazide diuretics, but they spare potassium from being lost, as occurs with thiazide medications.

■ Loop diuretics are the most potent of the three classifications. These medications act on the loop of Henle to inhibit the reabsorption of sodium and chloride. This effect, in turn, causes less water to be reabsorbed into the blood and is thus excreted into the urine, to reduce blood volume. Examples of loop diuretics include bumetanide (Bumex), ethacrynic acid (Edecrin, Sodium Edecrin), furosemide (Lasix), and torsemide (Demadex).

When thiazide and loop diuretics work effectively, the patient may lose valuable potassium, so potassium is usually prescribed as a supplement to prevent imbalances that could lead to severe arrhythmias, seizures, and death. Although diuretics relieve heart failure symptoms and decrease blood pressure, they can also significantly disrupt the lives of patients by necessitating frequent trips to the bathroom. A patient may need assistance in planning activities around dosing.

Calcium channel blockers block calcium from passing into the heart muscle and the blood vessel walls. Calcium allows muscles and blood vessels to contract and narrow, thus increasing blood pressure. These medications decrease the level of contraction in the muscles in the arteries and trigger a series of responses: dilation of the arteries, decreased peripheral vascular resistance, reduced workload for the heart, and, ultimately, reduced blood pressure. Calcium channel blockers are used to treat angina and certain tachyarrhythmias, as well as hypertension. Drugs in this class that are indicated for the treatment of hypertension include amlodipine (Norvasc), diltiazem (Cardizem, Dilacor, Tiazac, Diltia XL), nifedipine (Procardia XL, Adalat), and verapamil hydrochloride (Isoptin, Calan, Verelan, Covera-HS). Additional calcium channel blocker medications are included in the Master the Essentials table.

Methods to decrease or regulate blood pressure without medications include losing weight, ceasing tobacco use, decreasing salt (sodium) intake, limiting alcohol, reducing stress, and exercising.

 CRITICAL THINKING

What do you think is the role of stress in hypertension?

Medications for Heart Failure

Chronic high blood pressure can place great stress on the heart muscle. The muscle can weaken and fail to push a normal amount of blood around the body, thus leading to a condition called **congestive heart failure (CHF).** When this happens, the kidneys do not receive enough blood, and fluid that would normally be flushed out of the body builds back up in the blood. This additional fluid puts even greater strain on the heart and leads to worsening heart failure.

Although CHF has no cure, some drugs can decrease the symptoms caused by the weakened heart muscle. Drugs used to treat heart failure include vasodilators, which decrease the amount of pressure the heart has to exert to pump blood through the vascular system, and cardiac glycosides, which help the heart to beat more strongly and more efficiently. ACE inhibitors, angiotensin receptor blockers, beta blockers, and diuretics, discussed earlier in the chapter, are also used for the treatment of CHF. They work to slow the heart rate, relax the blood vessels, and decrease the amount of blood that the heart has to push through the vascular system.

Signs and symptoms of CHF are anxiety, restlessness, cyanotic and clammy skin, tachycardia, lower leg edema, tachypnea, persistent cough, and a forward-leaning posture.

In addition to taking medications, patients can decrease their symptoms and risk for complications by smoking cessation, exercising, reducing weight, decreasing salt consumption, and minimizing stress. The nicotine in tobacco contracts the blood vessels and increases blood pressure. Exercise decreases stress and causes increased blood flow to the tissue. Reducing body fat reduces the workload required to move an overweight body. With salt goes water; therefore, if the patient retains salt, water is also retained. Increased fluid retention raises blood pressure. Decreasing stress reduces the fight-or-flight mechanism and thus lowers blood pressure.

Vasodilators

Vasodilators taken by mouth, such as isosorbide dinitrate (Dilatrate-SR, Iso-Bid, Isonate, Isorbid, Isordil, Isotrate, Sorbitrate), isosorbide mononitrate (IMDUR), and hydralazine (Apresoline), decrease oxygen demand on the heart by decreasing resistance in the vessels (vascular resistance), thereby making it easier for the heart to pump more effectively. In essence, blood vessels open, blood pressure drops, and there is less pressure on the heart. Phosphodiesterase inhibitors, a type of vasodilator, cause vasodilation and increase the force of contraction by blocking the enzyme phosphodiesterase.

Cardiac Glycosides

Cardiac glycosides, which are made up of three sugars, called glycosides, strengthen the heart's contractility. In a fight-or-flight situation, constricting peripheral blood vessels would reduce blood loss if injury occurred. However, this is not a desired effect in the presence of cardiovascular disease. Cardiac glycosides increase the strength of heart contractions, whereas other drugs relax the resistance in the peripheral vessels (reduce afterload). Therefore, combining these drugs makes the cardiovascular system more efficient. Cardiac glycosides such as digoxin (Cardoxin, Digetek, Lanoxicaps, Lanoxin) and digitoxin come from plants, such as purple and white foxglove (Drug Spotlight 16.2).

Drugs for Abnormal Heart Rhythms

Dysrhythmias (heart rhythm irregularities) can be caused by increased blood pressure, cardiac valve disease, coronary artery disease, decreased or increased potassium consumption, heart failure, diabetes mellitus, stroke, MI, and certain medications (Fast Tip 16.3).

Drug Spotlight 16-2 *Digoxin (Lanoxin)*

Availability and History	Tablet. Used since the 1700s; obtained from the foxglove plant; chemists have been able to obtain purified drug from the plant so that the dosage and additives can be controlled for better safety
Indications	Mainly for congestive heart failure
Action	Helps the heart to beat more slowly and more strongly
Adverse Reactions/ Side Effects	Nausea, vomiting, diarrhea, stomach pain, slow heart rate, greenish halo around lights are signs of toxicity
Contraindications/ Precautions	Digoxin has a narrow therapeutic window; therefore, checking blood levels routinely is necessary
Patient education	Must include checking the pulse before taking medication, and if less than 60 beats per minute, do not take medication and call prescriber; call physician if any symptoms of toxicity occur; have blood levels drawn as advised; bulk laxatives and antacids containing aluminum will decrease digoxin levels in body, so avoid these

Fast Tip 16.3 Do Not Miss Dysrhythmias

Be sure you accurately check a patient's pulse for 1 full minute so you do not miss a dysrhythmia that would prevent the patient from benefiting from medication therapy.

Drugs used to treat dysrhythmias are classified by how they act to improve the heart rhythm.

- Sodium channel blockers (Class I antiarrhythmics)
- Beta-adrenergic blockers (Class II antiarrhythmics)
- Potassium channel blockers (Class III antiarrhythmics)
- Calcium channel blockers (Class IV antiarrhythmics)

Each class of medications is described here.

Sodium Channel Blockers (Class I)

Sodium channel blockers slow the rate of electrical conduction by inhibiting sodium. Sodium is necessary to facilitate nerve impulses and muscular contraction. Blocking sodium transfer therefore inhibits irregular rhythms. Sodium also is the main contributor to osmotic pressure and hydration. Class I antiarrhythmic medications are used to treat those irregular heartbeats that originate above the ventricles; these are also called supraventricular rhythms. Some medications in Class I include flecainide (Tambocor™), propafenone (Rythmol), and quinidine (Cardioquin, Quinaglute Dura-Tabs, Quinidex). All these medications are taken orally. In the case of emergencies with a life-threatening ventricular arrhythmia, lidocaine (Xylocaine) may be administered via the IV route to decrease the sensitivity of the heart muscle.

Beta-Adrenergic Blockers (Class II)

Beta-adrenergic blockers slow electrical conduction in the heart and return the heart rhythm to normal. They can also be used to decrease oxygen demands for the heart by decreasing the fight-or-flight response. This is the same class of medications discussed earlier under medications that lower blood pressure. Some Class II medications include atenolol (Tenormin), esmolol, and propranolol (Inderal).

Potassium Channel Blockers (Class III)

Potassium channel blockers are very successful in treating both ventricular and supraventricular arrhythmias. Patients with internal defibrillators are prescribed this class of medications if they are at high risk for sudden cardiac arrest because these medications will reduce the occurrence and severity of arrhythmias. Potassium channel blockers change the heart rhythm by affecting potassium, a necessary element for contraction of cardiac muscle. If too much potassium is lost through the use of diuretics or a poor diet, the patient may need to take potassium supplements or eat foods high in potassium, such as oranges, sweet potatoes, and bananas. Examples of Class III antiarrhythmics include amiodarone (Cordarone), bepridil, bretylium tosylate, dofetilide (Tikosyn), ibutilide (Corvert), and solatol (Betapace).

Calcium Channel Blockers (Class IV)

As discussed earlier, calcium channel blockers block calcium ions, dilate heart vessels, and thus decrease the workload of the heart. This class of antiarrhythmics is generally used for patients with very rapid arrhythmias. The specific calcium channel blocker medications used for arrhythmias include diltiazem (Cardizem, Tiazac) and verapamil (Covera, Isoptin, Calan).

Medications for Shock

Shock is the collapse of the cardiovascular system, and it can be of cardiogenic origin (heart stops pumping), hypovolemic origin (loss of blood volume), neurogenic origin (central nervous system fails leading to vasodilation), or septic origin (invasion of a microorganism). Treatment of shock primarily targets the underlying causes, as well as supports the cardiovascular system while that cause is treated. Signs and symptoms of shock affect every portion of the body. In the early stages, the metabolism slows, causing the temperature to drop and the patient to complain of thirst. The skin becomes cold, clammy, and pale. Urine output diminishes because of the lack of circulating blood volume. As blood pressure lowers, the patient's heart rate becomes rapid and thready as the heart attempts to pump more blood to the periphery. Respirations become rapid and shallow. The patient experiences anxiety, confusion, lethargy, and restlessness because the lack of oxygen and blood affect the brain. If the process is not reversed, the heart will eventually stop pumping, and the patient will die.

Drug therapy for shock includes IV vasopressors such as epinephrine, norepinephrine (Levophed), and dopamine (Intropin) to increase blood pressure and inotropic drugs such as dobutamine (Dobutrex) to strengthen the contraction of the heart and increase cardiac output. In addition, IV antibiotics are used to treat the infection that caused septic shock, and plasma expanders such as albumin human (Albutein) may be administered by the IV route in the treatment of hypovolemic shock.

Anaphylactic shock is another type of shock caused by the body's overactive response to a threat such as an allergen. Signs and symptoms include breathing difficulty, bronchoconstriction, decreased cardiac output, edema, increased heart rate, hives, itching, and vasodilation. It is treated with the vasopressor epinephrine (EpiPen). Patients with life-threatening allergies are advised to carry their EpiPens with them at all times and administer an injection as needed. Epinephrine can also be given via injection or by the IV route by a health-care professional.

MEDICATIONS FOR LIPID DISORDERS

Many Americans have a diet that is high in fat. Excess fat can be deposited on or in the walls of the blood vessels to cause **hyperlipemia.** Plugged vessels can lead to atherosclerosis, hypertension, and CHF.

Not all lipids or fats are the same. **High-density lipoproteins (HDLs)** act as street sweepers and clean out blood vessels. **Low-density lipoproteins (LDLs)** are more like snowflakes, depositing fat in the vessels. **Very low-density lipoproteins (VLDLs)** are the worst fats. Because they are so small, they actually wedge themselves inside the blood vessel walls and are difficult to clear.

You can help your patients by teaching them about nonpharmacological approaches for managing lipidemia, such as those mentioned in Fast Tip 16.4.

Some patients' lipid and cholesterol levels remain elevated even after making dietary and lifestyle changes. These patients have a high genetic risk factor regardless of lifestyle. For these patients, HMG-CoA (3-hydroxy-3-methyl-glutaryl-coenzyme A) reductase inhibitors, commonly referred to as statins, decrease blood levels of lipids. These drugs encourage the liver to make less cholesterol and increase the number of LDL receptors in the liver. Increased LDL receptors grab the circulating LDL from the blood. Examples of HMG-CoA reductase inhibitors are atorvastatin (Lipitor), cerivastatin (Baycol), fluvastatin (Lescol, Lescol XL), lovastatin (Altocor, Altoprev, Mevacor), pitavastatin (Livalo), pravastatin (Pravachol), rosuvastatin (Crestor), and simvastatin (Zocor).

In patients who have very high cholesterol levels, these medications are often not sufficient and require the help of bile acid sequestrants to decrease serum lipid levels. Bile acid sequestrants such as cholestyramine (Questran, Questran Light, Prevalite, Cholestyramine Light, Locholest, Locholest Light), colesevelam (Welchol), and colestipol (Colestid, Colestid Flavored) lower LDL blood levels by forming complexes with bile acids and thus cause the liver to make more bile acids from cholesterol.

Fibric acid derivatives such as fenofibrate (Antara, Fenoglide, Lipofen, TriCor, Triglide), fenofibric acid (Tilipix, Fibricor), and gemfibrozil (Lopid) are used mainly to lower triglyceride levels by inhibiting

 Fast Tip 16.4   Nonpharmacological Treatment of Lipidemia

Nonpharmacological ways to decrease lipids include smoking cessation, decreasing dietary fats and cholesterol, avoiding stress, exercising, maintaining a healthy weight, and periodic blood cholesterol screening to gauge the patient's success.

the liver from producing VLDL. In addition, these medications help speed up the removal of triglycerides from the blood. Patients taking any of these medications to lower their lipid levels must have their liver function tested on a routine basis because of the associated risk for liver damage.

●●● SUMMARY

■ The cardiovascular system, consisting of the heart and blood vessels, delivers nutrients such as oxygen, hormones, and immune and clotting factors to every part of the body. The system also carries waste products such as carbon dioxide out of the cells.

■ The heart's four chambers, the left and right atrium and the left and right ventricles, contract and relax in a coordinated rhythm.

■ During the pulmonary circulation sequence, the rhythmic pumping of the heart sends blood to the lungs via the pulmonary artery to obtain oxygen. Oxygen-rich blood returns to the heart via the pulmonary veins.

■ The oxygenated blood is sent to the upper and lower parts of the body via the aorta, which subdivides into a system of arteries.

■ The blood, now depleted of oxygen and rich in carbon dioxide, returns to the heart via a network of veins, where it is pumped to the lungs to exchange the carbon dioxide for more oxygen.

■ Myocardial infarction (MI) or heart attack, cerebrovascular accident (CVA) or stroke, and clots all cause damage when blood flow is impeded to the chest, brain, or lungs.

■ Chest pain can be a symptom of a total lack of oxygen, called anoxia, or significantly reduced oxygen, called hypoxia, in the heart muscle.

■ Antianginal medications can decrease chest pain.

■ Anticoagulants interrupt the clotting process and ensure that blood flows smoothly through the vessels.

■ Antiplatelet medications prevent platelets from clumping together to form clots.

■ Thrombolytics dissolve clots that have already formed.

■ Antifibrinolytic medications help form clots to provide hemostasis.

■ Hematopoietic stimulant medications stimulate the growth of blood cells to treat anemias.

■ Antihypertensives reduce hypertension, which can lead to congestive heart failure (CHF). Antihypertensives include ACE inhibitors, angiotensin blockers, diuretics, and calcium channel blockers.

■ Vasodilators decrease oxygen demand on the heart.

■ Antiarrhythmics are used to treat dysrhythmias and restore normal rhythm.

■ Cardiac glycosides strengthen the heart's contractility.

■ Vasosuppressors and epinephrine treat the symptoms of shock.

■ Statins, bile acid sequestrants, and fibric acid derivatives are used to reduce the level of fats in the blood.

■ Many of the medications prescribed to treat disorders of the cardiovascular system have potent effects that can potentially damage internal organs and have serious side effects. Therefore, education of the patient is extremely important in preventing these problems.

Master the Essentials: Cardiovascular Medications

This table shows the various classes of cardiovascular medications and key side effects, contraindications and precautions, interactions, and examples of each class.

Class	Indications for Use	Side Effects	Contraindications and Precautions	Interactions	Examples
Nitrates	Angina	Blurred vision, dry mouth, flushing, headache, hypersensitivity reaction, postural hypotension	Severe anemia, GI disease, glaucoma, intracranial pressure, hypotension	Alcohol, Viagra	Nitroglycerin (Nitrolingual, Nitroquick, Nitrostat, Nitro-Bid, Nitro-Dur), nitroglycerin topical (Nitro-Bid or Nitrol Appli-Kit)
Anticoagulants	Prevention of heart attack and stroke by preventing blood clots in veins and arteries	Increased bleeding; blood irregularities; GI, liver, and kidney disease	Uncontrolled bleeding, heparin (an anticoagulant does not cross the placenta but is used during pregnancy with caution)	Acetaminophen, alcohol, anabolic steroids, anti-infectives, barbiturates, chloral hydrate, corticosteroids, estrogen, NSAIDs, tricyclic antidepressants, thyroid drugs	Warfarin (Coumadin), heparin, enoxaparin (Lovenox)
Antiplatelet agents	History of heart attack and/or stroke, to prevent further clots	Diarrhea, dizziness, flushing, headache, nausea, rash, vomiting, weakness	Other medications that increase bleeding	ACE inhibitors, anticoagulants, anticonvulsants, NSAIDs, beta blockers, diuretics, methotrexate, oral hypoglycemics	Aspirin, ticlopidine (Ticlid), clopidogrel (Plavix), abciximab (ReoPro), eptifibatide (Integrilin), tirofiban (Aggrastat)
Thrombolytics	Stroke symptoms, clotted central venous devices	Allergic reactions, bleeding, respiratory depression	Active bleeding, CVA within 2 months, recent intracranial or intraspinal surgery, intracranial neoplasm, uncontrolled hypertension	Antiplatelet agents, anticoagulants	**Tissue plasminogen activators (tPAs):** tenecteplase (TNKase), alteplase (Cathflo Activase), reteplase (Retavase)
Antifibrinolytics	Bleeding caused by aplastic anemia, cirrhosis of the liver, placental abruption, cancer	Allergic reaction, anaphylaxis, dyspnea, confusion, bradycardia, rash	Known hypersensitivity, active intravascular clotting	Oral contraceptives	Aminocaproic acid (Amicar), tranexamic acid (Cyklokapron)

Continued

Master the Essentials: Cardiovascular Medications—cont'd

Class	Indications for Use	Side Effects	Contraindications and Precautions	Interactions	Examples
Hematopoietics	Anemia	Gastric irritation, liquid iron preparations can stain teeth, allergic reactions	Known hypersensitivity, primary hemochromatosis, hemosiderosis, and hemolytic anemia (iron)	Antacids, tetracycline, H₂ blocker (iron); alcohol, neomycin, colchicines (vitamin B₁₂)	Ferrous sulfate (Feosol, Fer-in-Sol, Ferra-TD), cyanocobalamin (vitamin B₁₂)
ACE inhibitors	Hypertension	Blood irregularities, decreased blood pressure, light sensitivity, increased potassium, rash, decreased taste	Children (increased risk for side effects), collagen disease, kidney impairment, lactation, pregnancy, vessel swelling	Antacids, digoxin, diuretics, lithium, NSAIDs, vasodilators	Benazepril (Lotensin), captopril (Capoten), enalapril (Vasotec), fosinopril (Monopril), lisinopril (Prinivil, Zestril), moexipril (Univasc), perindopril (Aceon), quinapril (Accupril), ramipril (Altace), trandolapril (Mavik)
Beta-adrenergic blockers	Angina, hypertension, cardiac arrhythmias, acute MI	Bronchodilation, uterine relaxation, vasodilation	Bronchospasm, heart failure, heart block, bradycardia, some valvular diseases; use with caution in diabetes mellitus, lactation, liver disease, pregnancy	Bronchodilators, cimetidine, diabetes medications, digoxin	Acebutolol (Sectral), atenolol (Tenormin), betaxolol (Kerlone), bisoprolol (Zebeta), carvedilol (Coreg), esmolol, metoprolol (Toprol, Lopressor), nadolol (Corgard), nebivolol (Bystolic), propranolol (Inderal LA), timolol (Blocadren)
Diuretics	Hypertension, congestive heart failure, renal disease	Hypotension, hyponatremia, hypokalemia, anorexia, nausea	Known hypersensitivity, anuria, breastfeeding, pregnancy	Oral hypoglycemics, lithium, corticosteroids, cardiac glycosides, NSAIDs	**Thiazide diuretics:** bendroflumethiazide (Naturetin), chlorthalidone (Thalitone), chlorothiazide (Diuril, Diuril Sodium), hydrochlorothiazide (HydroDIURIL, Aquazide H, Esidrix, Microzide), indapamide (Lozol methyclothiazide (Aquatensen, Enduron), metolazone (Mykrox, Zaroxolyn), polythiazide (Renese) **Potassium-sparing diuretics:** amiloride (Midamor), spironolactone (Aldactone), triamterene (Dyrenium) **Loop diuretics:** bumetanide (Bumex), ethacrynic acid (Edecrin, Sodium Edecrin), furosemide (Lasix), torsemide (Demadex)

Class	Uses	Side effects	Contraindications	Interactions	Examples
Calcium channel blockers	Angina, hypertension	Hypotension, constipation, bradycardia, edema	Children, lactation, liver or kidney disease, pregnancy	ACE inhibitors, barbiturates, diuretics, lithium, rifampin, salicylates, sulfonamides	Amlodipine (Norvasc), diltiazem (Cardizem, Dilacor, Tiazac, Diltia XL), felodipine (Plendil), isradipine (Dynacirc), nicardipine (Cardene), nifedipine (Procardia XL, Adalat), nisoldipine (Sular), verapamil (Isoptin, Calan, Verelan, Covera-HS)
Phosphodiesterase inhibitors	Congestive heart failure	Arrhythmias, nausea, vomiting, headache, fever, chest pain, hypotension	Known hypersensitivity, severe aortic or pulmonic valvular disease	Disopyramide, potassium-wasting diuretics	Inamrinone (Inocor)
Cardiac glycosides	Congestive heart failure, arrhythmias	Arrhythmias, dizziness, electrolyte imbalances, GI upset, headache, irritability, lethargy, muscle weakness, tremors, seizures	Hypothyroidism, lactation, MI, pregnancy, impaired renal function; monitor for high or low potassium, irregular rhythm, severe bradycardia; if noted, discontinue drug	Adrenergics, antacids, antiarrhythmics, diuretics, neomycin, phenobarbital, rifampin, sulfa drugs	Digoxin (Cardoxin, Digetek, Lanoxicaps, Lanoxin), digitoxin
Angiotensin receptor blockers	Hypertension, vasodilation	Dizziness, upper respiratory tract infection, palpitations	Known hypersensitivity, volume depletion, children	Cimetidine, fluconazole, digoxin, phenobarbital	Candesartan (Atacand), eprosartan (Teveten), irbesartan (Avapro), losartan (Cozaar), olmesartan (Benicar), telmisartan (Micardis), valsartan (Diovan)
Sodium channel blockers	Ventricular and atrial arrhythmias	New or worsened arrhythmia, dizziness, nausea, headache, fatigue, palpitations, dyspnea	Breastfeeding, heart block, pregnancy, known hypersensitivity, severe renal or liver disease	Other antiarrhythmics, anticholinergics, digoxin, warfarin, cimetidine	Disopyramide (Norpace), flecainide (Tambocor), lidocaine (Xylocaine) (emergency IV use only), mexiletene (Mexitel), phenytoin (Dilantin), procainamide (Procainimide HCl, Procan, Procanabid, Pronestyl), propafenone (Rythmol), quinidine (Cardioquin, Quinaglute Dura-Tabs, Quinidex), tocainide (Tonocard)

Continued

Master the Essentials: Cardiovascular Medications—cont'd

Class	Indications for Use	Side Effects	Contraindications and Precautions	Interactions	Examples
Potassium channel blockers	Life-threatening ventricular arrhythmias	Hypotension, nausea, anorexia, malaise, fatigue, tremor, pulmonary toxicity	Known hypersensitivity, severe sinus node dysfunction, second- or third-degree heart block, severe aortic stenosis, severe pulmonary hypertension	Sympathomimetics, antihypertensives, warfarin, digoxin, procainamide	Amiodarone (Cordarone), bepridil, bretylium tosylate, dofetilide (Tikosyn), ibutilide (Convert), sotalol (Betapace)
Vasopressors	Hypotension	Angina, apnea, dyspnea, dizziness, headache, necrosis, pallor, palpitations, tremor, weakness, arrhythmias	Ventricular arrhythmias, hypoxia, acidosis	MAOIs, phenytoin, tricyclic antidepressants, oxytocic drugs	Epinephrine, norepinephrine (Levophed), dopamine (Intropin)
Inotropic agents	Cardiac decompensation	Increased blood pressure, increased heart rate, premature ventricular beats, allergic reactions	Hypersensitivity, caution with pregnancy and breastfeeding, children	Beta blockers, nitroprusside	Dobutamine (Dobutrex)
Vasodilators	Hypertension, angina pectoris	Nausea, vomiting, loss of appetite, diarrhea, constipation, headache, dizziness, anxiety, muscle or joint pain, runny or stuffy nose, mild itching or skin rash	Hypersensitivity, coronary artery disease, rheumatic heart disease	Dizoxide, MAOIs, erectile dysfunction medications	Isorbide dinitrate (Dilatrate-SR, Iso-Bid, Isonate, Isorbid, Isordil, Isotrate, Sorbitrate), isosorbide mononitrate (IMDUR), hydralazine (Apresoline)

HMG-CoA reductase inhibitors	Hyperlipidemia	Weakness, headache, abdominal pain, nausea, vomiting, constipation, diarrhea, myalgia, rash	Known hypersensitivity, liver disease, elevated liver enzymes, pregnancy, lactation	Itraconazole, erythromycin, protease inhibitors, nefazodone, cyclosporine, antacids, cimetidine	Atorvastatin (Lipitor), cerivastatin (Baycol), fluvastatin (Lescol, Lescol XL), lovastatin (Altocor, Altoprev, Mevacor), pitavastatin (Livalo), pravastatin (Pravachol), rosuvastatin (Crestor), simvastatin (Zocor)
Bile acid sequestrants	Hyperlipidemia	Constipation, abdominal pain, nausea, vomiting, headache, dizziness	Complete biliary obstruction, known hypersensitivity, pregnancy, lactation	Anticoagulants, corticosteroids, cardiac glycosides, iron	Cholestyramine (Questran, Questran Light, Prevalite, Cholestyramine Light, Locholest, Locholest Light), colesevelam (Welchol), colestipol (Colestid, Colestid Flavored)
Fibric acid derivatives	Hyperlipidemia	Hypersensitivity, adverse GI effects similar to bile acid sequestrants, arrhythmias, gallstones with prolonged use	Gallbladder disease, hepatic or renal dysfunction, pregnancy, peptic ulcer disease, breastfeeding	Anticoagulants, sulfonylureas	Clofibrate (Atromid-S), fenofibrate (Antara, Fenoglide, Lipofen, Lofibra, TriCor, Triglide), fenofibric acid (Tilipix, Fibricor), gemfibrozil (Lopid)

ACE, angiotensin-converting enzyme; CVA, cerebrovascular accident; GI, gastrointestinal; HMG-CoA, 3-hydroxy-3-methyl-glutaryl-coenzyme A; MAOI, monoamine oxidase inhibitor; MI, myocardial infarction; NSAID, nonsteroidal anti-inflammatory drug.

Activities

To make sure that you have learned the key points covered in this chapter, complete the following activities.

True or False
Write true if the statement is true. Beside the false statements, write false, and correct the statement to make it true.

1. Anticoagulents increase clot formation. _____

_____

2. Antianginals destroy clots. _____

_____

3. HDLs are the best kind of lipids. _____

_____

4. Diet can decrease blood lipid levels. _____

_____

5. Infarction is tissue death. _____

_____

Multiple Choice
Choose the best answer for each question.

1. Which keep platelets from aggregating and forming clots?
   A. Anticoagulants
   B. Antiplatelets
   C. Antifibrinolytics
   D. Thrombolytics

2. Aspirin is an _____.
   A. Antipyretic
   B. Anticoagulant
   C. Analgesic
   D. All of the above

3. Which are used to treat hypertension?
   A. Anticoagulants
   B. Diuretics
   C. Anti-infectives
   D. Thrombolytics

4. **Which drug is indicated within 60 minutes of the onset of stroke symptoms?**
    A. Digoxin
    B. Lasix
    C. tPA
    D. Cozaar

5. **Antihypertensives include which of the following?**
    A. ACE inhibitors
    B. Calcium channel blockers
    C. Beta blockers
    D. A and B

6. **Nicotine has what effect on blood pressure?**
    A. Decreases
    B. Increases
    C. Has no effect
    D. Stabilizes

7. **Digoxin has been in use since the _____.**
    A. 1400s
    B. 1500s
    C. 1600s
    D. 1700s

8. **Dysrhythmias can be caused by all of the following EXCEPT _____.**
    A. Hypertension
    B. Cardiac disease
    C. Potassium level alterations
    D. Hernia

9. **All of the following are types of lipids EXCEPT _____.**
    A. HDL
    B. CDL
    C. LDL
    D. VLDL

10. **Which of the following does not affect blood pressure?**
    A. Heart rate
    B. Stroke volume
    C. Peripheral resistance
    D. Temperature

Respond to the following situations.

1. Sherrie has just had a stroke. Although she agrees to take the medications the physician prescribes, she asks you what behaviors she could adopt to reduce the risk for another stroke. What would you teach her? _____

_____

_____

2. Henry has just been given a prescription for Lipitor. Does he need to make lifestyle changes?

_____

_____

3. Richard has just been hospitalized for a pulmonary embolism. He wants to know why he has to wear such tight stockings and also take medications. What would you tell him about his antiembolic stockings and medication therapy? _____

_____

_____

4. Anthony has congestive heart failure. He has been prescribed Digoxin. What are some of the symptoms to watch for closely as an indication of toxicity? _____

_____

_____

5. Barbara has been prescribed a diuretic and is now having heart arrhythmias. She asks why this is happening and what she can do to prevent this. What would you tell her? _____

_____

_____

Essentials Review

For further study and practice with drug classifications learned in this chapter, complete the following table to the best of your ability. Use resources such as the *PDR,* the Internet, or printed drug guides for help.

Classification	Purpose	Side Effects	Contraindications and Precautions	Examples	Patient Education
Anticoagulants					
Antiplatelet agents					
ACE inhibitors					
Diuretics					
Calcium channel blockers					
Vasopressors					

ACE, angiotensin-converting enzyme.

1. Visit the American Heart Association website (www.heart.org), and find a support group for heart patients in your area and information that will allow you to create an educational tool to decrease behaviors that could lead to heart attacks.

2. Search the Internet for a list of side effects of cancer medications on blood cells. Print the list, and bring it to class for discussion.

3. Locate a drug information website, and record the classifications of the following drugs: Lasix, Apresoline, Lanoxin, Nitrobid, Zocar, Streptase, Plavix, Inderal, quinidine, and heparin sodium.

Immunological System Medications

A healthy immune system means a healthy body. The immunological system protects the body from disease. Specialized cells attack invading microbes and then eliminate the damaged cells. Most often, medications are used to enhance or strengthen the body's immune system; however, at other times, drugs are used to suppress an immune response, such as in allergic reactions and rejection of transplanted organs. Educating patients and their families about these medications and their possible complications will ensure safety for all: the health professional, the patient, and the family.

LEARNING OUTCOMES

At the end of this chapter, you should be able to:

17.1 Define key terms.

17.2 Discuss five categories of anti-inflammatory medications, when they are used, and their actions in the body.

17.3 Differentiate among the five classifications of anti-infectives, and describe when each is used and their actions in the body.

17.4 Compare natural and acquired immunity and how they occur.

17.5 Identify at least three types of antineoplastic medications, and describe when each is used and their actions in the body.

17.6 Discuss the toxic effects of antineoplastic medications on patients and health-care workers, including the proper handling of both medications and patients' secretions.

KEY TERMS

Active artificial immunity
Active natural immunity
Aerobe
Anaerobes
Antibodies
Antigen
Autoimmune
Bactericidal

Bacteriostatic
Benign
Chemotherapy
Culture and sensitivity
  (C & S)
Host
Inflammation
Malignant

Metastasis
Nosocomial
Passive artificial
  immunity
Passive natural
  immunity
Pathogenic
Superinfection

■ THE IMMUNE RESPONSE

When microbes or other **antigens** (foreign substance) invade the body, the body responds by attacking the antigen. The natural response against any microbial invasion is **inflammation,** which helps limit the spread of microbes or injury (Fig. 17-1). The four signs of inflammation are redness, swelling, heat, and pain. Several phases occur during this attack.

The first response occurs at the site of the invasion (e.g., a cut), where chemicals are released, such as bradykinin (a vasodilator that causes pain), complement, (a protein that destroy antigens), and three chemicals released by mast cells: histamine and leukotrienes, both of which cause smooth muscle contraction, blood vessel dilation, and itching; and prostaglandins, which increase capillary permeability, attract leukocytes to the inflammation site, and increase pain.

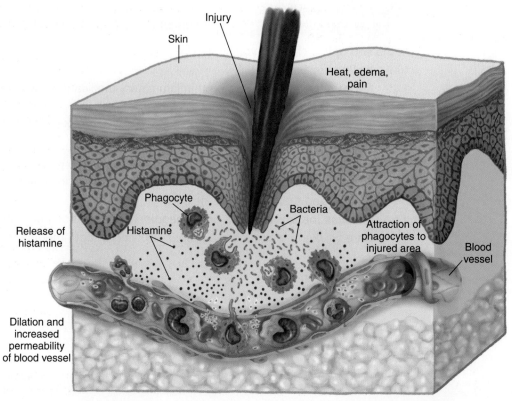

FIGURE 17-1: The inflammatory response. When bacteria or other antigens invade the body, the first response is inflammation, which helps limit the spread of the invading microorganisms.

The second phase occurs as the immune system launches an attack throughout the body by secreting **antibodies** (immunoglobins that fight antigens) that are specific to the invading antigen. During this phase phagocytic cells are sent to the site of infection. These cells protect the body by ingesting any foreign bodies, bacteria or dead and dying cells, that are harmful to the body.

Additionally, some B cells (memory cells) record the attack and help guard against those particular microbes if they enter the body again. Vaccines are administered to encourage the production of these memory cells.

T cells (CD cells) are lymphocytes and do not produce antibodies but instead create cytokines. Some cytokines create inflammation, and others attack the invader directly.

MEDICATIONS THAT AFFECT THE IMMUNE SYSTEM

Medications are used to support or inhibit the immune response, depending on the patient's condition. Various anti-inflammatory medications may be given to suppress the immune response when a patient is faced with allergies, asthma attacks, or autoimmune disorders. Anti-infective medications may be given to combat bacterial infections. Antitoxin, antifungal, antiviral, and antiparasitic medications fight off other invading microorganisms. Vaccines are given from birth to very old age in an effort to prevent microorganisms from causing disease. The last category of medication discussed in this chapter comprises antineoplastic medications, more commonly known as chemotherapy. Chemotherapy is used to combat cancer (see the Master the Essentials table for descriptions of the most common immunological system drugs).

Anti-Inflammatory Medications

Anti-inflammatory medications shut off or reduce the body's inflammatory response. They may be used in patients with **autoimmune** disorders, in which the body's immune system attacks itself and must be stopped to halt the damage caused by this attack. Examples of autoimmune disorders include ankylosing spondylitis, rheumatoid arthritis, ulcerative colitis, Crohn's disease, dermatitis, type 1 diabetes mellitus, glomerulonephritis, Hashimoto's thyroiditis, multiple sclerosis, peptic ulcers, and systemic lupus erythematosus.

Allergies are an overresponse of the body's defense to substances (allergens) that may not be an actual threat to the body. Examples of sensitizing substances are pollen, animal dander, mold, mildew, dust, and cigarette smoke. Patients may also have allergic reactions to food or medications.

Signs and symptoms of a mild allergy, such as allergic rhinitis, are sneezing, nasal congestion, and watery eyes. Patients who have serious reactions, such as anaphylactic shock (the most serious reaction), may experience urticaria (hives), swelling, itching, or difficulty breathing, all of which can be fatal if the patient is not given immediate, proper treatment. Medications used to treat allergic reactions include antihistamines, glucocorticoids, nasal decongestants, nonsteroidal anti-inflammatory drugs (NSAIDs), and immunosuppressants.

Antihistamines

Antihistamines, such as diphenhydramine (Benadryl), loratadine (Claritin, Tavist), and cetirizine (Zyrtec), block the histamine response (allergy symptoms) and thereby decrease swelling, itching, and congestion. All these medications are routinely taken by mouth for allergy symptoms associated with seasonal and environmental allergies. In addition, diphenhydramine can be administered by the intravenous (IV) route for severe allergic reactions. These medications are also referred to as H_1-receptor antagonists. The effects include relaxation of the respiratory, vascular, and gastrointestinal (GI) smooth muscle.

Glucocorticoids

Glucocorticoids are steroid-like compounds that suppress the body's inflammatory response. Glucocorticoids such as beclomethasone (Beconase), budesonide (Entocort), and fluticasone (Flovent) are administered intranasally to combat allergic rhinitis. Medications such as hydrocortisone are administered topically for minor inflammation. Methylprednisolone is a medication that is given systemically, usually in IV form, for acute or severe inflammation such as in spinal cord injury. Because of the serious side effects and danger of long-term suppression of the immune system, glucocorticoids must be used only as prescribed and discontinued gradually. (For a more complete list of glucocorticoids commonly used, please refer to the Master the Essentials table.)

Nasal Decongestants

Nasal decongestants such as tetrahydrozoline nasal (Tyzine Nasal) can alleviate nasal congestion intranasally by drying secretions. Nasal decongestants such as phenylpropanolamine are taken orally to produce the desired effects. They cause vasoconstriction on the adrenergic receptors in the nose by affecting the sympathetic tone of the blood vessels. The mucous membranes shrink as a result, thereby promoting drainage. These medications are typically used for only 3 to 5 days; otherwise, "rebound" nasal congestion occurs, and the patient continues to suffer.

Nonsteroidal Anti-Inflammatory Drugs

NSAIDs are by definition medications that reduce inflammation and do not contain steroids. They are the most common treatments for inflammation. In addition, NSAIDs also have antipyretic (fever reduction) and analgesic (pain reduction) properties. They accomplish these effects by inhibiting prostaglandin synthesis. Prostaglandins are substances responsible for producing inflammation, fever, and pain. NSAIDs such as ibuprofen (Advil, Motrin) and naproxen (Aleve, Naprosyn) can be purchased over the counter (OTC) and are taken by mouth. Other oral NSAIDs such as diclofenac (Zorvolex) and celecoxib (Celebrex) are available by prescription only for the treatment of conditions such as arthritis. Ketorolac (Toradol) is an NSAID that is given by the IV route for moderate to severe pain. As with all medications, NSAIDs must be taken as directed. Many medications in this class have similar mechanisms, but the patient's response varies. A patient may respond poorly to one NSAID but report great relief from another.

Immunosuppressants

Immunosuppressants are typically used for long-term therapy of inflammatory diseases, such as rheumatoid arthritis, psoriasis, and Crohn's disease. Rheumatoid arthritis is treated with immunosuppressants such as azathioprine (Imuran, Azasan) and cyclosporine (Neoral, Sandimmune, and Gengraf). Psoriasis (see Chapter 11) is treated with cyclosporine and sirolimus (Rapamune) for a short time (up to several months), alternating with other therapies. Crohn's disease is treated with oral doses of azathioprine (Imuran, Azasan). Corticosteroids are sometimes prescribed for short periods of time to speed up the suppression of the immune system and thus the healing process in inflammatory diseases. Because long-term suppression of the immune system renders the body vulnerable to infection and certain cancers, the immunosuppressants listed here are used on a long-term basis only to prevent or treat rejection in relation to organ transplants.

Anti-Infective Medications

Anti-infective medications are classified by their mechanisms of action or chemical structure. They target the processes of the **pathogenic** (disease-causing) microorganism. Some medications target protein synthesis, others inhibit DNA or RNA synthesis, and still others destroy the cell wall. Anti-infective medications include antibiotics, antitoxins, and antifungal, antiviral, and antiparasitic medications. These medications are discussed in the following subsections.

Antibiotics

Antibiotics are prescribed to treat bacterial infections. Bacterial organisms have special characteristics: they do not require a **host** (e.g., person or animal) to reproduce, they can change or mutate, and all are potentially vulnerable to antibiotics. Bacteria are characterized and named based on their shapes and ability to retain stains, either gram negative or gram positive (A Closer Look 17.1). Common antibiotic categories include penicillins, cephalosporins, tetracyclines, macrolides, and aminoglycosides. A broad-spectrum antibiotic, one that is effective against many types of bacteria, is prescribed if the bacteria have not yet been identified.

    One drawback of antibiotics is that when they kill the bacteria, they also kill healthy or normal flora that are usually present in the human body and are beneficial in helping us fight off infection and in aiding digestion. When these healthy bacteria are destroyed, a **superinfection** can arise. In other words,

CHECK UP 17.1

Review the following Immune Response terms, and explain how each contributes to the immune response.

1. B-cells _____

2. T-cells _____

3. Phagocytes _____

4. Mast cells _____

5. Histamine _____

6. Leukotrienes _____

7. Prostaglandins _____

A CLOSER LOOK 17.1: All About Bacteria

Bacteria are characterized by their shape, how they stain, and whether they need oxygen to survive (Fig. 17-2).

Shape. Bacteria shaped like rods are called bacilli. An example of a rod-shaped bacterium is gonorrhea. Bacteria shaped like spheres are called cocci. Strep throat is caused by streptococci. Spiral-shaped bacteria are called spirilla. Syphilis and Lyme disease are illnesses caused by spirilla.

Coccus

Coccobacillus

Bacillus

Spirillum

FIGURE 17-2: Bacteria shapes.

Staining. When stained with violet dye in the laboratory, some bacteria with thick cell walls hold onto the purple color (Fig. 17-3). They are known as gram-positive bacteria. Those with thinner walls do not retain the stain and so are called gram-negative bacteria. Different medications are used for these two types.

Continued

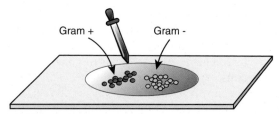

FIGURE 17-3: Gram stains.

Oxygen. Some bacteria like to live in oxygen-rich environments (e.g., the lungs), and others do not. Oxygen-loving microbes are known as **aerobes.** Those that prefer to live without oxygen are **anaerobes.** They inhabit other parts of the body (e.g., gastrointestinal tract), where oxygen is not as prevalent as it is in the lungs.

the normal flora that helps us fight off infection is destroyed, and a new infection occurs. One of the most common examples of this is when a woman is taking antibiotics and the normal flora in the vagina is destroyed, allowing a yeast infection to occur. Thus, not only does she have the original infection to treat, but also the yeast infection, which requires a different antifungal medication.

Because of the wide range of bacteria, it is vital to prescribe the correct antibiotic. A **culture and sensitivity (C & S)** test can help determine which microorganism is present and which antibiotic would be most effective against it (Fig. 17-4). Once the laboratory has these test results, the broad-spectrum antibiotic may be changed to one that is more suitable. Antibiotics may be either **bactericidal** (kill bacteria), such as penicillins, or **bacteriostatic** (inhibit growth), such as tetracyclines.

Penicillins

Penicillins such as ampicillin, amoxicillin (Amoxil), and penicillin are among the oldest antibiotics. They have been used in various forms since World War II. These medications are used orally, topically, and via injection to treat many common infections, such as strep throat and otitis media. They kill gram-positive and gram-negative bacteria by destroying cell walls (A Closer Look 17.2). Because of the length of time they have been in use, they tend to be the least expensive antibiotics available. Unfortunately, many people are allergic to the penicillins, so other, more expensive antibiotics are needed. (For a more extensive list of penicillin medications, see the Master the Essentials table.)

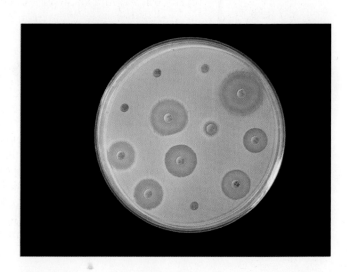

FIGURE 17-4: Disk diffusion method. Disks infused with antibiotics are placed on the culture plate to determine which antibiotic will be most effective in killing the bacteria. Clear spaces around the disk represent those antibiotics that are effective against growth of the microorganism.

Cephalosporins

Cephalosporins are similar to penicillins. They are more expensive but are useful for people who cannot tolerate penicillins. Cephalosporins are organized into four generations, based on their activity: First-generation cephalosporins such as cefazolin (Ancef, Kefzol) and cefadroxil are used mainly for patients who are allergic to penicillin. They act against gram-positive bacteria such as group B streptococci, which can cause pneumonia. Second-generation cephalosporins such as cefprozil and cefuroxime (Zinacef) are commonly used to treat **nosocomial** (infection acquired in a health-care facility) pneumonia and pelvic or intra-abdominal infections. Third-generation cephalosporins such as ceftriaxone (Rocephin) and ceftizoxime (Cefizox) act against gram-negative bacteria such as *Escherichia coli* (*E. coli*), a common cause of intestinal illnesses. Fourth-generation cephalosporins such as cefepime (Maxipime) are given by the IV route for severe nosocomial surgical infections.

This group of medications is used to both treat and prevent infections in many patients. The use of alcohol or alcohol-containing substances should be avoided during treatment because of associated abdominal side effects.

A CLOSER LOOK 17.2: Drug-Resistant Bacteria

Sometimes a specific bacterium is resistant to antibiotics and is therefore difficult to treat. Resistance to antibiotics occurs when a bacterium becomes weakened but does not die. The bacterium may then develop an ability to resist this antibiotic the next time it is given. This situation occurs when a medication is not taken for the full time it is ordered. Examples of drug-resistant bacteria that may be encountered are methicillin-resistant *Staphylococcus aureus* (MRSA), vancomycin-resistant *Staphylococcus aureus* (VRSA), and vancomycin-resistant *Enterococcus* (VRE).

Tetracyclines

Tetracyclines were commonly used during the 1950s and 1960s, but many bacteria have since become resistant to them. The main function of this class of medication is to prevent bacteria from making protein (protein synthesis), which interrupts the reproduction of bacteria. Tetracyclines such as doxy-cycline (Vibramycin), minocycline (Solodyn), and tetracycline (achromycin V) are useful against both gram-negative and gram-positive microbes that cause bacterial infections such as gonorrhea, chlamydia, anthrax, and urinary tract infections. These medications are not used in children or pregnant women because permanent staining occurs on the teeth of the child or fetus.

Macrolides

Macrolides such as erythromycin (E.E.S. Granules, Ery-Tab, Erythrocin Stearate Filmtab), clarithromycin (Biaxin), and azithromycin (Zithromax, Zithromax Z-Pak) are prescribed both orally and by injection for infections that are resistant to penicillins. These drugs function by inhibiting the bacterium's protein synthesis. These classes of medications are used for upper and lower respiratory tract infections, skin infections, pertussis, diphtheria, pelvic inflammatory disease, syphilis, Legionnaires' disease, strep throat, sinus infections, chronic bronchitis, pneumonia, and otitis media.

Aminoglycosides

Aminoglycosides such as amikacin (Amikin), gentamicin (Cidomycin, Garamycin, Septopal), kanamycin (Kantrex), neomycin (Mycifradin, Neo-Fradin, Neo-Tab), paromomycin (Humatin, Paromycin), and tobramycin (Nebcin, Tobi) are more toxic than other antibiotics. They are ideal against aerobic gram-negative bacteria such as *Pseudomonas,* which require oxygen to grow, mycobacteria (tuberculosis), and some protozoans, which are one-celled organisms. Aminoglycosides are administered topically via ointments, eye or ear drops, or as an IV injection. Patients taking aminoglycosides systemically should have blood levels of the antibiotic monitored periodically for efficacy and toxicity. These medications are used only when no other suitable anti-infective is available, because of the risks for damage to the patient's hearing and kidney function.

Quinolones

Quinolones such as ciprofloxacin (Cipro) and ofloxacin (Floxin) are bacteriostatic (Drug Spotlight 17.1). Quinolone medications are considered broad-spectrum antibiotics because they are effective against a wide variety of microorganisms. In view of some very serious, although rare, side effects such as ruptured tendons, these medications tend to be reserved for more antibiotic resistant strains of bacteria. These drugs can be given by the IV route, ophthalmically, or orally. Oral quinolones are very useful in the treatment of chronic urinary tract infections. (Refer to the Master the Essentials table for a more complete list of quinolone medications.)

Sulfonamides

Sulfonamides are among the earliest classes of antibiotics. Drugs such as sulfadiazine, sulfamethizole (Thiosulfil Forte), sulfamethoxazole (Gantanol), sulfasalazine (Azulfidine), and sulfisoxazole (Gantrisin), as well as combination sulfonamide medications such as trimethoprim-sulfamethoxazole (Septra, Bactrim) and erythromycin-sulfisoxazole (Pediazole), are used to kill bacteria by interrupting their metabolism. Because these "sulfa drugs" tend to collect in the bladder before they are excreted, they are very effective in treating urinary tract infections. Many patients are allergic to sulfonamides and develop various severities of skin reactions, liver and kidney injuries, breathing difficulties, and decreased levels of red blood cells, white blood cells, and platelets. For this reason, it is important to pay close attention to any history of a sulfonamide antibiotic allergy when administering medications.

Antituberculosis Agents

Tuberculosis antibiotics treat the disease caused by *Mycobacterium tuberculosis,* which mainly affects the lungs. Tuberculosis was very well controlled until the 1980s, when the appearance of acquired immunodeficiency syndrome (AIDS) preceded a resurgence of the disease related to the increased numbers of patients with compromised immune systems. Tuberculosis is treated with a mixture of two to four daily medications simultaneously for up to 1 year. Each drug eradicates the mycobacterium in a different way. One of the medications is cycloserine (Seromycin), which prevents the tuberculosis bacteria from growing in the body. Rifampin (Rifadin, Rimactane) is another antibiotic commonly used to treat or prevent tuberculosis. This medication has one unique side effect of which patients and health-care workers must be aware: it turns body secretions, including sweat, tears, urine, feces, and saliva, red orange. If the patient wears contact lenses, this drug will permanently stain them. In addition, rifampin may render hormonally based birth control ineffective. (See the Master the Essentials table for a more complete list of antituberculosis agents.)

Antitoxins

Many bacterial diseases are caused by the toxins that the bacteria produce. Diphtheria, tetanus, and botulism are toxin-related diseases. Antitoxins are antibodies that are created in response to specific toxins. The antitoxins are able to counteract that toxin in a person at high risk for the disease or

---

Drug Spotlight 17-1 *Cipro (ciprofloxacin hydrochloride)*

Definition	Anti-infective used for bacterial infections; approved for use in patients exposed to the inhaled form of anthrax; used by thousands because of the anthrax by letter attacks in Washington, DC, Florida, and New York in 2001
Side effects	CNS effects: dizziness, confusion, tremors, hallucinations, depression; allergic reactions; pain or rupture of tendon; severe inflammation of the colon; increased sensitivity to sunlight
Special considerations	FDA discourages widespread use because of the risk of the development of drug-resistant microorganisms

CNS, central nervous system; FDA, Food and Drug Administration.
  From Information on Cipro (Ciprofloxacin Hydrochloride) for Inhalation Anthrax for Consumers: Questions and Answers (11/14/2001). U.S. Department of Health and Human Services, Washington, DC, 2001.

condition. For example, an antitoxin is given to a person who has been exposed to a toxin but who does not have adequate immunity to combat the toxin-producing bacteria. An example is a landscaper who received a puncture wound while mowing lawns. Because *Clostridium tetani* live in soil and a puncture wound could conceivably allow the soil and bacteria into his body, he is at risk of developing a life-threatening tetanus infection. He should be administered the tetanus vaccine booster, but this will not provide immediate protection against the invasion. For that, he may receive a tetanus immune globulin (Baytet, HyperTET S/D) injection to provide immediate neutralization of the tetanus toxin (tetanospasmin) in his system with antibodies specific to the toxin.

Antifungal Medications

Antifungal medications treat fungal infections such as tinea pedis (commonly known as athlete's foot) or candidiasis (yeast infection). Fungi can live on the skin or inside the body. Unlike bacteria, fungi can be single-cell organisms or multicellular organisms with a complex structure. The human body can usually fight off fungal infections. Patients whose immune system is compromised by the human immunodeficiency virus (HIV), other microbes, or medical treatments are especially vulnerable to fungal infections.

Topical antifungal medications such as ketoconazole (Extina, Nizoral) and miconazole (Desenex, Micatin) can treat fungal infections on the skin such as athlete's foot. If the infection is in the oral and GI mucosa (a condition known as thrush), the medication nystatin (Mycostatin) is used because it is not absorbed but coats the mouth and stomach. If the fungi are growing in the body, or if skin infections are worsening, systemic antifungal medications such as fluconazole (Diflucan), itraconazole (Sporanox), and ketoconazole (Nizoral) are given to combat the infection. These systemic medications can be given orally or as an injection. Amphotericin B (Fungizone) is an IV medication reserved for potentially life-threatening fungal infections such as histoplasmosis, which can affect the lungs and other organs. The side effects of Fungizone are very serious and can affect the kidney, liver, blood counts, and electrolytes.

Medications that Fight Viruses

Viruses are microorganisms that require a host to reproduce themselves. Hosts can be humans, plants, or animals. Viruses, which are smaller than other microorganisms, insert their genetic material into this host and take over the host's cells to use them as a breeding facility. AIDS, cytomegalovirus (CMV) infection, rabies, smallpox, chickenpox, shingles, influenza, the common cold, and herpes are all caused by viruses. Even some types of cancer have been linked to viruses. The human body reacts to most viruses by developing antibodies to fight the invading microorganisms naturally. When the body needs help to fight off a viral infection, antiviral and antiretroviral medications are used. The choice is based on the type of virus infecting the patient.

Antiviral Medications

Antiviral therapy is the use of medications to inhibit the reproduction of a virus. Antiviral therapy is difficult because viruses replicate (reproduce) and mutate rapidly. Unlike antibiotics that kill the invader, antiviral drugs eliminate the materials that the virus needs to reproduce and flourish. This can be done in several ways. The virus can be blocked from entering the host cell, thus preventing the implantation of the virus DNA. Some antiviral medications target the enzymes and proteins the virus needs to replicate and function properly. Another way the virus is stopped is by strengthening the host's ability to fight the infections. Antiviral medications such as acyclovir (Acivir, Acivirax, Cyclovir, Herpex, Zovirax, and Zovir) are used to treat the viruses that cause herpes, chickenpox, and shingles. Zanamivir (Relenza) and oseltamivir (Tamiflu) are used to treat influenza type A and B. Also used to treat influenza type A is amantadine (Symmetrel). Relenza is an inhaled medication, whereas Tamiflu is an oral medication. CMV infection of the eye associated with AIDS and the smallpox virus can be treated with cidofovir. Ribavirin (Virazole) is use in fighting the hepatitis C virus and respiratory syncytial virus (RSV).

Antiretroviral Medications

Antiretroviral medications refer specifically to a group of medications used to fight retroviruses such as HIV. Retroviruses are different in that they have an RNA blueprint. The name implies that they use RNA to synthesize DNA, which is the opposite of the normal process. This allows genetic material from a retrovirus to become a permanent part of the genes of an infected cell. This embedding of the retrovirus into the genetic material makes it difficult to combat. HIV specifically attacks the assembling T4, or CD4, cells. Because these cells are the body's defensive soldiers, the host is rendered powerless to fight reproduction of the HIV. The term *HIV* is also used to refer to the virus's presence in the body. When the virus grows stronger and lowers T4 cell levels significantly, the patient develops AIDS. At this point, the patient begins to suffer from many viral, bacterial, and fungal infections. Therefore, the key is to prevent or delay this development as long as possible with the use of antiretroviral medications. Because HIV mutates easily, it is imperative that patients with AIDS take several medications according to a specific regimen to fight the retrovirus, prevent its reproduction, and protect their own immune system. These medications are classified according to where in the RNA-to-DNA process they are effective and include the following: nucleoside reverse transcriptase inhibitors (NRTIs), nonnucleoside reverse transcriptase inhibitors (NNRTIs), protease inhibitors (PIs), fusion inhibitors, entry inhibitors, and HIV integrase strand transfer inhibitors. (The Master the Essentials table includes more detail on these medications.)

Antiparasitic Medications

Parasites are organisms that live on or in another organism (host) and that often cause diseases. Common parasitic diseases include malaria, ascariasis (roundworm infection), pediculosis (lice infestation), and scabies. Although some parasitic diseases (e.g., malaria) are not commonly contracted in North America because of the cooler climate, purified drinking water, and advanced septic systems, knowing the types of medications used to treat them is important because you may encounter a patient who, for instance, develops a parasitic disease after traveling abroad. The following classes of medications are used to treat parasitic infections and disease.

- Antimalarials: Antimalarial medications such as atovaquone/proguanil (Malarone), chloroquine (Aralen), mefloquine (Lariam), and primaquine are taken to prevent a patient from contracting malaria as well as to treat the disease. These medications work by inhibiting the growth of the malaria parasite in the red blood cells of the body. To prevent malaria, these medications should be combined with the use of personal protection, such as long sleeves and pants and insect repellent.

- Antiprotozoals: Protozoan microorganisms differ from bacteria and fungi in that they do not have a cell wall. Therefore, the antibiotics effective against bacteria have very little effect on protozoans. Medications such as metronidazole (Flagyl, Metro I.V.) and trimethoprim-sulfamethoxazole (Bactrim, Septra, Sulfatrim) are given orally or by the IV route to combat vaginal infections such as trichomonas, giardiasis (infection of the intestines), and *Pneumocystis carinii* (causes pulmonary disease). These medications disrupt the strands of DNA and thus prevent the reproduction of this infection. Metronidazole is also the drug of choice in giardiasis (infection of the intestines).

- Anthelmintics: Tapeworms, roundworms, and flukes are all treated with anthelmintics, which affect the nervous system of the worm and paralyze it or prevent the worm from absorbing glucose. Tapeworms do not enter the tissue of their host and are treated with albendazole (Albenza) and praziquantel (Biltricide) orally. Roundworms enter the tissue and thus are more difficult to kill. Ivermectin (Stromectol) is prescribed for the treatment of roundworms. Mebendazole (Vermox), pyrantel (Antiminth, Ascarel), and praziquantel (Biltricide) are given orally for the treatment of hookworms, whipworms, pinworms, and flukes.

- Pediculicides: Lice are parasites that live on the blood found on the body, scalp, and pubic area. Head lice spread easily among children who are in close proximity during play. Body lice is the only type known to spread disease, and this type is spread through close contact in crowded conditions, such as seen with homeless people. Pubic lice are spread through sexual contact. Treatment consists of shampoos and lotions that either attack the nervous system of the louse or suffocate them. These medications containing permethrin (Acticin, Elimite, and Nix), piperonyl butoxide/pyrethrins (Licide, RID), and spinosa (Natroba) can be purchased OTC without a prescription. Prescription lotions and shampoos include malathion (Ovide), benzyl alcohol lotion (Ulesfia), and lindane. All treatment for lice must include treatment of close contacts, as well as cleaning of bedding and any clothing or hair care items used on the patient.

- Scabicides: Scabies are caused by itch mites that burrow in the webbing of the fingers and toes, as well as the axillary area. They are spread by skin-to-skin contact, sometimes as brief as a handshake. Medication consists of topical pesticide lotions such as crotamiton (Eurax), lindane, and permethrin (Acticin, Elimite). It is again important to clean the bedding because the mite can live for a period when not on the body.

CHECK UP 17.2

Review what you have learned. What is the mechanism of action of each of the anti-infective category of medications (how do they treat the infection)?

1. Antibiotics

2. Antitoxins

3. Antifungals

4. Antivirals

5. Antiparasitics

Vaccines

Vaccines offer immunity from a disease (Check Up 17.1). The two types of immunity are natural and acquired. Natural immunity is the ability humans have to resist infection through normal body functions. The natural immune system can respond immediately to invasion by any pathogen. Prior exposure to the foreign substance is not required. Acquired immunity occurs in a variety of ways. **Active natural immunity** is created when a microbe invades the body, and the body learns to fight it, such as the childhood disease chickenpox. Once a child contracts the disease, he or she will develop antibodies to fight it, and those antibodies will remain in the system to guard against any further attacks. This immunity is permanent. **Passive natural immunity** results from the transfer of antibodies from one person to a nonimmune person; for example, when a mother passes her immunity to her fetus through the placenta. This mother to fetus immunity generally lasts for about 3 to 6 months.

Active artificial immunity is acquired when a patient is given a vaccination of live attenuated (weakened) or dead bacteria, viruses, or toxoids, and the patient's body forms antibodies. This protection may be semipermanent (i.e., years) or permanent. **Passive artificial immunity** occurs when antibodies from a donor are directly given to a patient to teach the patient's immune system how to fight. This protection is temporary.

Vaccines act by provoking memory B cells to prepare for a future attack from a similar microbe. Boosters (later doses given for the semipermanent vaccines) are given to boost the immune system into continuing its protection. A blood titer, or level, may determine whether the body has produced enough antibodies in response to a vaccination.

Some vaccines have side effects, including fever and redness and pain at the injection site. Severe reactions, called anaphylaxis, are possible, and patients must always be observed for at least 15 minutes after a vaccination. Assess the patient for rash or difficulty breathing. Document your observations even if the patient tolerated the procedure well.

Antineoplastic Medications (Chemotherapy)

Cancer is a disease caused by a disorderly and uncontrolled division of cells. Many chemicals, such as nicotine and alcohol, can trigger a cell to begin dividing abnormally. Although in most cases, the body can spot an abnormal cell and eliminate it, in some individuals the body cannot make that identification, so the abnormal cell remains, and cancer results.

Cancer cells typically divide much more rapidly than normal, healthy cells and can spread to surrounding or distant body areas, a process called **metastasis.** For instance, cancers of the breast frequently metastasize to the brain, bones, or liver (A Closer Look 17.3).

Sarcomas (Fig. 17-5), carcinomas, and other malignant cancers must be completely eliminated, or they can return. For this reason, a powerful treatment, chemotherapy, is often prescribed. **Chemotherapy,** usually a combination of several antineoplastic (anticancer) and cytotoxic (destruction to cells) medications, is frequently given in several doses for maximum effectiveness. These terms are often used

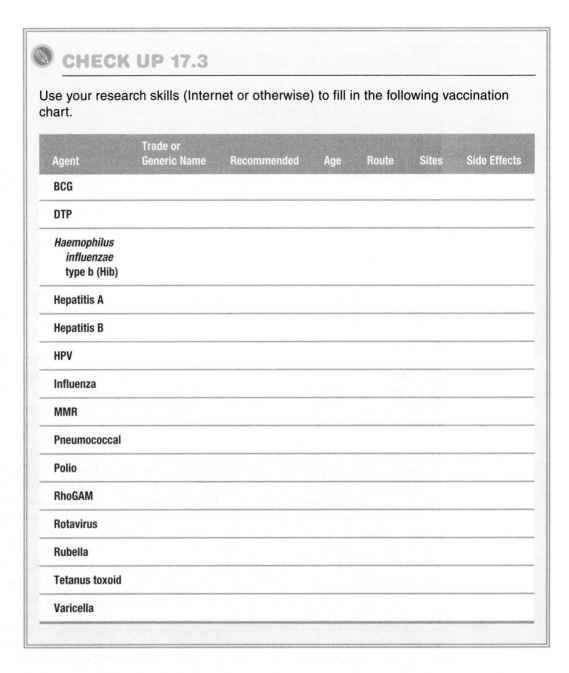

CHECK UP 17.3

Use your research skills (Internet or otherwise) to fill in the following vaccination chart.

Agent	Trade or Generic Name	Recommended	Age	Route	Sites	Side Effects
BCG						
DTP						
Haemophilus influenzae type b (Hib)						
Hepatitis A						
Hepatitis B						
HPV						
Influenza						
MMR						
Pneumococcal						
Polio						
RhoGAM						
Rotavirus						
Rubella						
Tetanus toxoid						
Varicella						

A CLOSER LOOK 17.3: Types of Tumors

Tumors are classified as benign or malignant. Tumors that are not fatal are called **benign.** Benign tumors grow slowly and do not metastasize. They may be removed if they impede the function of surrounding tissues; they do not usually grow back when removed.

Malignant tumors are cancerous. They must be treated, or the patient will die. They spread as nonfunctional tissues that compete with healthy tissue for the blood and nutrient supply. Malignant cancers are treated with surgery, radiation, and/or chemotherapy unless the patient decides not to be treated.

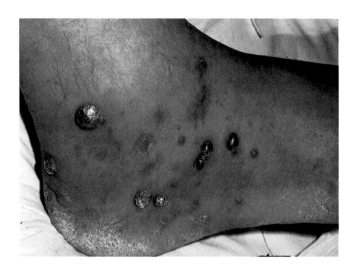

FIGURE 17-5: Kaposi's sarcoma. This skin tumor is related to AIDS. *(Reprinted from Goldsmith, LA, Lazarus, GS, and Tharp, MD: Adult and Pediatric Dermatology: A Color Guide to Diagnosis and Treatment. F.A. Davis, Philadelphia; 1997.)*

interchangeably and in the remainder of this chapter antineoplastic medications will be the term used. These medications act as toxins, or poisons, to the malignant cells. Each patient receives a highly individualized combination of medications because no two cancers or persons are identical. In addition, the drugs are given on an intermittent basis, never continuously.

Among the antineoplastic medications available for treating cancer are alkylating agents, antimetabolites, antitumor antibodies, plant extracts, hormones, biological response modifiers, monoclonal antibodies, immunomodulators, and radioactive isotopes. These agents are usually given parenterally by the intramuscular (IM), subcutaneous (SC), IV, or intrathecal route. In some instances, creams and gels are administered topically for mild forms of skin cancer.

Alkylating Agents

Alkylating agents are among the oldest categories of antineoplastic medications. They work by attaching to DNA and altering its shape, thus preventing it from reproducing normally. Alkylating agents are effective during all phases of the cell cycle. These medications are ideal for treating leukemia because blood and bone marrow cells are especially sensitive to them. Examples of oral and IV alkylating agents are chlorambucil (Leukeran), cisplatin (Platinol), cyclophosphamide (Cytoxan, Neosar), dacarbazine (DTIC-Dome), mechlorethamine (Mustargen) (Drug Spotlight 17.2), oxaliplatin (Eloxatin), stretozocin (Zanosar), and thiotepa (Thioplex). (For a more complete list, see the Master the Essentials table.) An effect of these drugs is the possibility of permanent infertility in both male and female patients.

Antimetabolite Medications

Antimetabolites disrupt critical cell pathways. Normally, cells take up metabolites to create substance the cell needs function. Cancer cells mistake the antimetabolites for metabolites, and the drugs kill the cells. These drugs are used to treat ovarian, breast, and GI tumors. They can also be used to treat some cases of leukemia. Antimetabolite medications include 6-mercaptopurine, cladribine (Cladribine NovaPulse, Leustatin), cytarabine (Cytosar-U, Tarabine PFS), fluorouracil (Efudex, Adrucil), leucovorin (Wellcovorin), methotrexate (Rheumatrex, Trexall), and thioguanine (Tabloid). They can be administered orally, topically, or through an IV line.

Antitumor Antibiotics

Bacteria found in soil are used to create antibiotics that can kill cancer cells. Many of these agents cause cell death by altering the DNA molecules and breaking the actual DNA strands. Although these medications have properties of antibiotics, they are used for their cytotoxic effects. Bleomycin (Blenoxane) is an example of an antitumor antibiotic that is used primarily in combination with other antineoplastic medications to treat Hodgkin's lymphoma and testicular cancer. Another antitumor antibiotic is dactinomycin (Cosmegen), which is used to treat cancers of the kidneys, uterus, testicles, bones, muscles, joints, and soft tissues. The factor that limits the use of this class of medications is that in damaging the cancer cells, lung cells are also injured.

Drug Spotlight 17-2 *Mustargen (mechlorethamine hydrochloride)*

Definition and history	Commonly known as nitrogen mustard; one of the first chemotherapeutic agents; some originally produced as chemical weapons in the early part of the 20th century; these agents blister the skin
Indications	Used to treat cancers such as Hodgkin's disease and some blood and lung cancers
Adverse Reactions/ Side Effects	These most common side effects are temporary: • Nausea and vomiting • Hair loss • Mouth sores • Discoloration of infusion veins Infertility may be permanent
Route of administration	Given via IV route; very damaging to tissue, thus given with extreme care
Special considerations	No antidote exists for this drug, which is considered a poison; if exposed: • Contact poison control • Remove clothing, cutting off any clothes that must be removed over head • Place all clothes in plastic bag • Wash off skin

Plant Extracts (Alkaloids)

Plant extracts, or alkaloids, called mitotic inhibitors, prevent cell division. Plants used for this purpose include periwinkle, the mandrake plant, the Pacific yew, and a shrub called *Camptotheca acuminata*. These drugs are called mitotic inhibitors because they prevent formation of the mitotic spindle. The cells cannot complete mitosis and the cells die. Cancers treated with plant alkaloids include soft tissue, breast, ovarian, testicular, stomach, prostate, head, neck, and lung cancers, Wilms' tumor, leukemia, Hodgkin's disease, and non-Hodgkin's lymphoma. Examples include docetaxel (Docefrez, Taxotere), etoposide (VePesid, Toposar), irinotecan (Camptosar), paclitaxel (Onxol, Taxol), teniposide (Vumon), topotecan (Hycamtin), vinblastine (Velban), vincristine (Oncovin, Vincasar PFS), and vinorelbine (Navelbine).

Hormones

Hormones can help the brain communicate with other organs in the body (see Chapter 15) and can tell them when to grow and how to function. Some hormones such as testosterone, estrogen, and luteinizing hormone are powerful and can significantly impair the growth of some tumors. Tumors that depend on hormones for growth can be eradicated by large amounts of an opposing hormone. For example, tumors that thrive under the effects of estrogen, such as breast cancer, can be killed by injections of fluoxymesterone (Androxy, Halotestin), testolactone (Teslac), or testosterone (Andro LA 200, Delatestryl, DepAndro 100, and Depo-Testosterone). Conversely, a patient with prostate or testicular cancer may be treated with oral doses of antiandrogens such as bicalutamide (Casodex), flutamide (Eulexin), or nilutamide (Nilandron), which block testosterone production, or with estrogen, such as or Cenestin, Enjuvia, Premarin, or estradiol (Estrace, Femtrace, Gynodiol), which makes the environment unfavorable for tumor growth. (See the Master the Essentials table for a more complete list of hormonal medications used as antineoplastic agents.)

Biological Therapy

Biological therapy involves assisting the body's immune system, rather than destroying the cancer cells. However, biological therapy also alters the nature of the response and often produces severe side effects. Three drug classes fall under this heading: biological response modifiers, monoclonal antibodies, and immunomodulators.

Biological response modifiers boost the immune system. The exact mechanisms by which these medications exhibit antitumor effects are not clear. Biological response modifiers include the interleukins, which stimulate the growth of blood cells important to the immune system. Interferon alfa-2a (Roferon-A) is used to treat leukemia and AIDS-related Kaposi's sarcoma. Interferon alfa-2b (Intron A) is used to treat leukemia, malignant melanoma, AIDS-related Kaposi's sarcoma, and hepatitis B and C.

Monoclonal antibodies are substances that specifically target tumor cells. Whereas toxic substances are nonselective and kill any rapidly growing cells (both diseased and healthy), monoclonal antibodies attack cancer cells only. They attach themselves to the tumor antigens and make them easily recognizable to the body's immune system. Monoclonal antibody medications such as alemtuzumab (Campath), bevacizumab (Avastin), cetuximab (Erbitux), gemtuzumab (Mylotarg), ibritumomab (Zevalin), panitumumab (Vectibix), rituximab (Rituxan), tositumomab (Bexxar), and trastuzumab (Herceptin) are used in the treatment of colon, lung, head, neck, and breast cancers, as well as leukemia and non-Hodgkin's lymphoma.

A third form of biological therapy uses immunomodulatory cytokines, which are messenger proteins that deliver messages within the cells. In some patients with cancer, these cytokines are not functional. Immunomodulators such as lenalidomide (Revlimid) and thalidomide (Thalomid) stimulate the immune system in patients with multiple myeloma. The use of thalidomide carries a high risk of birth defects, as was seen in the 1950s and 1960s. Those patients prescribed thalidomide are encouraged to use multiple methods of birth control to prevent pregnancy.

Radioactive Isotopes

Radiation can also be used to kill cancer cells. Radiation in some form is used to treat roughly half of all patients with cancer patients. Tumors are the target of radiation therapy. In addition to external irradiation, radioactive isotopes can be swallowed as capsules or solutions, or they can be implanted. Iodine-125, iridium-194, palladium-103, and thulium-170 are radioactive isotopes implanted in the form of seeds. This procedure is called brachytherapy, and the seeds emit radiation to shrink the tumor. Always be extremely careful when handling these substances because they are dangerous. Follow your facility's policy about isolating the patient and the patient's body fluids after administering radioactive isotopes because they will emit radiation for a period of time after implantation.

Adverse Effects of Chemotherapy

Healthy cells that also rapidly divide in the body, such as hair follicles and the mucous membranes of the GI tract, are affected by chemotherapy because the medication's main function is to target rapidly dividing cells. As the healthy cells are damaged or killed in addition to the malignant cells, patients often become sick and weak, and they experience negative side effects of the medications. The most common side effects of chemotherapy are nausea and vomiting, alopecia (hair loss), and decreased blood counts.

Most chemotherapy is administered via the IV route over a period of time. Whether health professionals are allowed to administer IV chemotherapy varies according to state, facility, and level of training. Because chemotherapy is usually a long process, patient education regarding IV therapy, care of venous lines, and recognition of signs and symptoms of infection is vital. Infiltration, or accidental leakage of medication into surrounding tissue, is always a risk with IV therapy. These substances are particularly toxic if they infiltrate tissues. Always assess the IV site for swelling or coolness. The potential for infiltration increases when the rate of the IV infusion is increased too quickly or when pressure is put on the vein. If infiltration occurs, the IV catheter must be removed, and a new IV line must be started in a different location.

If the patient complains of burning pain or aching in the vein, the chemotherapy may have irritated or damaged the vein wall, with resulting phlebitis and thrombosis. You may need to obtain an order to dilute the strength of the medication, lower the infusion rate, or change the site.

Because of the caustic nature of these medications, it is common practice to insert a central line or port (see Chapter 10) to administer chemotherapeutic agents into a larger vein, with less risk to surrounding tissues.

Other complications result from the destruction of hematopoietic cells. The first is a suppressed immune system, leading to infections that quickly become overwhelming because of the patient's inability to fight the invading microorganisms. In addition, patients may have difficulty with bleeding as a result of low platelet counts and anemia from low red blood cell counts. For these reasons, patients must be protected from injury and infectious visitors or health-care workers who may endanger their health.

BOX 17.1 Special Handling of Chemotherapeutic Drugs

Always give as ordered, and have another colleague double-check the order.

Frequently assess the IV site.

Help the patient with oral hygiene as needed.

Assess for malnutrition related to nausea, vomiting, and diarrhea.

Administer an antiemetic, as ordered.

Encourage soft, mild foods.

Offer cool liquids.

Measure input and output.

Inquire about pregnancy, and perform a test as ordered before administering to women.

Assess for complications.

Use standard precautions to decrease infection in the patient and to protect yourself.

Assess vital signs, as ordered.

Educate the patient about the effects of the therapy.

Dispose of chemotherapeutic products according to facility standards.

Major organ damage can result from the toxic effects of these drugs. Therefore, the patient must be closely observed for any signs of organ compromise, such as decreased urine output, change in skin color, or change in blood test results.

Antineoplastic agents are toxic to cells, but they can also be dangerous or even fatal to persons who administer them and thus require special handling. Exposure to chemotherapy poses risks to reproductive health in men and women, as well as other problems. For that reason, gloves should be worn while administering, handling, or transporting antineoplastic agents, so that agents are not absorbed through the skin. Ensure that packages of hazardous drugs are well labeled and secured properly. Although protocols vary by location, follow all safety measures, and do not perform any task outside your scope of practice. All staff members handling these drugs should be required to complete specialized training to protect themselves, their patients, and the patients' families. Regulations always include wearing protective clothing, strictly following safety measures, and rigidly observing protocols for drug preparation and delivery (Box 17-1).

●●● SUMMARY

- The immune system functions to maintain health by blocking or fighting foreign invaders.
- Medications are used to support or inhibit the immune response, depending on the patient's condition.
- When the immune system is overstimulated by conditions such as allergies or autoimmune disorders, anti-inflammatory medications are used to suppress the immune system.
- Anti-inflammatory medications shut off or reduce the body's inflammatory response to treat inflammation, autoimmune disorders, and allergies.
- The five categories of anti-inflammatory medications are antihistamines, glucocorticoids, nasal decongestants, NSAIDs, and immunosuppressants.
- Anti-infective agents assist in fighting infections and include antibiotics, antitoxins, antifungals, antivirals, and antiparasitics.
- Viruses are smaller than other microorganisms and insert their genetic material into hosts to reproduce.
- Vaccines assist in preventing infections.

■ The two types of immunity are natural and adaptive (acquired). Natural immunity is the ability humans have to resist infection through normal body functions. Acquired immunity is produced through vaccines or when antibodies from a donor are directly given to a patient.

■ Malignant (cancerous) tumors spread as nonfunctional tissues that compete with healthy tissue for the blood and nutrient supply.

■ Chemotherapy usually consists of a combination of several antineoplastic and cytotoxic medications.

■ Antineoplastic medications include alkylating agents, antimetabolites, antitumor antibodies, plant extracts, hormones, biological response modifiers, monoclonal antibodies, immunomodulators, and radioactive isotopes.

■ Antineoplastic agents must be carefully handled, administered, and disposed of because of their toxicity and hazards to the health professional and to all persons coming into contact with the patient or their secretions or waste.

■ Educating patients and their families about immunological system medications and their possible complications will ensure safety for all: the health professional, the patient, and the family.

Master the Essentials: Immunological System Medications

This table shows the various classes of immunological medications and key side effects, contraindications and precautions, interactions, and examples of each class.

Class	Indications for Use	Side Effects	Contraindications and Precautions	Interactions	Examples
Antihistamines	Allergies, prophylactic use before medications likely to cause allergic reaction	CNS depression (sedation, dizziness, muscle weakness), epigastric distress, dry mouth	Known hypersensitivity, breastfeeding, MAO inhibitors, glaucoma, hypertension	CNS depressants, anticholinergics, aminoglycosides, salicylates, epinephrine	Diphenhydramine (Benadryl), loratadine (Claritin, Tavist), cetirizine (Zyrtec)
Glucocorticoids	Suppression of immune response; severe inflammation	Behavioral changes, hyperglycemia, increased susceptibility to infection, osteoporosis, hypertension	Known hypersensitivity, systemic fungal infection	Phenytoin, salicylates, NSAIDs, vaccines, estrogen, antihypertensives	Beclomethasone (Beconase, Qvar, Vanceril, Vanceril DS), budesonide (Entocort EC), ciclesonide (Omnaris), flunisolide (AeroBid, AeroBid-M), fluticasone (Flovent), triamcinolone (Aristocort), dexamethasone (Decadron), hydrocortisone (Solu-Cortef), methylprednisolone (Medrol, Solu-Medrol), prednisolone (Pediapred, Prelone), prednisone
Nasal decongestants	Nasal congestion	Arrhythmias, hypertension, headaches, nausea, sneezing, dryness (topical)	Known hypersensitivity, MAO inhibitors, hypertension	Beta blockers, MAO inhibitors, tricyclic antidepressants	Phenylephrine (Dimetapp Cold Drops, PediaCare Children's Decongestant, Sudafed PE Quick Dissolve, Triaminic Thin Strips Cold, Lusonal, Nasop), phenylpropanolamine, propylhexedrine (Benzedrex), pseudoephedrine (Sudafed, Suphedrin), tetrahydrozoline (Tyzine Nasal)
NSAIDs	Inflammation, pain, fever	Nausea, vomiting, hypersensitivity reactions, vertigo, insomnia, rash	Known hypersensitivity, renal disease, GI bleeding, allergic reaction to sulfonamides	ACE inhibitors, fluconazole, phenobarbital, phenobarbital, cyclosporine, corticosteroids, anticoagulants	Aspirin, celecoxib (Celebrex), diclofenac, diflunisal (Dolobid), etodolac (Lodine), ibuprofen (Advil, Motrin, Nuprin, Haltran), indomethacin (Indocin), ketoprofen (Actron, Orudis, Oruvail), ketorolac (Toradol), nabumetone (Relafen), naproxen (Aleve, Anaprox, Naprosyn), oxaprozin (Daypro), piroxicam (Feldene), salsalate (Amigesic, Disalcid Salsitab, Marthritic), sulindac (Clinoril), tolmetin (Tolectin)

	Uses	Side Effects	Contraindications	Interactions	Examples
Immunosuppressants	Autoimmune diseases such as lupus or rheumatoid arthritis; organ transplant	Leukopenia, thrombocytopenia, nephrotoxicity, hyperkalemia, hypertension, diarrhea, nausea	Known hypersensitivity, pregnancy, breastfeeding	Allopurinol, aminoglycosides, other immunosuppressants, calcium channel blockers, cardiac glycosides	Azathioprine (Imuran, Azasan), corticosteroids, cyclosporine (Neoral, Sandimmune, Gengraf), sirolimus (Rapamune)
Penicillins	Common infections with gram-positive and gram-negative bacteria	Blood changes, CNS effects, diarrhea, hypersensitivity, kidney and liver disorders, nausea, vomiting	Known hypersensitivity, decreased renal function, electrolyte imbalances	Antagonizes antacids and foods; probenecid potentiates penicillin; may decrease the action of oral contraceptives	Ampicillin, amoxicillin (Amoxil), carbenicillin (Geocillin), dicloxacillin (Dycill, Dynapen), nafcillin (Nallpen, Unipen) oxacillin (Bactocill), penicillin, penicillin g benzathine/potassium/sodium (Bicillin), piperacillin, ticarcillin (Ticar)
Cephalosporins	**First generation:** gram-positive bacterial infections in patients' allergic to penicillins **Second generation:** nosocomial pneumonia **Third generation:** gram-negative bacterial infections **Fourth generation:** severe nosocomial surgical infections	Bleeding, diarrhea, hypersensitivity, liver dysfunction, kidney disease, nausea, phlebitis, respiratory distress, seizures, vomiting, vaginal itching or discharge, headache	Known hypersensitivity, children, kidney impairment, lactation, pregnancy; not for long-term use	Alcohol and diuretics	**First generation:** cefazolin (Ancef, Kefzol), cefadroxil, cephalexin (Biocef, Keflex), cephalothin (Keflin), cephapirin, cephradine (Velosef) **Second generation:** cefaclor (Ceclor, Raniclor), cefprozil (Cefzil), cefotetan (Cefotan), cefuroxime (Ceftin, Zinacef), cefoxitin (Mefoxin), loracarbef (Lorabid) **Third generation:** cefdinir (Omnicef), cefditoren (Spectracef), cefixime (Suprax), cefoperazone (Cefobid), cefotaxime (Claforan), cefpodoxime (Vantin), ceftazidime (Ceptaz, Fortaz, Tazicef), ceftibuten (Cedax), ceftriaxone (Rocephin), ceftizoxime (Cefizox) **Fourth generation:** cefepime (Maxipime)
Tetracyclines	Gram-negative and/or gram-positive bacterial infections	Allergic hypersensitivity, CNS malfunction, diarrhea, decreased bone growth in a fetus or child, discolored teeth in fetus or child, light sensitivity, thrombophlebitis, nausea, superinfection, vomiting	Children, direct sunlight, esophageal illness, kidney and liver disease, lactation, pregnancy	Antacids, antidiarrheal agents, calcium, dairy products, iron, magnesium, oral contraceptives, zinc	Doxycycline (Adoxa, Alodox, Avidoxy, Doryx, Monodox, Oracea, Oraxyl, Periostat, Vibramycin, Morgidox), minocycline (Dynacin, Minocin, Myrac, Solodyn, Vectrin), tetracycline (Ala-Tet, Panmycin)

Continued

Master the Essentials: Immunological System Medications—cont'd

Class	Indications for Use	Side Effects	Contraindications and Precautions	Interactions	Examples
Macrolides	Bacterial infections resistant to penicillin	Anorexia, cramps, diarrhea, nausea, superinfection, urticaria, vomiting	Alcoholism and liver damage	Cyclosporine, digoxin Halcion, Tegretol, theophylline, warfarin	Erythromycin (E.E.S. Granules, Ery-Tab, Erythrocin Stearate Filmtab), clarithromycin (Biaxin), azithromycin (Zithromax, Zithromax, Z-Pak)
Aminoglycosides	Aerobic gram-negative bacteria, mycobacteria, or some protozoal infections	Blurred vision, CNS symptoms, ear damage, kidney disease, paralysis (including respiratory paralysis) rash urticaria	Decreased kidney function, dehydration, infancy, high-frequency hearing loss, lactation, pregnancy, tinnitus, vertigo	Antiemetics, general anesthesia, ototoxic drugs	Amikacin (Amikin), gentamicin (Cidomycin, Garamycin, Septopal), kanamycin (Kantrex), neomycin (Mycifradin, Neo-Fradin, Neo-Tab), paromomycin (Humatin, Paromycin), tobramycin (Nebcin, Tobi)
Quinolones	Chronic urinary tract infections	CNS effects, diarrhea, toxicity in sunlight, nausea, superinfections, vomiting	Cardiovascular disorders, children, kidney disease, lactation, pregnancy	Antacids, calcium, Coumadin, iron, magnesium, probenecid, theophylline, zinc	Ciprofloxacin (Ciloxan Ophthalmic, Cipro), enoxacin (Penetrex), gatifloxacin (Tequin), levofloxacin (Levaquin, QUIXIN Ophthalmic), lomefloxacin (Maxaquin), moxifloxacin (Avelox), norfloxacin (Chibroxin Ophthalmic, Noroxin Oral), ofloxacin (Floxin, Ocuflox Ophthalmic), sparfloxacin (Zagam), trovafloxacin (Trovan)
Sulfonamides	Acute urinary tract infections	Fever, crystalluria, nausea, vomiting, diarrhea, rash, photosensitivity	Known hypersensitivity, impaired kidney or liver function, lactation, pregnancy	Anticoagulants, antidiabetics, local anesthesia, cyclosporine	Erythromycin-sulfisoxazole (Pediazole), sulfadiazine, sulfamethizole (Thiosulfil Forte), sulfamethoxazole (Gantanol), sulfasalazine (Azulfidine), sulfisoxazole (Gantrisin), trimethoprim-sulfamethoxazole (Septra, Bactrim)
Antitoxins	Exposure to toxin in at-risk patient	**Diphtheria:** Fever, inflammation of joints, muscle aches, reddening of skin around ears, swollen lymph glands, weakness **Tetanus:** Pain at injection site, hypersensitivity	Known hypersensitivity, caution in pregnancy and breastfeeding	None reported	Botulism antitoxin (Heptavalent (HBAT), diphtheria antitoxin tetanus immune globulin (Baytet, HyperTET S/D)

Classification	Use	Side Effects	Contraindications/Precautions	Interactions	Medications
Antituberculosis Agents	Tuberculosis infection and/or exposure	Allergic reaction, dizziness, seizures, numbness or tingling in extremities, rash, confusion, tremors, headache, drowsiness, irritability, fatigue, red/orange urine, stool, tears, sweat, saliva (rifampin, rifabutin), liver damage (INH), nausea, vomiting, anorexia	Epilepsy, psychiatric disorders, kidney disorder, alcoholism, children, lactation, liver or kidney disease, pregnancy	Ethionamide, rifampin may make birth control pill less effective; alcohol, anticoagulants, corticosteroids, digoxin, estrogen, phenytoin	Cycloserine (Seromycin), ethambutol (Myambutol), ethionamide (Trecator SC), isoniazid (Nydrazid), pyrazinamide, rifabutin (Mycobutin), rifampin (Rifadin, Rimactane)
Antifungals	Fungal infections	Anemia, chills, hypotension, dizziness, fever, headache, hypokalemia, kidney damage, malaise, muscle and joint pain and weakness, tachycardia, photosensitivity	Children, liver damage, penicillin hypersensitivity, pregnancy, porphyria	Alcohol, anticoagulants, oral contraceptives, phenobarbital	**Topical:** amphotericin B (Fungizone), benzoic acid/salicylic acid (Bensal HP), ciclopirox (CNL8 Nail, Loprox, Penlac), clotrimazole (Canesten, Lotrimin, Mycelex), econazole (Spectazole), haloprogin (Halotex), ketoconazole (Extina, Nizoral, Xolegel), miconazole (Aloe Vesta, Baza, Dermagran AF, Desenex, Lotrimin, Micatin, Monistat, Zeasorb-AF), miconazole/zinc oxide (Vusion), naftifine (Naftin), nystatin (Mycostatin, Pedi-Dri), oxiconazole (Oxistat), sertaconazole (Ertaczo), sulconazole (Exelderm), terbinafine (Lamisil), tolnaftate (Absorbine, Aftate, Blis-To-Sol, Tinactin), undecylenic acid (Blis-To-Sol Powder, Cruex, Trifungol) **Systemic:** amphotericin B (Fungizone), caspofungin (Cancidas), flucytosine, fluconazole (Diflucan), itraconazole (Sporanox), ketoconazole (Nizoral), miconazole (Monistat I.V.)
Antivirals	Viral infections	Confusion, diarrhea, headache, kidney disease, nausea, rash, urticaria, vomiting	Children, dehydration, lactation, kidney disease, neurological disease, pregnancy	Probenecid, nephrotoxic agents, cytotoxic agents, anticholinergics	Acyclovir (Acivir, Acivirax, Cyclovir, Herplex, Zovirax, Zovir), amantadine (Symmetrel), cidofovir, oseltamivir (Tamiflu), ribavirin (Copegus, Rebetol, RibaPak, Ribasphere, Ribatab, Virazole), zanamivir (Relenza)
Antiretrovirals	HIV infection	Fat redistribution, hypoglycemia, GI upset, kidney stones	Known hypersensitivity, breastfeeding, pregnancy, kidney or liver impairment	Alcohol, oral contraceptives	**Multiclass combination medications:** efavirenz/emtricitabine/tenofovir (Atripla), emtricitabine/rilpivirine/tenofovir (Complera) **Nucleoside reverse transcriptase inhibitors (NRTIs):** abacavir/lamivudine (Epzicom), abacavir sulfate/ABC (Ziagen), abacavir/zidovudine/

Continued

Master the Essentials: Immunological System Medications—cont'd

Class	Indications for Use	Side Effects	Contraindications and Precautions	Interactions	Examples
					lamivudine (Trizivir), emtricitabine/FTC (Emtriva), didanosine/dideoxyinosine (Videx), lamivudine/zidovudine (Combivir), lamivudine/3TC (Epivir), stavudine/d4T (Zerit), tenofovir disoproxil, fumarate/emtricitabine (Truvada), tenofovir disoproxil fumarate (Viread), zidovudine/azidothymidine (Retrovir) **Nonnucleoside reverse transcriptase inhibitors (NNRTIs):** delavirdine (Rescriptor), efavirenz (Sustiva), etravirine (Intelence), nevirapine (Viramune), rilpivirine (Edurant) **Protease inhibitors:** amprenavir (Agenerase), atazanavir sulfate (Reyataz), darunavir (Prezista), indinavir (Crixivan), fosamprenavir calcium (Lexiva), lopinavir/ritonavir (Kaletra), nelfinavir mesylate (Viracept), ritonavir (Norvir), saquinavir mesylate (Invirase), tipranavir (Aptivus) **Fusion inhibitors:** enfuvirtide (Fuzeon) **Entry inhibitors-CCR5 coreceptor antagonist:** maraviroc (Selzentry) **HIV integrase strand transfer inhibitors:** raltegravir (Isentress), delavirdine (Rescriptor), nelfinavir (Viracept), ritonavir (Norvir)
Antimalarials	Prevention and treatment of malaria	Visual disturbances, hearing changes, nausea, vomiting, diarrhea, anorexia, muscle weakness, rash	Known hypersensitivity, pregnancy, breastfeeding, kidney disease, liver disease, uncontrolled vomiting or diarrhea	Cimetidine, kaolin, magnesium trisilicate	Atovaquone/proguanil (Malarone), chloroquine (Aralen), mefloquine (Lariam), primaquine

Classification	Use	Side effects	Contraindications	Interactions	Examples
Antiprotozoal drugs	Treatment of protozoal infection	Altered blood glucose levels both high and low; taste changes, diarrhea, nausea, vomiting	Diabetes, heart problems, kidney disease, pancreatic disease, asthma, recent radiation or chemotherapy, caution with pregnancy, breastfeeding	Azathioprine, carbamazepine, antibiotics, NSAIDs, chemotherapy, birth control pills, antihypertensives, antidiabetics, metoclopramide	Metronidazole (Flagyl, Metro I.V.), pentamidine (Nebupent, Pentam 300), trimethoprim-sulfamethoxazole (Bactrim, Septra, Sulfatrim)
Anthelmintics	Treatment of tapeworms, roundworms, hookworms, pinworms, and flukes	Headache, dizziness, nausea, mild fever, skin rash, fatigue	Known sensitivity, caution with pregnancy and breastfeeding, patients less than 2 years of age	Cimetidine, chloroquine, itraconazole, ketoconazole, dexamethasone, erythromycin, barbiturates, HIV medications, antiseizure medications	Albendazole (Albenza), praziquantel (Biltricide), ivermectin (Stromectol), mebendazole (Vermox), pyrantel (Antiminth, Ascarel), praziquantel (Biltricide)
Pediculicides	Lice treatment	Allergic reactions, stinging or skin irritation, dizziness, drowsiness	Known hypersensitivity, nonintact skin, HIV/AIDS, risk factors for seizures	None reported	Permethrin (Acticin, Elimite, and Nix), piperonyl butoxide/pyrethrins (Licide, RID), spinosad (Natroba), malathion (Ovide), benzyl alcohol lotion (Ulesfia), lindane
Scabicides	Scabies treatment	Mild itching, burning or skin	Known hypersensitivity, caution with pregnancy and breastfeeding, HIV/AIDS, risk factors for seizures	None reported	Crotamiton (Eurax), lindane, permethrin (Acticin, Elimite)
Alkylating agents	Leukemia, solid tumors	Allergic reactions, nausea, vomiting, diarrhea, bone marrow suppression, pulmonary fibrosis, hepatotoxicity	Known hypersensitivity, pregnancy, breastfeeding	Anticoagulants, phenobarbital, digoxin	Bendamustine (Treanda), busulfan (Busulfex, Myleran), carboplatin (Paraplatin), carmustin (BiCNU, Gliadel), chlorambucil (Leukeran), cisplatin (Platinol), cyclophosphamide (Cytoxan, Neosar), dacarbazine (DTIC-Dome), ifosfamide (Ifex), lomustine (CeeNU), mechlorethamine (Mustargen), melphalan (Alkeran), oxaliplatin (Eloxatin), streptozocin (Zanosar), temozolomide (Temodar), thiotepa (Thioplex)

Continued

Master the Essentials: Immunological System Medications—cont'd

Class	Indications for Use	Side Effects	Contraindications and Precautions	Interactions	Examples
Antimetabolites	Lung, metastatic breast, pancreatic, and ovarian cancer, GI tumors	Alopecia, bone marrow depression, diarrhea, nausea, neurotoxicity, rash, reproductive ability loss, pulmonary fibrosis, vomiting	Pregnancy, breastfeeding, hepatic impairment	Probenecid, NSAIDs, alcohol, salicylates	6-Mercaptopurine, cladribine (Cladribine NovaPulse, Leustatin), cytarabine (Cytosar-U, Tarabine PFS), fluorouracil (Efudex, Adrucil), leucovorin (Wellcovorin), methotrexate (Rheumatrex, Trexall), thioguanine (Tabloid)
Antitumor antibiotics	Testicular tumors, Hodgkin's lymphoma, tumors of kidney, uterine, bone, muscle, soft tissue cancers	Alopecia, anorexia, bone marrow suppression, cardiotoxicity, nausea, pneumonitis, rash and scaly skin, ulceration of the skin and mouth, vomiting	Known hypersensitivity, pregnancy, renal impairment, heart disease, breastfeeding	Cyclophosphamide, myelosuppressive drugs, hepatotoxic medications, digoxin, phenytoin, oxygen, vitamin E, NSAIDs, warfarin, clopidogrel, ticlopidine	Bleomycin (Blenoxane), dactinomycin (Cosmegen)
Plant alkaloids	Soft tissue tumors, Wilms tumor, leukemia, Hodgkin's disease, non-Hodgkin's lymphoma	Alopecia, constipation, diarrhea, nausea, necrosis, neurotoxicity, rash, sensitivity to light, ulcers in the mouth or GI system, vomiting, white blood cell deficiency	Pregnancy, breastfeeding, bacterial infection, severe granulocytopenia, liver impairment	Mitomycin, phenytoin, erythromycin, digoxin	Docetaxel (Docefrez, Taxotere), etoposide (VePesid, Toposar), irinotecan (Camptosar), paclitaxel (Onxol, Taxol), teniposide (Vumon), topotecan (Hycamtin), vinblastine (Velban), vincristine (Oncovin, Vincasar PFS), vinorelbine (Navelbine)
Hormones	Breast, ovarian, testicular, prostate cancer	Hot flashes, decreased sex drive, nausea, vomiting, headache, dizziness, depression	Pregnancy, thromboembolic disorders, breastfeeding, undiagnosed vaginal bleeding	Warfarin, bromocriptine, insulin, corticosteroids, Parlodel, cimetidine, rifampin, heart, hypertension medications, HIV/AIDS medicine, psychiatric medications,	Aminoglutethimide (Cytadren), anastrazole (Arimidex), bicalutamide (Casodex), estradiol (Estrace, Femtrace, Gynodiol), estramustine (Emcyt), estrogen (Cenestin, Enjuvia, Premarin), exemestane (Aromasin), flutamide (Eulexin), fluoxymesterone (Androxy, Halotestin), goserelin acetate (Zoladex), hydroxyprogesterone caproate (Delta-Lutin, Duralutin, Hylutin, Hyprogesterone, Makena, Prodrox), letrozole (Femara), leuprolide acetate (Eligard, Lupron, Viadur), medroxyprogesterone acetate

Category	Uses	Side effects	Contraindications	Interactions	Drugs
				migraine medications, narcotics	(Provera), megestrol (Megace), mitotane (Lysodren), nilutamide (Nilandron), raloxifene (Evista), tamoxifen (Soltamox), testolactone (Teslac), testosterone (Andro LA 200, Delatestryl, DepAndro 100, Depo-Testosterone), toremifene (Fareston), triptorelin (Trelstar)
Biological response modifiers	Leukemia, malignant melanoma, AIDS-related Kaposi's sarcoma hepatitis B and C	Anemia, bleeding, difficulty breathing, fever, muscle aches and pain, mouth infection, nausea, vomiting, diarrhea, malnutrition, anorexia, alopecia, damage to ear and peripheral nervous system, kidney and heart disease, tingling, loss of reflexes, confusion, personality changes, bone marrow suppression, GI upset	Known hypersensitivity, pregnancy; because of intense side effects, antiemetics may be needed to prevent vomiting	Protease inhibitors, antihypertensives, corticosteroids	Interferon alfa-2a (Roferon-A), interferon alfa-2b (Intron A)
Monoclonal antibodies	Colon, lung, head, neck, and breast cancer, leukemia, non-Hodgkin's lymphoma	Infusion reactions, arrhythmias, angina, renal failure, bleeding, nausea, thrombocytopenia, rash, abdominal pain, malaise	Known hypersensitivity, pregnancy, breastfeeding	Anticoagulants	Alemtuzumab (Campath), bevacizumab (Avastin), cetuximab (Erbitux), gemtuzumab (Mylotarg), ibritumomab (Zevalin), panitumumab (Vectibix), rituximab (Rituxan), tositumomab (Bexxar), trastuzumab (Herceptin)
Immunomodulators	Multiple myeloma	Headache, fever, nausea, vomiting, fatigue, myalgia, depression	Known hypersensitivity, depression, kidney or liver disease, autoimmune disorders	Theophylline; neurotoxic, hematotoxic, or cardiotoxic drugs	Lenalidomide (Revlimid), thalidomide (Thalomid)
Radioactive isotopes	Prostate, lung, cervical, endometrial, bile duct cancer	Radiation sickness, nausea, vomiting, rash, fatigue, low blood counts, difficulty swallowing, changes in taste, anorexia	Pregnancy, breastfeeding	None reported	Brachytherapy seeds: iodine-125, iridium-194, palladium-103, thulium-170

ACE, angiotensin-converting enzyme; CNS, central nervous system; GI, gastrointestinal; INH, isoniazid; MAO, monoamine oxidase; NSAIDs, nonsteroidal anti-inflammatory drugs.

Activities

To make sure that you have learned the key points covered in this chapter, complete the following activities.

True or False

Write true if the statement is true. Beside the false statements, write false, and correct the statement to make it true.

1. Bacteria are identified by their shape and ability to retain a dye. _____

_____

2. Anticancer drugs work against slowly dividing cells. _____

_____

3. Tetracycline is the antibiotic of choice for pregnant women and small children. _____

_____

4. Antiretrovirals are given to fight HIV infections. _____

_____

5. Only the person actually administering chemotherapy must follow safety rules. _____

_____

6. Some antituberculosis agents turn body secretions red/brown. _____

_____

7. Malaria is caused by a parasite. _____

_____

8. Anti-inflammatory medications are used when the immune system is not active enough.

_____

9. C cells, which are known as memory cells, are the part of the immune system that record

attacks of microorganisms. _____

_____

10. Antibiotics are considered anti-infective medications. _____

_____

Multiple Choice

Choose the best answer for each question.

1. Which class of medications treats worms?
   A. Antimalarials
   B. Anthelmintics
   C. Antiprotozoals
   D. Pediculicides

2. Which is NOT a side effect of Cipro?

A. Severe inflammation of the colon

B. Increased sensitivity to sunlight

C. CNS effects: dizziness, confusion, hallucinations

D. Nasal congestion

3. Which vaccine is given for rubella?

A. Varicella

B. MMR

C. DTP

D. Pneumococcus

E. HiB

4. Which immunity provides immunity to a fetus?

A. Active natural immunity

B. Active artificial immunity

C. Passive natural immunity

D. Passive artificial immunity

5. Which of the following healthy cells are harmed along with cancer cells by chemotherapy?

A. Hair follicles

B. Hematopoietic cells

C. Mucous membranes

D. All of the above

6. Which of the following antineoplastic medications was developed after its use in World War I?

A. Mustargen

B. Cisplatin

C. Methotrexate

D. Leucovorin

7. Tinea pedis is more commonly known as _____.

A. Ringworm

B. Yeast infection

C. Athlete's foot

D. None of the above

8. The class of drugs used to treat HIV infections is _____.

A. Antivirals

B. Antiretrovirals

C. Antifungals

D. Antibiotics

9. Which of the following are types of worms?

    A. Round

    B. Tape

    C. Pin

    D. All of the above

10. What is an example of an active natural immunity?

    A. Patient has the measles

    B. Patient is given antibodies

    C. Patient is given a live attenuated vaccine

    D. Mother passes immunity to infant

Application Exercises

Respond to the following situations.

1. Harvey has injured his foot on a dirty nail. What vaccine will most likely be ordered? Why? _____

_____

_____

2. Beth has been prescribed an antibiotic for 10 days and calls to say that she is feeling better and is discontinuing it because it gives her an upset stomach. Explain to her why she should continue her medication despite feeling better and having side effects. _____

_____

_____

3. Holly brings her baby in for vaccinations. She is concerned that her baby needs so many shots and asks whether it is really necessary. How do you respond? _____

_____

_____

4. Beverly has cervical cancer and is to begin treatment with a radioactive isotope implant. What teaching should be done before beginning therapy? _____

_____

_____

5. Larry has come in because the antifungal spray is not working on his athlete's foot, and now a few of his toenails are becoming thick and painful, signs indicating that the infection is worsening. What will the prescriber most likely order for him? _____

_____

_____

For further study and practice with drug classifications learned in this chapter, complete the following table to the best of your ability. Use resources such as the *PDR,* reliable websites on the Internet, or printed drug guides for help.

Trade Name	Generic Name	Classification	Purpose	Side Effects	Contraindications and Precautions	Examples	Patient Education
Bicillin							
Nydrazid							
Flagyl							
Zovirax							
Platinol							
Blenoxane							

Internet Research

1. Using your favorite search engine, research medications currently used for patients with AIDS. Discover the average number of pills these patients must take in a day, and develop a schedule to assist a patient in implementing this regimen.

2. Using your favorite search engine:
   Download a patient teaching aid for cancer.
   Print a list of common side effects of cancer medications.

18

Pulmonary System Medications

The body depends on the respiratory, or pulmonary, system to bring oxygen to the cells and dispose of carbon dioxide. If this system works improperly, immediate medication may be needed. The fastest method for conveying medication to the lungs is through inhalation.

LEARNING OUTCOMES

At the end of this chapter, you should be able to:

18.1 Define all key terms.

18.2 Describe how the respiratory system functions to exchange oxygen and carbon dioxide.

18.3 Discuss the actions of mast cell stabilizers, bronchodilators, anticholinergics, xanthines, and beta-adrenergic agonists used in the treatment of asthma and other respiratory disorders.

18.4 Describe two medications that may be used to treat a viral respiratory illness.

18.5 Compare and contrast antitussive and expectorant medications and when each is appropriate to use.

18.6 Discuss tuberculosis and how it is treated.

KEY TERMS

Alveoli
Apnea
Chronic obstructive
   pulmonary disease
   (COPD)

Dyspnea
Expiration
Hypoxia
Inspiration
Latent tuberculosis (TB)

Purified protein derivative
   (PPD)
Respiration
Respiratory syncytial
   virus (RSV)

■ THE PULMONARY SYSTEM

The pulmonary system is responsible for **respiration**—the process of inhaling oxygen (O_2) into the bloodstream and exhaling the waste in the form of carbon dioxide (CO_2). It works with the musculoskeletal system during this process. To survive, the muscles need O_2 supplied and CO_2 removed. The diaphragm, the large muscle under the stomach, facilitates breathing. When the diaphragm contracts, the lungs are compressed, and CO_2 is expelled up through the bronchial tubes and trachea, out of the mouth, and into the air. This outward movement of air is known as **expiration.** The now mostly empty lungs inhale O_2 from the air; the inward movement of air is called **inspiration.** Both require energy (Fig. 18-1).

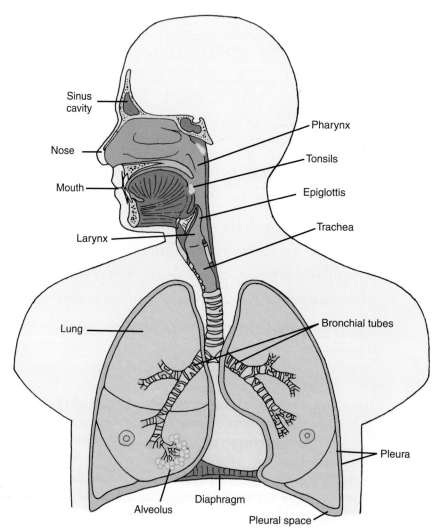

FIGURE 18-1: Respiratory system.

The brain regulates the rate and depth of breathing, depending on the needs of the body. For example, when you exercise, your body requires more O_2, and therefore you breathe more rapidly.

The exchange of CO_2 and O_2 occurs at the level of the **alveoli** (tiny air sacs in the lungs). Any time alveolar function is impaired, CO_2 builds up, and oxygenation declines. Changes in alveolar function occur with smoking and in diseases such as asthma.

O_2 is vital to every cell in the body, and the brain needs O_2 to function. Even 4 to 6 minutes without breathing can cause death. The lack of O_2 can cause the heart to stop beating or have serious implications for other systems that can lead to failure. Often, it is a medical emergency when someone either stops breathing or presents with **dyspnea** (trouble breathing) (Fast Tip 18.1).

 Fast Tip 18.1 Fast Relief for Dyspnea

Pulmonary medications are usually administered via inhalation for quick action. Examples of this route are the nebulizer and the inhaler.

Diseases such as asthma, **chronic obstructive pulmonary disease (COPD),** and tuberculosis (TB) can cause dyspnea or impair the lung's ability to function. Pulmonary medications can improve pulmonary function in these patients (Table 18-1).

PULMONARY MEDICATIONS

The medications used to treat pulmonary infections or disease are determined by the part of the pulmonary system that is affected. Some medications liquefy secretions, and others dry them up. Some medications act locally, whereas others act systemically (see the Master the Essentials table for descriptions of the most common pulmonary system drugs).

Mast Cell Stabilizers

Mast cell stabilizers inhibit allergens binding to mast cells (a type of white blood cell) from bursting open and releasing substances that cause inflammation. These medications are used to prevent or decrease the occurrence of asthma attacks. They do not cure the disease or help during an acute attack, but rather they decrease the body's reaction to asthma triggers, such as air pollutants, respiratory infections, chemicals, food allergies, pollen, dust, mold, animal dander, and stress.

Cromolyn sodium (Intal) and nedocromil sodium (Tilade) are examples of mast cell stabilizers. These medications should not be used for acute asthma attacks, but as a preventive measure. They take 2 to 6 weeks to start working. They are administered via a nebulizer or metered-dose inhaler most commonly, but they also come in an intranasal form for seasonal allergies.

TABLE 18.1 Common Pulmonary Diseases

Pulmonary Disease	Overview	Symptoms	Medications
Asthma	Asthma is a disease caused by an increased reaction of the tracheobronchial tree to stimuli that results in episodic narrowing and inflammation of the airways. Although the cause is not always known, the airways are chronically inflamed.	Breathlessness, air hunger (pursing of lips, gasping for air), coughing, and dyspnea are common symptoms. If asthma continues for a long time, status asthmaticus, or an asthma attack that does not stop, becomes a medical emergency.	Antiasthmatic medications target both the bronchoconstriction and the inflammation.
Chronic obstructive pulmonary disease (COPD)	The main COPD diseases are chronic bronchitis and emphysema. Chronic bronchitis is an inflammation of the bronchial tree. In response to irritation, mucus floods the bronchi and impairs breathing. Emphysema occurs after years of chronic inflammation, when the bronchioles lose elasticity and the alveoli dilate beyond effectiveness. COPD is usually caused by tobacco smoking, both direct and second-hand. Irritants and pollutants in the air can also cause COPD. There is no cure for COPD.	Dyspnea and coughing occur, particularly a cough that is productive (one that brings up mucus).	A patient with COPD needs a variety of drugs to treat infections because the lungs, and their defenses, have been damaged. The patient also needs drugs to decrease the bronchospasm that is created by the chemical irritation and to control the chronic cough that comes from irritating the pharynx. Mucolytics and expectorants are usually indicated, along with oxygen therapy. Oxygen must be given only at low levels (4 L/min maximum). Higher levels may lead to dangerous CO_2 levels and cause the patient to stop breathing.

Continued

TABLE 18.1 Common Pulmonary Diseases—cont'd

Pulmonary Disease	Overview	Symptoms	Medications
Cystic fibrosis	Cystic fibrosis is a genetic disease that affects the respiratory and digestive systems. In the respiratory system, thick secretions are excreted into the lungs, and patients require vigilant respiratory care to keep the lungs clear and free from infection.	Patients have persistent productive cough, frequent infections in the lungs, wheezing, shortness of breath, failure to gain weight, salty-tasting skin, and GI difficulties.	Mucolytic medications assist in breaking up thick secretions, and antibiotics treat lung infections.
Tuberculosis	Tuberculosis (TB) is an infection caused by *Mycobacterium tuberculosis*, a gram-positive bacterium.	Patients have a persistent cough, night sweats, and weight loss.	The TB bacterium is gram-positive but frequently resists treatment with traditional antibiotics. Consequently, it is often treated with a combination of drugs. Treatment must continue for as long as 6 to 12 months.

GI, gastrointestinal.

Antitussives and Expectorants

Antitussives stop coughs by blocking the cough reflex. If a cough is dry and thus not productive, an antitussive may be prescribed to allow the patient to rest, especially at night. Some narcotic analgesics, such as codeine, are effective antitussives in low dosages.

When secretions are present, expectorants are used to increase the body's ability to clear the lungs and upper airway by thinning the secretions. Expectorants such as guaifenesin (Duratess, Mucinex, Robitussin) can also soothe respiratory tract mucous membranes. These medications are given by mouth as a syrup, tablet, or capsule.

Antibiotics

Many respiratory illnesses either are caused by or are accompanied by bacterial infections, and antibiotics are therefore prescribed to combat or prevent the infections as appropriate (see Chapter 17). Intravenous antibiotics may be administered for serious infections requiring hospitalization, such as pneumonia. The usual treatment for most other respiratory infections consists of oral antibiotics for a period of 10 to 14 days. Occasionally, a patient is given an injection of an antibiotic, followed by an oral medication course. This injection jump-starts the healing process without the need for IV infusions and hospitalization.

One bacterium in particular, *Mycobacterium tuberculosis,* causes the highly contagious TB infection. Tubercles remain in a patient's body for a lifetime and can become active in patients with compromised immune systems if the infection is not treated. For this reason, many patients with **latent tuberculosis (TB)** (infected with TB, but without the disease) who contract other immunologic disorders such as acquired immunodeficiency syndrome (AIDS) can die of TB. Pharmacological treatment of TB requires exact adherence to a regimen of several drugs over 6 to 12 months because TB heals very slowly. These medications can also be given to close companions of infected patients to prevent infection. The most common combination of drugs consists of INH (isoniazid) and Rifadin (rifampin), but usually a combination of up to four antibiotics is used. In addition, those patients with latent tuberculosis are treated with one antibiotic for 6 to 12 months to prevent them from developing the disease at some point later in life. Patients with latent TB are not contagious. Rifampin has a unique side effect of which patients must be made aware. Tears, urine, perspiration, and other body fluids will turn orange yellow. This can be scary for a patient who is unaware of this side effect (see A Closer Look: Tuberculosis Diagnosis).

A CLOSER LOOK: Tuberculosis Diagnosis

What is the difference between having the disease and having latent TB? When a person is given a TB test **(purified protein derivative [PPD]),** the skin test result is positive in both TB disease and latent TB. The difference is that those patients with latent TB do not have any signs of active disease such as changes to their chest radiographs. They have been exposed to the disease and the tubercles are in their bodies but are not making them sick. Prophylactic administration of antibiotics helps to keep the disease from becoming active.

Antiviral Medications

As discussed in Chapter 17, antiviral medications are used to prevent the growth of a virus. Although a virus cannot be killed, its replication can be inhibited. Antibiotics cannot kill a virus and may actually cause harm by increasing the patient's risk of developing an infection resistant to antibiotic treatment. Antiviral medications are usually administered to decrease the duration of a viral illness and/or minimize the symptoms. Medications can ease the signs and symptoms of influenza. These medications are usually taken for 2 to 5 days. Although prevention of influenza through vaccination is preferred, anti-influenza agents can reduce the severity of influenza symptoms and shorten the duration of the illness. Examples of drugs used to treat influenza include zanmivir (Relenza) and oseltamivir phosphate (Tamiflu). Relenza is a powder that is delivered via an inhaler, and Tamiflu is taken by mouth as a capsule or liquid. These medications do not cure influenza or prevent patients from spreading it to others.

In addition, **respiratory syncytial virus (RSV)** is a common virus that affects premature and other small infants adversely because of the extremely thick secretions associated with this viral illness. Small infants who have other risk factors, such as being immunocompromised or those with congenital birth defects, may be at risk of developing complications such as pneumonia or bronchiolitis. These infants are therefore given an antiviral drug called ribavirin (Virazole) (Drug Spotlight 18.1). This drug is given as an aerosol treatment continuously for approximately 3 to 5 days. Exposure to these medications has serious side effects, so visitors and health-care workers must be educated and monitored closely during administration of this medication.

Drug Spotlight 18-1 *Ribavirin (Virazole)*

Classification	Antiviral
Indications	Respiratory syncytial virus (RSV). Used primarily in infants and children at risk for developing complications such as pneumonia from underlying chronic illness or prematurity
Adverse Reactions/ Side Effects	Thickened secretions leading to potential respiratory distress, rash, eye irritation
Contraindications/ Precautions	Possible risk to developing fetus, so women who are possibly pregnant or trying to become pregnant (including parents and health-care workers) should avoid being in room where drug is administered
Implementation	Aerosol treatment administered via a tent for 3 to 5 days
Special instructions	Remove contact lenses before entrance into the room because of the possibility of damage to the contacts and increased eye irritation

Bronchodilator Medications

Bronchodilators relieve acute bronchospasm and include anticholinergics, xanthines (methylxanthines), and beta-adrenergic agonists. They relax the smooth muscle of the bronchi and allow the patient to breathe more easily. When inhaled, these drugs work immediately on the pulmonary system. When they are taken orally, it takes longer for the patient to feel the effect, but the action is of longer duration, and side effects may last longer as well.

Anticholinergics

Parasympatholytics or anticholinergics dilate bronchi by blocking the action of acetylcholine, which causes bronchospasm. These medications when taken orally are used to prevent bronchospasms, not to treat those already in progress.

Because these drugs stimulate the sympathetic nervous system, the patient can expect a fight-or-flight response, including increased heart rate and blood pressure. This effect also dries up lung secretions and thereby decreases congestion and improves pulmonary function. Examples of anticholinergic bronchodilators include ipratropium bromide (Atrovent) and tiotropium (Spiriva). Both these medications are administered via inhalation and are prescribed for patients with bronchitis, emphysema, or COPD. Atrovent is inhaled as a mist, and Spiriva is inhaled in powder form.

Xanthines (Methylxanthines)

Xanthines, also called methylxanthines, include theophylline and aminophylline. These medications relax smooth muscle and relieve bronchospasm. Asthma is the most common illness for which these medications are used. Because patients metabolize them at different rates, the dosage must be carefully adjusted based on the patient's reaction. These medications have a narrow safety margin. In other words, there is a small difference between the amount of medication needed to be effective and the amount that produces toxic effects in the patient. Careful monitoring is essential. IV aminophylline may be given as a continuous infusion for serious asthma attacks when the patient is hospitalized. Oral forms such as aminophylline (no brands available, only generic) and theophylline (Elixophyllin, Theo-Dur Sprinkles) should be taken on an empty stomach with a full glass of water, for faster absorption. However, taking this medication on a full stomach decreases gastric upset.

Beta-Adrenergic Agonists

Beta-adrenergic agonists are bronchodilators that are commonly used for treating asthma (Fig. 18-2). They stimulate beta-2 receptor sites in the sympathetic nervous system and result in bronchial dilation. Short-acting agents include albuterol (Proventil, Ventolin), bitolterol (Tornalate), levalbuterol (Xopenex), isoproterenol (Isuprel), metaproterenol (Alupent, Metaprel), pirbuterol (Maxair), and

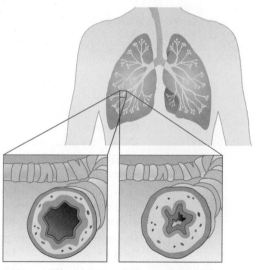

FIGURE 18-2: Asthma.   Normal bronchiole   Asthmatic bronchiole

terbutaline (Brethaire, Brethine, Bricanyl); they are mainly used as needed. A long-acting agent, such as formoterol (Foradil) or salmeterol (Serevent), is used to control asthma.

Additionally, epinephrine (Adrenalin) is given as a subcutaneous injection in episodes of severe dyspnea associated with asthma. This acts as a bronchodilator and opens up the airways when other drugs do not create the desired response in an emergency situation. Other forms are found in multidose inhalers (MDIs) as a part of a combination of drugs to help with milder asthma attacks.

Decongestants

Decongestants cause the blood vessels in the nasal mucous membranes to constrict, thus reducing nasal passage drainage. They are available as nasal sprays and oral medications that are combined with different medications to treat cold and allergy symptoms. The main decongestant medications include phenylephrine (Dimetapp, Neo-Synephrine, PediaCare, Sudafed PE Quick Dissolve, Triaminic) and pseudoephedrine (Chlor-Trimeton, Contac Cold, Drixoral, Triaminic). Use of the topical form provides immediate relief of nasal mucosal swelling and congestion. These medications must be used on a short-term basis only, to avoid rebound congestion problems. They should never be given to children younger than 2 years old. In addition, because many of these medications are mixed with antipyretics and analgesics in cold and allergy remedies, dosages of medications such as acetaminophen and ibuprofen need to be monitored closely, to avoid overdose situations.

Glucocorticoids

Glucocorticoids suppress the immune system, which means inflammation is decreased. When the risk of asthma exacerbation increases (e.g., pollen counts are high), medications such as beclomethasone (Vanceril, Beclovent), budesonide (Pulmicort), flunisolide (Aerobid), fluticasone (Flovent), mometasone furoate (Asmanex), and triamcinolone (Azmacort) are usually taken daily in an oral or inhaled form as prophylaxis, but they are not used for acute episodes. To treat acute asthma episodes or other respiratory illnesses such as croup, short periods of oral steroids such as dexamethasone sodium phosphate (Decadron, Dexone), prednisone (Deltasone, Orasone, Prednicot), prednisolone (Orapred), and methylprednisolone (Medrol) may be prescribed in an oral form. In severe acute episodes, medications such as methylprednisolone (Solu-Medrol) may be used in an intravenous form in much higher doses, to dilate the airways and allow respirations to ease.

As discussed previously (see Chapter 17), glucocorticoids should be taken only in the short term. If taken for more than 10 days, oral glucocorticoids may have severe adverse effects resulting from immune system suppression. Medications in this class should be taken at the lowest effective dose for the least amount of time as possible.

Mucolytics

Mucolytics liquefy very thick lung secretions so the secretions can be excreted through coughing. These drugs do this by changing the composition of the mucus. Combined with expectorants, mucolytic agents help remove irritating substances from the lungs. Acetylcysteine (Mucomyst) is an example of a mucolytic. This type of drug is most commonly used as an aerosol treatment in patients with cystic fibrosis. This genetic disease causes the respiratory secretions to be extremely thick and difficult to cough up. With frequent daily mucolytics as part of their respiratory care, these patients are able to remove the secretions through coughing and thus decrease the occurrence of lung infections.

Oxygen

O_2 is used as therapy for low oxygenation, or **hypoxia.** Long-term use includes management of COPD; acute use is needed to treat dyspnea and carbon monoxide poisoning. O_2 can be delivered by nasal cannula, mask, endotracheal tube, hood, or tent.

O_2 is considered a drug, and there must be an order to administer it. It is important not to give more O_2 than ordered. For instance, patients with COPD tend to retain CO_2. This leads to higher than normal levels of CO_2 and lower than normal levels of O_2 in the blood (Fig. 18-3). Normally, the body reacts to higher levels of CO_2 by prompting the lungs to breathe more deeply and rapidly to exhale the excess CO_2. In patients with COPD, however, the body has adapted to the long-term higher levels of CO_2, so these patients have lowered O_2 levels as the trigger to breathe. Giving a patient with COPD more O_2

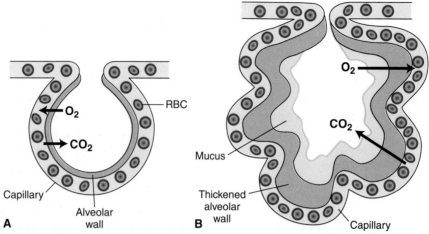

FIGURE 18-3: Chronic obstructive pulmonary disease (COPD). (A) Normal alveoli. (B) Destructive changes of COPD.

than is prescribed can actually shut off this adaptive mechanism and cause the patient's breathing to stop or slow markedly, thus further lowering the O_2 level in the blood.

Additionally, too much O_2 can damage the eyes, especially those of premature infants. Therefore, we give the lowest levels of O_2 that produce the results that the prescriber desires.

Respiratory Stimulants

For patients who have problems with **apnea** (periods of breathing cessation), medications to stimulate the respiratory center of the brain may be prescribed. The typical patient is a premature infant whose brain is not developed to the degree of a normal newborn. These infants require a nudge to breathe, and that is done with medications such as caffeine citrate (Cafcit) or theophylline. Many premature infants take these medications for many months after release from the neonatal intensive care unit. In the adult patient, the reason for sleep apnea is usually a structural problem causing an obstruction. Medication has not been demonstrated to help with this situation. Surgery, lifestyle change such as weight loss, or an assistive breathing apparatus used to open the obstructed airway are common interventions.

Smoking Cessation

Because tobacco smoking is addictive and causes so many illnesses (e.g., emphysema, lung cancer, and bronchitis) in both smokers and those around them, medications have been developed to facilitate smoking cessation. Combined with hypnosis and behavioral therapy, these medications can be extremely effective. It is very difficult to quit completely and suddenly ("cold turkey"); therefore, smoking cessation aids, which contain the drug nicotine, deliver small, consistent doses of nicotine to help the individual gradually withdraw from nicotine use. This treatment is usually administered via a transdermal patch (NicoDerm) or in gum (Nicorette). Be sure to educate patients and reinforce for them that they cannot smoke while using nicotine patches, to avoid a nicotine overdose. In addition, patients should not wear nicotine patches when they are inside magnetic resonance imaging (MRI) equipment because patients have been reported to suffer burns at the site of the patch. Other routes for nicotine include inhalation (Nicotrol) and nasal spray (Nicotrol).

Another drug that may be prescribed as an oral medication is bupropion hydrochloride (Budeprion, Wellbutrin, Zyban). This drug was originally developed as an antidepressant, but it has been found to have significant benefit in the battle to stop smoking. However, it has serious risks of suicidal ideation and completion. The potential benefits of this medication should therefore be weighed heavily against the risks when this drug is considered. Patient education must be thorough with each prescription of this drug.

A newer oral medication used with behavior modification that works to convince your brain that smoking is not pleasurable is varenicline (Chantix). The patient may smoke during treatment but slowly loses the desire to do so.

● ● ○ S U M M A R Y

- The pulmonary system is responsible for respiration and works with musculoskeletal systems. The pulmonary system must function properly to maintain health.

- Respiration is the process of inhaling oxygen (O_2) into the bloodstream and exhaling the waste in the form of carbon dioxide (CO_2). This outward movement of air is known as expiration. The inward movement of air into the lungs is called inspiration.

- The exchange of CO_2 and O_2 occurs at the level of the alveoli.

- Antitussives stop coughs by blocking the cough reflex. Expectorants increase the body's ability to clear the lungs and upper airway by thinning the secretions.

- Antiviral drugs, such as ribavirin, zanmivir, and oseltamivir phosphate, reduce the severity of viral infections but do not kill the viruses.

- Bronchodilators, such as anticholinergics, xanthines, and beta-adrenergic agonists, are used to treat the bronchospasms associated with asthma and other respiratory disorders.

- Many decongestants, nucolytics, glucocorticoids, antibiotics, and antivirals exist to help heal a malfunctioning system and work by opening the bronchi, drying secretions, decreasing the histamine response, treating infections, conveying O_2 to the lungs, stopping coughs, loosening mucus, and forcing out secretions.

- Tuberculosis is caused by *Mycobacterium tuberculosis*; therefore, it is treated with an extensive program of antibiotics.

- O_2 is used as therapy for hypoxia (low oxygenation) such as seen in COPD.

- Patients who have problems with apnea can use respiratory stimulants (caffeine citrate, theophylline) to stimulate the respiratory center.

- Smoking cessation drugs help patients stop a habit that could lead to significant complications, as well as death.

Master the Essentials: Respiratory Medications

This table shows the various classes of respiratory medications and key side effects, contraindications and precautions, interactions, and examples of each class.

Class	Indications for Use	Side Effects	Contraindications and Precautions	Interactions	Examples
Mast cell stabilizers	Prevention of asthma attacks	Throat irritation, bad taste, wheezing, cough	Hypersensitivity	None reported	cromolyn sodium (Intal), nedocromil (Tilade aerosol)
Anti-influenza agents	Reduction of influenza symptoms	Anorexia, bronchitis, diarrhea, dizziness, dry mouth, headache, insomnia, nervousness, urinary retention	Hypersensitivity, kidney or liver impairment, pregnancy, breastfeeding, underlying respiratory disease	Acetaminophen, aspirin, cimetidine	zanamivir (Relenza), oseltamivir (Tamiflu)
Antitussives	Coughing cessation	Constipation, dizziness, respiratory depression, sedation, urinary retention	Asthma, COPD, addiction-prone patients, hypersensitivity	MAO inhibitors, other CNS depressants	dextromethorphan (Robitussin Cough, Triaminic long acting cough), codeine

Continued

Master the Essentials: Respiratory Medications—cont'd

Class	Indications for Use	Side Effects	Contraindications and Precautions	Interactions	Examples
Expectorants	Achievement of a more productive cough	Vomiting, diarrhea, abdominal pain	Hypersensitivity	None reported	guaifenesin (Duratuss, Mucinex, Robitussin)
Anticholinergics	Dilation of the bronchi	Agitation, confusion, dizziness, drowsiness, headache, increased heart rate, thickened secretions, bronchitis	Hypersensitivity, cardiac instability, glaucoma, prostatic hypertrophy	Use with other anticholinergics not recommended	ipratropium (Atrovent), tiotropium (Spiriva)
Xanthines (methylxanthines)	Relief of asthma symptoms	Dysrhythmias, CNS stimulation, GI distress, increased blood glucose and heart rate, urinary frequency	Diabetes mellitus, glaucoma, peptic ulcer, pregnancy, hypersensitivity	Barbiturates, hydantoins, ketoconazole, loop diuretics, beta blockers, calcium channel blockers, oral contraceptives	Aminophylline, theophylline (Elixophyllin, Theo-Dur Sprinkles)
Beta-adrenergic agonists	Dilation of the bronchi	CNS stimulation; increased appetite, blood glucose, and blood pressure	CV disorders, diabetes mellitus, hyperthyroidism, kidney problems, seizure disorders	MAO inhibitors, tricyclic antidepressants, cardiac glycosides, beta blockers	albuterol (Proventil, Ventolin), bitolterol (Tornalate), epinephrine (Adrenalin), formoterol (Foradil), levalbuterol (Xopenex), isoproterenol (Isuprel), metaproterenol (Alupent, Metaprel), pirbuterol (Maxair), salmeterol (Serevent), terbutaline (Brethine)
Decongestants	Removal of fluid buildup in the respiratory passages	Hypersensitivity reactions, anxiety, decreased cardiac output, decreased urine output, electrolyte imbalances, headaches, nervousness, racing heart rate, seizures, tremor	CV disorders, diabetes mellitus, hyperthyroidism, lactation, pregnancy, hypersensitivity	Other sympathomimetics, MAO inhibitors, beta blockers, methyldopa	Phenylephrine (Dimetapp, PediaCare, Sudafed PE Quick Dissolve, Triaminic), pseudoephedrine (Chlor-Trimeton, Contac Cold, Drixoral, Triaminic)
Glucocorticoids	Decrease of inflammation	Cough, dry mouth, hoarseness, oral fungal infection, throat irritation, headache, dizziness	Viral, bacterial, or fungal infections, heart failure, cirrhosis, diabetes mellitus, hypertension,	Barbiturates, phenytoin, oral contraceptives	beclomethasone (Vanceril, Beclovent), budesonide (Pulmicort), dexamethasone sodium phosphate

Master the Essentials: Respiratory Medications—cont'd

Class	Indications for Use	Side Effects	Contraindications and Precautions	Interactions	Examples
			hypothyroidism, renal failure		(Decadron, Dexone), flunisolide (Aerobid), fluticasone (Flovent), methyl-prednisolone (Medrol, Solu-Medrol), mometasone furoate (Asmanex), triamcinolone (Azmacort), prednisone (Deltasone, Prednicot), prednisolone (Orapred)
Mucolytics	Loosening or breaking up of thick mucus	Drowsiness, mouth inflammation, runny nose, bronchospasm, nausea, vomiting	CV disease, diabetes mellitus, ineffective cough, lactation, pregnancy, thyroid abnormalities	Activated charcoal	acetylcysteine (Mucomyst)
Oxygen	Provision of additional needed oxygen to the lungs	Alveolar changes, blindness in premature infants, confusion, hypoventilation	Avoidance of high doses in patients with COPD	None reported	Oxygen
Respiratory stimulants	Treatment of apnea	Abdominal pain, blood in stools, seizure, fever, bradycardia or tachycardia, sleep problems, fussiness, loss of appetite	Hypersensitivity, seizure disorders, heart, kidney or liver disease, hyperglycemia or hypoglycemia	Caffeine-containing foods (chocolate, cola)	theophylline, caffeine citrate (Cafcit)
Smoking cessation aids	Smoking cessation; decrease in symptoms of nicotine withdrawal such as a tight chest	**Nicotine:** cardiac irritability, local irritation, headache **Bupropion:** nausea, vomiting, constipation, appetite changes, headache, insomnia **Varenicline:** nausea, constipation, unusual dreams	Hypersensitivity, pregnancy, breastfeeding, epilepsy, anorexia, bulimia	Alcohol, benzo-diazepines, beta blockers, insulin, MAO inhibitors	bupropion (Wellbutrin, Zyban), nicotine (Nicorette), varenicline (Chantix)

CNS, central nervous system; COPD, chronic obstructive pulmonary disease; CV, cardiovascular; GI, gastrointestinal; MAO, monoamine oxidase.

Activities

To make sure that you have learned the key points covered in this chapter, complete the following activities.

True or False

Write true if the statement is true. Beside the false statements, write false, and correct the statement to make it true.

1. Glucocorticoids are used during severe asthma attacks. _____

_____

2. Mucolytics are used to suppress cough. _____

_____

3. Cystic fibrosis is treated with antiviral medications. _____

_____

4. Apnea is most common in athletes. _____

_____

5. Alveoli are where O_2 and CO_2 are exchanged. _____

_____

Multiple Choice

Choose the best answer for each question.

1. Asthma medications can be given via which of the following routes?

   A. Oral

   B. Inhalation

   C. Intravenously

   D. All of the above

2. Caffeine is given to prevent _____.

   A. Asthma

   B. Pneumonia

   C. Apnea

   D. COPD

3. Which class of pulmonary medications suppresses coughing?

   A. Antitussives

   B. Mucolytics

   C. Expectorants

   D. Mast cell stabilizers

4. Which class of medications is given to prevent asthma attacks?

   A. Antitussives

   B. Mucolytics

   C. Expectorants

   D. Mast cell stabilizers

5. Which of the following medications are used in the treatment of tuberculosis?

    A. INH

    B. Rifampin

    C. Both A and B

    D. None of the above

Application Exercises

1. Harold calls the office complaining that ever since he was prescribed rifampin at the TB clinic, his urine is orange. How would you explain this to him, and is it of concern?

_____

_____

_____

2. Wilma has cystic fibrosis. She complains about the frequency of treatments and dislikes taking medication. She wonders why she has to take antibiotics if she is not sick. What would you tell her? _____

_____

_____

3. Sandi is a busy working mother. She is asking for antibiotics because she cannot afford to get sick and is quite angry that the physician will not prescribe them for her. What would you say to her? _____

_____

_____

4. Julian has COPD. He wants to know why, the more oxygen he uses, the worse he feels. What would you say to him? _____

_____

_____

5. Charlotte has a cold with a productive cough. She has been prescribed an antitussive to be used only at bedtime. She states that it helps so much that she is going to use it around the clock. How would you counsel her? _____

_____

_____

For further study and practice with drug classifications learned in this chapter, complete the following table to the best of your ability. Use resources such as the *PDR,* the Internet, or printed drug guides for help.

Trade Name	Generic Name	Classification	Purpose	Side Effects	Contraindications and Precautions	Examples	Patient Education
Spiriva							
Tamiflu							
Robitussin Cough							
Xopenex							
Sudafed							
Decadron							
Intal							
Mucomyst							
Cafcit							
Chantix							
Virazole							

Internet Research

Visit the American Lung Association's website, and find tips for smoking cessation to create a teaching plan for patients.

19

Gastrointestinal System Medications

*W*hen disorders of the GI system occur or when a need exists to control certain signs and symptoms, such as abdominal pain, heartburn, gas, nausea, diarrhea, vomiting, malnutrition, and blood or mucus in the feces, we must turn to medications to alleviate the discomfort.

The gastrointestinal tract is mainly a very long tube through which food passes, nutrients are absorbed, and waste is removed. The main organs of digestion include the stomach, small intestine, and large intestine. Accessory organs such as the liver and pancreas assist these organs by secreting enzymes to break down food into vital nutrients.

LEARNING OUTCOMES

At the end of this chapter, you should be able to:

19.1   Define all key terms.

19.2   Detail how the gastrointestinal (GI) system functions.

19.3   Identify medications used to treat constipation.

19.4   Identify medications used to treat diarrhea, and explain how the underlying cause should be treated.

19.5   Identify medications used to treat nausea and vomiting.

19.6   Compare the different types of medications used to treat gastroesophageal reflux disease (GERD) and gastric ulcers.

19.7   Discuss medications used for gallstones, obesity, hemorrhoids, flatulence, stomatitis, and fungal and parasitic infections of the GI tract.

19.8   Discuss how poisoning and overdoses are treated.

19.9   Identify populations of patients needing nutritional supplements or those needing assistance digesting their food and how each of these are treated.

```
KEY TERMS

Alimentary canal          Fissure                    Hydrochloric acid (HCl)
Calculus                  Flatulence                 Morbidly obese
Cathartic                 Gastroesophageal reflux    Nausea
Chyme                        disease (GERD)          Peristalsis
Constipation              Helicobacter pylori        Reflux
Diarrhea                  Halitosis                  Stomatitis
Digestion                 Heartburn                  Thrush
Emesis                    Hemorrhoid                 Ulcer
```

■ GASTROINTESTINAL SYSTEM

The gastrointestinal (GI), or digestive, system consists of a long tube called the **alimentary canal** that begins at the mouth and ends at the anus, with accessory organs attached (Fig. 19-1). The alimentary canal is responsible for the four major functions of the digestive system: ingestion, digestion, absorption, and excretion. The goal of each function is to allow nutrients from food to be used as cellular energy.

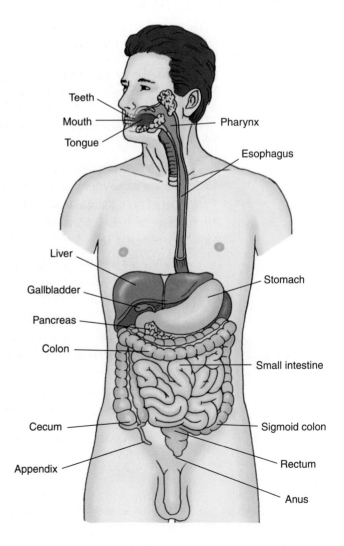

FIGURE 19-1: The gastrointestinal system.

Digestion is the process of converting food into chemical substances used by the body. Digestion begins in the mouth, where food is consumed and broken down into a usable form first by mechanical digestion (chewing) and then by chemical digestion (enzymes). Certain enzymes perform specific functions with respect to digesting the three complex organic molecules found in food: fats, proteins, and carbohydrates. These enzymes work at various sites along the GI tract. Food particles are chewed in the mouth and then swallowed, move through the oropharynx, and then the esophagus, into the stomach, and are then pushed through the small intestine and large intestine via **peristalsis** (wavelike movements). If this process is impeded, toxic substances can build up. Infection can develop when the normal flora living in the alimentary canal is disturbed.

Review Table 19-1 to understand the role of the major digestive organs more clearly.

The stomach's environment is high in **hydrochloric acid (HCl),** which helps it break down food for absorption. **Reflux** or backflow of HCl into the esophagus can lead to ulcers, or mucosal breakdown. When the mucosa is penetrated, it creates a prime environment for infection to spread because food moving through the digestive tract comes from outside sources that may carry harmful microorganisms. Although the HCl and normal flora of the digestive tract kill some organisms, the GI system can still be a major site of infection.

Depending on our food choices, we can damage our GI system. Bad or "junk" food can damage the system by overworking the pancreas, liver, and gallbladder. Extreme undereating can lead to anorexia nervosa, and extreme overeating can cause obesity. Other ways to damage the GI system include using medications that change the acidity of the stomach and eating food or other substances that contain harmful worms, viruses, or bacteria.

GASTROINTESTINAL MEDICATIONS

GI medications are used to treat specific disorders of the GI system or to control certain signs and symptoms, such as abdominal pain, change in bowel habits, heartburn, gas, weight loss, nausea, vomiting, difficulty swallowing, loss of appetite, and blood or mucus in the feces (see the Master the Essentials table for descriptions of the most common GI system drugs).

GI system drugs work to increase or decrease function by changing the muscle tone, replacing deficient enzymes, or increasing or decreasing the emptying time or rate of passage through the system. Some drugs such as Reglan serve to move food through the system at a more rapid rate when a patient is having difficulty with reflux or heartburn. Other medications such as pancreatic enzymes are given to patients with cystic fibrosis to aid in the process of digestion.

Timing of GI medication administration is important as well. Some medications are taken to coat the stomach lining or to reduce gastric acidity and must be ingested on an empty stomach. Other medications must be taken with food so they can be absorbed properly. Some foods such as grapefruit can affect the absorption of certain medications if they are eaten at the same time the medicine is taken. It is important to understand the effect of food and medications on the GI system.

The following sections detail the most common complaints and disorders of the GI system and the medications used to manage them.

TABLE 19.1 Functions of the Major Digestive Organs

Stomach	• Stores food • Mixes food with hydrochloric acid • Passes this mixture, called **chyme,** into the small intestine
Small intestine	• Carbohydrates, fats, and proteins broken down here • Pancreatic enzymes and bile from the liver aid digestion • End products of digestion absorbed into the bloodstream through mucous membranes
Large intestine	• Absorbs extra water and electrolytes • Eliminates waste products (feces)

Medications to Treat Constipation

Many of the medications discussed in previous chapters have a systemic effect and an effect on body systems other than the one for which the medication is prescribed. For example, medications that change smooth muscle tone to open up the respiratory tract in an asthmatic patient or that decrease the blood pressure in a cardiac patient can also affect the rate at which food moves through the body. When peristalsis slows, **constipation** or infrequent, hard stools can result. Some medications that contribute to constipation are diuretics, which remove fluid from the body and thereby cause hard stools. One such medication is furosemide (Lasix). As a result, the colon reabsorbs too much fluid, the feces become hard, and the alimentary canal does not clear. Laxatives are a class of medications that can help relieve constipation by promoting bowel movements. Laxatives can help diagnose GI disorders by cleansing the bowel to allow observation of the intestinal walls during examination. These medications should not be used for losing weight because they could lead to a dependency on them to have a bowel movement and may also cause electrolyte imbalances. A **cathartic** is a stronger medication that facilitates fast emptying of the colon. Laxatives are classified as bulk-forming agents, osmotics, stimulants, or stool softeners.

- **Bulk-forming laxatives.** Bulk-forming laxatives such as psyllium (Metamucil) increase bulk and water content of the stool because they resemble dietary fiber. This medication is available as a powder that can be added to liquid, as a capsule, and as a wafer to be eaten. Prunes and bran have the same effects. Bulk-forming laxatives are the best laxatives to take during pregnancy and if needed on a routine basis; they absorb water and create larger, softer stools. These larger stools stimulate peristalsis and thus purge the body of feces. These laxatives take 12 hours to 3 days to work.

- **Lubricant laxatives.** Lubricant laxatives such as mineral oil increase the water-to-fecal mass to ease the passage of stool and are usually taken as suppositories. Lubricant laxatives are typically oily. They take 6 to 8 hours to work.

- **Osmotic laxatives.** Osmotic laxatives, given rectally, such as glycerin or sorbitol exert an immediate action that draws water into the stool and irritates the bowel to increase peristalsis. The result is evacuation of stool, sometimes in the form of diarrhea, within 15 to 60 minutes. These laxatives are contraindicated in patients with hypertension, edema, or congestive heart failure because of the stress on the cardiovascular system caused by this rapid action. Milk of Magnesia is a mild osmotic laxative sometimes called a saline laxative. It increases the amount of water in the large intestine and usually works within 2 to 12 hours, depending on the dose. The salt ions in Milk of Magnesia can attract water molecules toward each other and thus lubricate the GI tract. Milk of Magnesia is therefore a safe option for patients with hypertension, edema, or congestive heart failure.

- **Stimulant laxatives.** Stimulant laxatives stimulate peristalsis because they act directly on the intestinal mucosa and irritate the bowel. They are typically effective within 6 to 8 hours. Some examples include bisacodyl, senna, aloe, cascara sagrada, and castor oil. Side effects include cramping, diarrhea, flatulence, and nausea. Senna, aloe, and cascara sagrada discolor urine. Castor oil should not be used during pregnancy because of the risk for premature labor or during lactation because it may cause diarrhea in the infant.

- **Stool softeners.** Stool softeners decrease the consistency of stool by reducing surface tension and attracting water and fat to the stool to soften it and improve its passage through the colon. Docusate (Colace) is a detergent stool softener. This type of laxative is typically used routinely in patients with limited mobility resulting from injury or chronic illness.

- **Bowel evacuators.** Bowel evacuators are cleansing solutions that are used to remove stool before diagnostic tests, such as colonoscopy. They are made as mixes similar to body fluids, so material held in the bowel is rejected. Typically, the patient is asked to drink 1 gallon of fluid mixed with a bowel evacuator within a 2- to 3-hour time frame. Side effects can include bloating, nausea, and fullness. Examples of bowel evacuants include polyethylene glycol electrolyte solution (Colyte, GoLYTELY, MoviPrep, NuLYTELY, PEG-3350 with Electrolytes, TriLyte) and polyethylene glycol 3350 (GlycoLax, MiraLax).

In addition to the previously mentioned pharmacological medications to treat constipation, some nonpharmacological treatments for constipation include exercising, laughing (because it massages the intestines and thus encourages peristalsis), increasing dietary fiber, drinking more fluids, decreasing consumption of dairy products, and drinking warmed prune juice.

 CRITICAL THINKING

Patients can become dependent on laxatives. Why is this problematic? What are some nonpharmacological treatments for constipation?

Medications to Treat Diarrhea

The opposite of constipation is **diarrhea,** which is an increase in the frequency and fluidity of bowel movements. Almost all individuals have diarrhea at one time or another, but if it occurs over several days, the body can lose too much fluid and too many electrolytes. This loss can occur within several hours in small children and infants.

Diarrhea is a symptom, not a disease. Certain chemicals, inflammation, infections, and other medications can cause diarrhea. Anti-infective therapy frequently causes diarrhea. Anxiety and circulatory disorders can cause diarrhea as well.

Stools of excessive volume and fluidity are more than just a bother. The cramping that frequently accompanies diarrhea can be very painful. Diarrhea can signal that the person has eaten spoiled or contaminated food and has an intestinal infection. In small children and the elderly, diarrhea can cause life-threatening loss of valuable fluid and electrolytes. Fortunately, several available medications, such as opioid-related antidiarrheals and absorbents, can help treat diarrhea.

Opioid-related antidiarrheal medications are highly effective and are used for the most serious cases of diarrhea. They work by inhibiting GI motility, decreasing peristalsis, and slowing the function of the GI system, thus allowing more time for water to be reabsorbed through the intestinal wall. An example is loperamide (Imodium), which is taken orally and is available over the counter (OTC), as well as by prescription. Another example is diphenoxylate with atropine (Lomotil), which comes in tablet form and is available only by prescription because of the addictive qualities of this drug. Side effects include dizziness, dry mouth, agitation, numbness, drowsiness, and tachycardia.

Absorbents

Absorbents, such as bismuth (Pepto-Bismol) (Drug Spotlight 19.1) or kaolin and pectin (Kaopectate), are taken after every bowel movement to absorb toxins or bacteria and to coat the walls of the GI tract. Because the treatment focuses on the cause of the diarrhea, medications may also include antibiotics, anti-inflammatories, or antiparasitics. The most common use of antibiotics for diarrhea occurs with "traveler's diarrhea." Exposure to contaminated water or food (often in less-developed countries with poor sanitation infrastructure) leads to bacterial, viral, or parasitic infections. Ciprofloxacin (Cipro), ofloxacin (Floxin), and azithromycin (Zithromax Z-Pak) are commonly used antibiotics, depending on the destination of the traveler. Ulcerative colitis is an example of inflammation that causes diarrhea and is treated with anti-inflammatory drugs such as sulfasalazine (Azulfidine), mesalamine rectal (Canasa, Rowasa), balsalazide (Colazal), and olsalazine (Dipentum). Antiparasitic medications are discussed later in this chapter (also see Chapter 17 for more information).

Medications to Treat Nausea and Vomiting (Antiemetics)

Nausea, although an uncomfortable feeling that vomiting is imminent, is not dangerous. Sometimes nausea is caused by unusual smells, pregnancy hormones, or emptiness of the stomach. **Emesis,** or vomiting, occurs when the patient ejects the contents of the stomach.

Antiemetics decrease nausea and vomiting and are also used to treat motion sickness. Examples of antiemetics include phenothiazines such as prochlorperazine (Compazine), antihistamines such as diphenhydramine (Benadryl) and meclizine (Antivert, Bonine), trimethobenzamide (Benzacot, Tigan, Ticon), cannabinoids, phosphorated carbohydrate solution (Emetrol), and 5-hydroxytryptamine-3 (5-HT$_3$, serotonin) receptor antagonists such as ondansetron (Zofran).

Drug Spotlight 19-1 *Bismuth subsalicylate (Pepto-Bismol, Kaopectate)*

Classification	Antidiarrheals, antiulcer agents, absorbents
Indications/Definition	The pink medicine that relieves five different gastrointestinal symptoms: heartburn, nausea, indigestion, upset stomach, and diarrhea
Availability	Suspension, tablets, and chewable tablets
Contraindications/ Precautions	• Salicylate in this medication may make gout symptoms worse • May make ulcer symptoms worse • May make bleeding problems worse • Taking other salicylate medications with this drug may lead to overdose • Mothers should not breastfeed while taking this medication
Special Concerns	• This drug used only in teenagers 12 years of age and older and adults; younger children are usually not given medication for diarrhea, but managed with fluid replacement therapy only; in addition, this drug should never be used in a child or teenager with a viral illness because of the unknown association between salicylates and Reye's syndrome • Elderly patients should check with their physician before using this medication
Adverse Reactions/ Side Effects	• Constipation • Tongue may turn black: normal, secondary to interaction of bismuth and the sulfides found in the digestive tract; subsides after discontinuation of medication • Stools turn black: same reason as tongue

Phenothiazines

Phenothiazines block dopamine receptors in the area of the brain that stimulates vomiting. Two examples, chlorpromazine (Thorazine) and prochlorperazine (Compazine), are used to control the nausea and vomiting that occur with chemotherapy and can be administered orally, by injection, or by the intravenous (IV) route. In addition, prochlorperazine may be given as a rectal suppository. These drugs tend to produce sedation while treating the nausea and vomiting. These medications are available by prescription only.

5-Hydroxytryptamine-3 Receptor Antagonists

5-HT$_3$ is more commonly known as serotonin. Therefore, these medications are known as serotonin antagonists and are also commonly used to prevent and treat the nausea and vomiting associated with chemotherapy. They block the chemical serotonin, which is produced in the brain and in the stomach. Examples of this class of medications include dolasetron (Anzemet), ondansetron (Zofran), granisetron (Kytril), and palonosetron (Aloxi). These medications are all administered either orally or by the IV route. Additionally, Zofran may be given as an injection. These medications are available by prescription only.

Antihistamines

The action of antihistamines in decreasing nausea and vomiting is unclear. It is believed that these medications block signals to the brain's movement center. Therefore, they tend to work best on the nausea associated with motion sickness. Dramamine (dimenhydrinate), diphenhydramine (Benadryl), meclizine (Antivert, Bonine), and promethazine (Adgan, Phenergan, Promethacon) are examples of this class of drugs used for nausea and vomiting. All of these medications are available to be taken orally, and dimenhydrinate, diphenhydramine, and meclizine may be purchased OTC. Dimenhydrinate, diphenhydramine, and promethazine may also be administered by injection or by the IV route. Promethazine may also be given by rectal suppository.

Anticholinergic Medications

As discussed in Chapter 13, anticholinergic medications block the effects of the neurotransmitter acetylcholine. It is thought to act on the brain's chemoreceptor trigger zone in an area of the medulla. This zone initiates vomiting and can be stimulated by blood-borne medications or hormones. Trimethobenzamide (Benzacot, Tigan, Ticon) is an anticholinergic that can be given orally, rectally, or by IM injection and is available by prescription only. Another prescription anticholinergic medication is scopolamine (Maldemar, Scopace, Transderm-Scōp), which can be given by the IV, IM, or subcutaneous route for nausea and vomiting. In addition, scopolamine can be used as a transdermal disc placed behind the ear before exposure to a motion sickness–causing event.

Cannabinoids

These are manufactured forms of cannabis. Marijuana is the herbal form of cannabis. An example of a cannabinoid is nabilone (Cesamet), and it works by affecting the area of the brain that controls the nausea and vomiting impulses. This medication has a high level of addiction possibility and therefore should be prescribed only when other antiemetics are unsuccessful for the patient receiving chemotherapy. In addition, the patient may suffer from altered thinking and thus should take this medication with care. Cesamet is taken orally before the start of chemotherapy and for a period of time during and after each chemotherapy dose. This drug and marijuana are controlled substances. According to the National Conference of State Legislatures, as of August 2017, a total of 29 states, the District of Columbia, Guam, and Puerto Rico now allow for comprehensive public medical marijuana and cannabis programs. There are varying laws in each state as to who can grow and dispense marijuana and what medical conditions are eligible. There are also some states that allow only cannabis oils with low THC and not the actual marijuana plant. It is important to check the most up-to-date regulations in your state if you are involved with patients that would benefit from medical marijuana.

A CLOSER LOOK: Illnesses Qualifying Patients for Medical Marijuana

The following list provides examples of the qualifying illnesses; the list may differ by state.

- Cancer
- Glaucoma
- HIV/AIDS
- Hepatitis C
- Amyotrophic lateral sclerosis
- Crohn's disease
- Alzheimer's disease
- PTSD
- Peripheral neuropathy
- Severe arthritis
- Chronic or debilitating diseases or treatments causing:
  - Wasting
  - Severe pain

Phosphorated Carbohydrate Solution

The trade name of phosphorated carbohydrate solution is Emetrol, and it contains dextrose, fructose (a type of sugar), and phosphoric acid. It decreases the hyperactivity of the smooth muscle of the gastric mucosa. This medication is contraindicated in patients with diabetes mellitus because of the fructose content. It is available OTC and is taken by mouth. It is thought to be safe to use during pregnancy, but, as always, the physician's advice should be sought before any medication is taken.

Medications to Treat Gastroesophageal Reflux Disease

If the cardiac sphincter is loose, stomach acid can move upward into the esophagus, thus causing irritation and damage to the mucosa. This can result in **gastroesophageal reflux disease (GERD)** (Fig. 19-2). The burning sensation that the patient feels when acid damages the esophagus is **heartburn.** Heartburn does not actually involve the heart, but pain is localized near the heart, and patients often report that it feels like their heart is burning. Several medications are available to alleviate the symptoms of GERD and also promote healing.

Antacids

Antacids, as the name implies, decrease the amount of hydrochloric acid (HCl) in the stomach. Antacids create a more alkaline environment, which neutralizes the acid and protects the vulnerable mucosa, thereby relieving the pain and destruction associated with GERD. Except for sodium bicarbonate (baking soda), antacids are not readily absorbed and do not alter the pH of the entire body. These medications contain aluminum, calcium, magnesium, sodium, or a combination of these active ingredients. Thus, the prescriber will choose an antacid based on which of these substances the patient would benefit from best and which should be avoided. For example, a woman with osteoporosis would benefit from a calcium-based antacid. Conversely, a patient suffering from calcium-based kidney stones should avoid dietary calcium, so another medication would be chosen.

Some antacids may need to be taken regularly to condition the stomach to decrease acid production. Timing of these medications is critical; they must be taken before food. Sometimes antacids are given in suspension form, which must be shaken, or chewable tablets. Chewable tablets are usually taken with a glass of water or milk. Action occurs within 30 minutes to 3 hours. H_2-receptor blockers are given 1 hour before or 3 hours after meals. Long-term use of antacids can increase acid secretion. Patients should be cautioned not to overuse sodium bicarbonate because of its systemic effect, and they should be told that changing gastric acid pH may affect absorption of other medications.

Antacids are also used to lower elevated acid levels resulting from spicy foods and to decrease the nausea related to pregnancy hormones. Many mild antacids, such as Tums and Rolaids, are available OTC.

Proton Pump Inhibitor Drugs

Proton pump inhibitors reduce the acidity of the stomach by binding to stomach enzymes. Because they block the enzymes that cause acid production, these medications tend to protect the stomach for a longer period of time than those medications that just counteract the acid. They inhibit hydrogen and potassium ions and are used as short-term treatment for GERD and benign peptic ulcers. Side effects include abdominal pain, headache, constipation, diarrhea, and nausea. Examples of proton pump inhibitors are esomeprazole (Nexium), lansoprazole (Prevacid), omeprazole (Prilosec), pantoprazole (Protonix), and rabeprazole (Aciphex). These medications are given by mouth and are mostly available by prescription, although some are beginning to be available in low doses OTC. In addition, all of these

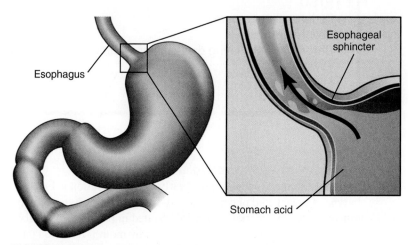

Esophagus

Esophageal sphincter

Stomach acid

FIGURE 19-2: Gastroesophageal reflux disease.

medications except pantoprazole may be given by the IV route when the patient is unable to tolerate the oral form.

Gastric Stimulants

Gastric stimulants or prokinetic agents stimulate gastric activity in the patient with decreased peptic activity. They decrease esophageal sphincter pressure and increase gastric emptying, which improves peristalsis. If a patient is at risk for aspiration of stomach contents, this drug may be given to decrease the amount of time the food is in the stomach and thus reduce the risk for aspiration pneumonia or choking. This quick emptying of the stomach has the added benefit of working as an antiemetic. An example of a GI stimulant is metoclopramide (Reglan). Reglan is given primarily by the IV route in the hospital setting, but it may also be given IM or by mouth. Side effects include drowsiness, restlessness, headache, dry mouth, menstrual period changes, and diarrhea.

Medications to Treat Peptic Ulcers

The stomach secretes HCl to break down food into amounts small enough to allow easy absorption. However, the stomach can create too much acid, which erodes the mucosal layer and can lead to a peptic **ulcer** (perforation of the mucosa) (Fig. 19-3). Acid from the stomach can spill into the duodenum and erode the mucosa there as well.

Patients at high risk for ulcers are those with type O blood, cigarette smokers, those infected with ***Helicobacter pylori (H. pylori),*** and those who do not cope well with stress. Alcohol, caffeinated foods and beverages, and certain drugs (corticosteroids, aspirin, nonsteroidal anti-inflammatory drugs [NSAIDs]) can also increase the risk for peptic ulcer.

H. pylori is associated with 75% of gastric ulcers and with 90% of duodenal ulcers. In the past, patients with peptic ulcers were encouraged to drink lots of milk because it was thought that ulcers were related

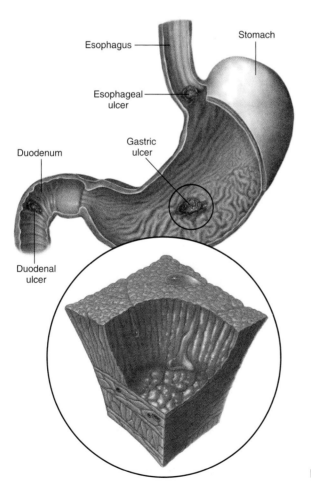

FIGURE 19-3: Peptic ulcers.

to the acidity of the stomach, and milk is alkaline. Now it is known that *H. pylori* grows very well in milk, and milk was perhaps one of the worst treatments to recommend. This is why it is important for health-care professionals to keep current on treatments supported by research. Some medications used to treat peptic ulcers include antibiotics, mucosal protectants, prostaglandins, antispasmodics, H_2-receptor antagonists, and proton pump inhibitors. Each is described in more detail here.

- **Antibiotics.** Antibiotics fight *H. pylori*. When the *H. pylori* is killed, the ulcer has a chance to heal. Antibiotics used to treat *H. pylori* include amoxicillin (Amoxil, Trimox), clarithromycin (Biaxin), metronidazole (Flagyl), and tetracycline. These agents are never used alone but in a combination of two antibiotics. This approach helps to avoid failure of treatment as well as antibiotic resistance. It is important that patients complete the entire 7- to 14-day regimen, even if they feel better, to remove the bacterium completely. Bismuth compounds can also be prescribed because they are bacteriostatic and stop *H. pylori* from sticking to the mucosa.

- **Mucosal protectants.** Mucosal protectants work to cover and protect the ulcer to promote healing. These oral medications must be taken on an empty stomach. Mucosal protectants such as sucralfate (Carafate), which is aluminum hydroxide and sulfated sucrose, are like a bandage protecting a wound from dirt and injury and allowing it to heal. Side effects include constipation and vitamin deficiency.

- **Prostaglandins.** Prostaglandins are hormone-like substances with a wide range of effects on the body, such as contraction and relaxation of smooth muscle, moderation of inflammation, and control of blood pressure. In the case of peptic ulcers, misoprostol (Cytotec) is a prostaglandin that inhibits gastric acid secretion and thus decreases the amount of acid in the stomach and protects the lining of the stomach. It is used to reduce the risk for NSAID-induced ulcers. This medication is taken orally, and side effects may include diarrhea, stomach cramps, and nausea during the first weeks of treatment; these side effects can be reduced by taking the medication with food. This drug must not be used during pregnancy because of the risk for miscarriage, premature labor, or possible birth defects.

- **Antispasmodics.** Antispasmodics (anticholinergics) decrease secretions and gastric mobility, reduce gastric spasm, and slow gastric motility. These effects decrease the exposure of the fragile gastric mucosa to HCl by keeping food in the stomach and reducing the amount of stomach acids produced. These medications are also used to treat GERD, ulcerative colitis, diverticulitis, biliary spasm, and irritable bowel syndrome. Examples include dicyclomine (Bentyl) and glycopyrrolate (Robinul). These are both available by prescription only. They may be administered orally but if needed can be given as an IM injection and, in the case of glycopyrrolate, as an IV dose.

- **H_2-receptor antagonists.** H_2-receptor antagonists are a group of drugs that block histamine from binding to parietal cells and prevent the parietal cells from secreting the gastric acid HCl. H_2-receptor antagonists include the drugs cimetidine (Tagamet), famotidine (Pepcid), nizatidine (Axid), and ranitidine (Taladine, Zantac). All of these medications are available both by prescription and in other forms OTC. Initial treatment of ulcers with cimetidine, famotidine, and ranitidine may be accomplished via IV therapy. Then, once the acute phase is treated, oral forms of the medications are begun. Nizatidine is only administered orally. In addition, ranitidine may be given as an IM injection. H_2-receptor antagonists can be taken with or without meals, but they are most effective if taken approximately 30 minutes before meals so that medications levels are optimal when acid is actively being produced. In addition, they should not be given within 1 hour of an antacid because the antacid may inhibit the absorption of the H_2-receptor antagonist. Side effects may include nausea, vomiting, diarrhea, dry mouth, dizziness, weakness, headache, and muscle cramps.

- **Proton pump inhibitors.** As discussed earlier in relation to GERD, these drugs reduce the acidity of the stomach and thus decrease exposure of the ulceration to acid. They are frequently combined with antibiotics to act against *H. pylori*.

Antacids and GI stimulants are also often used in the treatment of ulcers.

What risks for peptic ulcers involve lifestyle, not genetics? What lifestyle changes should a patient with a peptic ulcer make?

Medications to Treat Gallstones

Cholelithiasis, or the abnormal condition of having stones in the gallbladder, is caused when cholesterol or calcium forms a **calculus** (stone) (Fig. 19-4). Cholesterol cannot be seen on radiographs, but calcium stones can. Symptoms of gallstones are bloating, gas, and nausea. Most symptomatic patients undergo surgical removal of the stones and/or gallbladder. For patients who cannot tolerate surgery, medication such as ursodiol (Actigall, Urso) may be prescribed in oral form. Ursodiol is a naturally occurring bile acid that decreases the production of cholesterol and inhibits absorption of cholesterol by the intestines. Therapy can take up to 2 years, but if partial dissolution of the gallstones is not seen within 12 months, this treatment is likely to be unsuccessful. Side effects include flulike symptoms, stomach pain, dizziness, back pain, and headache.

Medications to Treat Obesity

Obesity rates in North America are increasing and are prompting many physicians to prescribe medications to decrease appetite. Many factors cause obesity: metabolic abnormalities, overeating, insulin resistance, and a sedentary lifestyle. A person is considered **morbidly obese** when he or she is 20% above ideal body weight. Obesity increases the workload of the pancreas, which helps digest carbohydrates, and the liver, which helps digest fats. It also causes increased workload on the circulatory system. Lifestyle changes are the best way to reduce obesity, but anorexiants (appetite suppressants) are sometimes necessary.

Appetite Suppressants

Appetite suppressants, also known as anorexiants, give a feeling of fullness. Suppressants can be used (with caution) to decrease food intake and thus decrease obesity potential. They mimic the sympathetic nervous system, so most are controlled substances. They are oral medications intended for short-term use only. Examples of these drugs include phentermine (Adipex-P, Oby-Cap, T-Diet, Zantryl). Taking phentermine concurrently with other diet medications can cause pulmonary hypertension, which can be fatal. In addition, phentermine can be habit-forming and affects cognitive function, so patients must be extremely cautious when taking this medication. Appetite suppressants sometimes create nausea.

Lipase Inhibitors

Lipase inhibitors such as orlistat (Alli, Xenical) can also be used to manage obesity. These drugs bind to the enzyme lipase, so the intestines cannot break down dietary fat. Instead, fats are eliminated in the feces. This reduces the amount of fat absorbed into the body and thereby reduces serum lipids. These medications are given by mouth and should not be taken by children or patients with chronic health

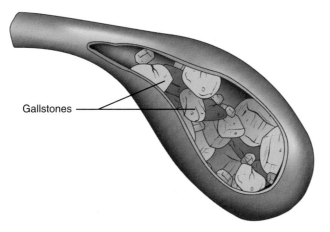

Gallstones

FIGURE 19-4: Cholelithiasis.

problems without close supervision by their physician. Xenical is available by prescription only, whereas Alli is the OTC version of this drug. Medication should not be taken more than three times a day or with a meal that does not contain fat. Meals with a high fat content will result in unpleasant GI side effects. Vitamin supplements may be suggested by the physician to compensate for any losses anticipated through use of this medication.

CRITICAL THINKING

What are some lifestyle changes that can lead to reduced weight?

Medications to Treat Hemorrhoids

Hemorrhoids are swollen varicose veins, and they usually occur if the anus, a sphincter at the end of the rectum, becomes irritated. **Fissures** are cracks in the same area. For these irritants, an anorectal preparation is often used to decrease swelling and soothe cracks. An example of a hemorrhoid cream is a combination of pramoxine, phenylephrine, glycerin, and petrolatum (Preparation H), which is applied topically to the hemorrhoids to shrink the swelling. Another medicated cream used for hemorrhoid treatment is pramoxine combined with zinc oxide (Anusol, Tronolane, Tucks). Pramoxine is an anesthetic to numb the pain and itching, whereas zinc oxide is a mineral that promotes healing. Some of these preparations contain lanolin or mineral oil, which act as an emollient to lubricate the anus and makes the passage of stool less traumatic. Anal fissures and hemorrhoids can be treated with rectal suppositories such as hydrocortisone acetate (Anusol-HC). This medication works by suppressing inflammation.

Medications to Treat Flatulence

Flatulence is gas released by the GI tract. Often, flatulence is caused by foods rather than by disease. Patients who complain of flatulence should be cautioned to decrease consumption of cabbage, onions, and beans and to use straws for drinking. Flatulence is more common in patients with air swallowing, diverticulitis, peptic ulcer, irritable bowel syndrome, and dyspepsia. Antiflatulents may also be used with gastroscopy and bowel radiography. The main drug in this class is simethicone (Flatulex, Gas-X, Genasyme, Mylicon). Many of these medications are available OTC, and all are oral medications. (See the Master the Essentials table for a more complete list of antiflatulent medications.) There are no reported adverse effects for this medication.

Medications to Treat Fungal Infections of the Gastrointestinal Tract

Oral candidiasis, **thrush,** is a fungal infection of the mucous membranes of the mouth (Fig. 19-5). Commonly, the only symptom is the presence of thick, white patches on the tongue and cheeks. These patches may extend into the esophagus and become painful and bleed if untreated. Nystatin (Bio-Statin, Mycostatin, Nilstat) is the main drug used to treat thrush. It is available as a suspension or a troche (lozenge). Regardless of the form used, it should be kept in the mouth as long as possible to coat the affected area. Troches should not be chewed or swallowed whole. Intestinal candidiasis is also treated with nystatin, but in tablet form. In this instance, the drugs should be swallowed whole. Because these medications are essentially topical applications and are not absorbed systematically, side effects are not expected to occur.

Medications to Treat Intestinal Parasites

Anthelmintics kill intestinal parasites, such as roundworms (ascariasis, hookworms, pinworms, strongyloidiasis, trichinosis, and whipworms) and tapeworms, by affecting the nervous system of the worm, paralyzing them, or preventing the worm from absorbing glucose. They also prevent newly hatched larvae from growing and multiplying. Roundworms may remain in the intestinal tract or enter other body tissues if untreated. Roundworms and tapeworms are treated with albendazole (Albenza), praziquantel (Biltricide), ivermectin (Stromectol), mebendazole (Vermox), pyrantel (Antiminth, Ascarel, Pin-X), and praziquantel (Biltricide). Laxatives may also be given at the same time to expel the dead parasites. Side effects are abdominal cramps, headaches, anorexia, nausea, and vomiting.

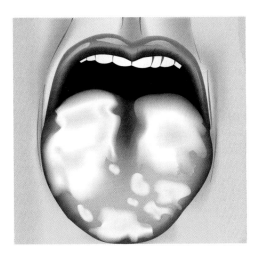

FIGURE 19-5: Oral candidiasis (thrush).

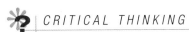 *CRITICAL THINKING*

Why is it important to cook chicken, beef, pork, and fish thoroughly?

Medications to Induce Vomiting and Treat Drug Overdose

Some medications are used to induce vomiting to rid the body of a harmful substance or toxin. Vomiting may or may not be beneficial, depending on the circumstance. If caused by food poisoning, vomiting is therapeutic because it helps rid the body of toxins. Antiemetics stop vomiting, and emetics promote it. Emetics, such as syrup of ipecac, induce vomiting in 80% to 90% of patients within 20 to 30 minutes. Syrup of ipecac has been widely used to induce vomiting in poisoning incidents outside the hospital. Now, however, parents are advised to destroy any syrup of ipecac that they have in the home because the benefits are inconclusive, and it may be dangerous. For instance, if it is given when a corrosive substance has been ingested, the substance will cause further damage when it is brought back up. Most poisonings and drug overdoses are treated with activated charcoal. Charcoal attracts the toxin and inactivates the poison as it travels the length of the GI tract in most instances. The poison is then excreted in the stool. Always call poison control anywhere in the United States at 1-800-222-1222 to receive the most current recommendations before acting to prevent further injury to a patient.

Because of the increase in drug overdoses in the United States, naloxone (Narcan) is becoming a standard medication available to many police departments and schools as well as EMS. Narcan blocks the effects of opioids and thus can reverse an overdose. It comes in a nasal spray for use outside of a medical facility as well as an injectable form that can be given as an injection or as a continuous IV drip.

Nutritional Supplements

Poor nutrition can result in poor health. Malnutrition can be caused by lack of availability of food, excessive dieting, poor dietary choices, or illnesses that reduce appetite. Medications that reduce nausea and vomiting can improve nutritional status. Furthermore, nutritional supplements such as a multivitamin can compensate for a lack of vitamins in food.

Nutritional supplements may not sound like drugs, but they are frequently prescribed to improve nutrition in patients who are malnourished. These supplements are more easily tolerated in a patient who is weak and possibly has a compromised immune system. Liquid nutritional supplements can help improve health. Examples include Boost and Ensure. Store brands are available, but be sure to ask the prescriber whether substitutions are allowed. Some prescribers want specific nutrients found only in certain supplements. The patient can usually choose the flavor of the supplement, however.

Digestants

In some instances, patients have difficulty digesting the food that they eat, most commonly because of a food allergy or possibly a genetic disorder such as cystic fibrosis. If a patient has no medical reason to avoid a certain food, medications can be given to assist with the digestion of the meal. One example is Lactaid, which is used in patients who are lactose intolerant to enable them to tolerate milk products. Patients with cystic fibrosis do not produce digestive enzymes in quantities sufficient to digest any food. Therefore, they require digestive enzymes (Enzymatic Digestant Oral) with every meal and snack that they ingest.

Mouthwashes and Other Oral Treatments

Mouthwashes or mouth rinses are used to decrease **halitosis** (bad breath) or **stomatitis** (inflammation of the mouth). Fluoride preparations can prevent tooth decay by hardening the tooth enamel. They are prescribed in tablets, drops, or mouth rinses. For a patient who does not produce saliva, saliva substitutes are prescribed. Oral topical anesthetics can be used for teething pain and mouth ulcers. Hydrogen peroxide is available OTC and acts as a weak antibacterial agent in the mouth. Dentifrices or toothpastes are used to clean teeth, decrease plaque, and prevent gum disease. Some have whitening elements as well.

●●● SUMMARY

■ For the gastrointestinal (GI), or digestive, system to function optimally, it is important to understand how the food we eat and drink affects it. Sometimes, what we consume can cause illness, pain, or discomfort.

■ The GI system consists of the alimentary canal, which is responsible for the four major functions of the digestive system: ingestion, digestion, absorption, and excretion.

■ Digestion is the process of converting food into chemical substances used by the body. Hydrochloric acid (HCl) in the stomach helps it break down food for absorption in the small intestine.

■ The GI system is vulnerable to bacterial and parasitic infection.

■ GI medications work to increase or decrease function by changing the muscle tone, replacing deficient enzymes, or increasing or decreasing the emptying time or rate of passage through the system.

■ The timing of GI medication administration is important for proper action or absorption.

■ GI medications have diverse purposes, including, but not limited to, coating the stomach, relieving nausea and vomiting, inducing vomiting, reducing acid in the stomach, protecting teeth, killing microbes, promoting good nutrition, reducing diarrhea and constipation, suppressing the appetite, and reducing gas.

Master the Essentials: Gastrointestinal Medications

This table shows the various classes of gastrointestinal medications and key side effects, contraindications and precautions, and interactions for each class.

Class	Indications for Use	Side Effects	Contraindications/ Precautions	Interactions	Examples
Antacids	Peptic ulcers, GERD, acid indigestion	Constipation, diarrhea (especially with magnesium compounds), electrolyte imbalances, flatulence, kidney stones, osteoporosis	Heart failure, dehydration, kidney or liver disease	Antibiotics, salicylates	Magnesium hydroxide (Dulcolax, Phillips Milk of Magnesia), magnesium oxide (Mag-ox 400, Uro-Mag), aluminum hydroxide gel (Alterna gel), calcium carbonate (Tums), aluminum-magnesium combinations (Maalox, Mylanta)
Anorexiants	Obesity	Palpitations, arrhythmias, dry mouth, hair loss, blurred vision, hypotension, dizziness, drowsiness	Arteriosclerosis, heart disease, hypertension, glaucoma, pregnancy	MAOIs, SSRIs, TCAs, alcohol, other diet medications	Phentermine (Adipex-P, Oby-Cap, T-Diet, Zantryl)
Antidiarrheals	Diarrhea	Nausea, vomiting, drowsiness; constipation (kaolin and pectin)	Hypersensitivity, bloody diarrhea	Alcohol, opiates, barbiturates, sedatives, metoclopramide, digoxin, allopurinol (kaolin and pectin)	Bismuth subsalicylate (Pepto-Bismol), diphenoxylate with atropine (Lomotil), loperamide (Imodium), kaolin and pectin (Kaopectate), *Lactobacillus acidophilus* (Lactinex, Bacid)
Antiemetics	Nausea, vomiting, motion sickness prophylaxis	Drowsiness, agitation, confusion, constipation, dry mouth, nausea, anorexia	Sensitivity, severe emesis, seizure disorder, pregnancy, prolonged QTc interval (5-HT$_3$ receptor antagonists)	Anticholinergics, lithium, CNS depressants	Chlorpromazine (Thorazine), prochlorperazine (Compazine), dolasetron (Anzemet), ondansetron (Zofran), granisetron (Kytril), palonosetron (Aloxi), dimenhydrinate (Dramamine), diphenhydramine (Benadryl), meclizine (Antivert, Bonine), promethazine (Adgan, Phenergan), trimethobenzamide (Benzacot, Tigan, Ticon), scopolamine (Maldemar, Scopace, Transderm-Scōp), nabilone (Cesamet), phosphorated carbohydrate solution (Emetrol), metoclopramide (Reglan)
Antiflatulents	Excessive intestinal gas	None reported	None reported	None reported	Simethicone (Alka-Seltzer Anti-Gas, Bicarsim, Equalize Gas Relief Drops, Flatulex, Gas Aid, Gas Free, Gas-X, Genasyme, Gerber Gas Relief Infantaire Gas Relief, Little Tummys, Maalox Anti-Gas, Mi-Acid Gas Relief, Mylanta Gas, Mylicon, Mytab Gas, Phazyme, SimePed)

Continued

Master the Essentials: Gastrointestinal Medications—cont'd

Class	Indications for Use	Side Effects	Contraindications/ Precautions	Interactions	Examples
Antifungals	Thrush	Nausea, vomiting, diarrhea	Hypersensitivity, pregnancy	None reported	Nystatin (Bio-Statin, Mycostatin, Nilstat)
Anthelmintics	Parasitic infection of GI tract	Abdominal pain, diarrhea	Hypersensitivity, pregnancy	Carbamazepine, hydantoins	Albendazole (Albenza), praziquantel (Biltricide), ivermectin (Stromectol), mebendazole (Vermox), pyrantel (Antiminth, Ascarel, Pin-X)
Antispasmodics	Irritable bowel syndrome, diverticulitis, peptic ulcer	Palpitations, vision disturbances, headache, nervousness	Hypersensitivity, glaucoma, bowel obstruction, urinary retention	Digoxin, phenothiazines, TCAs	Dicyclomine (Bentyl), glycopyrrolate (Robinul)
Bowel evacuants	Preparation for GI procedures (surgical and radiological) such as endoscopy, colonoscopy, sigmoid-oscopy	Nausea, abdominal fullness, bloating, cramping	GI obstruction, ileus, gastric retention, bowel perforation, pregnancy	Administration of oral drugs within 1 hour may be flushed from GI tract	Polyethylene glycol electrolyte solution (Colyte, GoLYTELY, MoviPrep, NuLYTELY, PEG-3350 with Electrolytes, TriLyte), polyethylene glycol 3350 (GlycoLax, MiraLax)
Gallstone-solubilizing agents	Gallstones	Headache, abdominal pain, diarrhea, dyspepsia, nausea	Hypersensitivity, intermittent acute cholecystitis, gallstone pancreatitis	Antacids, bile acid sequestrants, oral contraceptives	Ursodiol (Actigall, Urso)
GI stimulants (prokinetic agents)	GERD	Extrapyramidal symptoms, dizziness, drowsiness, fatigue, headache, insomnia, restlessness	GI hemorrhage, pheochromocytoma, sensitivity	Alcohol, cimetidine, cyclosporine, digoxin, levodopa, MAOIs, anticholinergics	Metoclopramide (Reglan, Metozolv ODT), cisapride (Propulsid)
H. pylori agents	Peptic ulcer	Diarrhea, tinnitus, infection, mild GI problems	Kidney or liver insufficiency	Salicylates, digoxin, anticoagulants	Amoxicillin (Amoxil, Trimox), clarithromycin (Biaxin), metronidazole (Flagyl), tetracycline

Drug class	Uses	Side effects	Contraindications	Drug interactions	Medications
H₂-receptor antagonists	Duodenal ulcer, gastric ulcer, GERD	Constipation, diarrhea, nausea, headache, malaise, rash	Hypersensitivity, liver impairment	Antacids, benzodiazepines, opioids, phenytoin, beta blockers, calcium channel blockers, cyclosporine	Cimetidine (Tagamet), famotidine (Pepcid), nizatidine (Axid), ranitidine (Zantac)
Laxatives and stool softeners	Constipation	Diarrhea, nausea, vomiting, cramping, bloating, flatulence	Hypersensitivity, nausea, vomiting, fecal impaction, intestinal obstruction	Antacids, H₂-receptor antagonists, proton pump inhibitors	Psyllium (Metamucil, Citrucel), mineral oil (Fleet Mineral Oil), magnesium hydroxide (Phillips Milk of Magnesia), docusate (Colace), senna with docusate bisacodyl (Peri-Colace, Dulcolax, Fleet), glycerine (Colace suppository), polyethylene glycol solution (MiraLax)
Lipase inhibitors	Obesity	Flatulence, fecal urgency, oily stool, incontinence, abdominal pain	Hypersensitivity, malabsorption syndrome, cholestasis	Prevastatin, warfarin	Orlistat (alli, Xenical)
Prostaglandins	Duodenal or gastric ulcer	Diarrhea, abdominal pain	Pregnancy, history of allergy to prostaglandins, heart disease	Antacids	Misoprostol (Cytotec)
Proton pump inhibitors	Active duodenal ulcers, GERD, benign gastric ulcers	Headache, abdominal pain, nausea, constipation, diarrhea	Hypersensitivity, liver disease	Clarithromycin, sucralfate, benzodiazepines, azole antifungals, digoxin, hydantoins	Esomeprazole (Nexium), lansoprazole (Prevacid), omeprazole (Prilosec), pantoprazole (Protonix), rabeprazole (Aciphex)
Mucosal protectant	Ulcers	Constipation, diarrhea, nausea, vomiting, flatulence, rash	Renal failure	Antacids, anticoagulants, digoxin, H₂-receptor antagonists, hydantoins	Sucralfate (Carafate)

CNS, central nervous system; GERD, gastroesophageal reflux disease; GI, gastrointestinal; 5-HT₃, serotonin; MAOI, monoamine oxidase inhibitor; SSRI, selective serotonin reuptake inhibitor; TCA, tricyclic antidepressant.

Activities

To make sure that you have learned the key points covered in this chapter, complete the following activities.

True or False

Write true if the statement is true. Beside the false statements, write false, and correct the statement to make it true.

1. Flatulence is intestinal gas. _____

_____

2. *H. pylori* is the bacterium responsible for causing GERD. _____

_____

3. Type AB blood is a risk factor for the development of ulcers. _____

_____

4. Anthelmintics are used to treat intestinal parasites. _____

_____

5. Halitosis means bad breath. _____

_____

6. High-fat meals are allowable when taking lipase inhibitors such as orlistat. _____

_____

7. Laxatives may be prescribed when a patient is taking anthelmintic medications. _____

_____

8. Cholelithiasis is a condition in which stones are present in the gallbladder. _____

_____

9. Medication taken for gallstones is effective within 6 weeks. _____

_____

10. Thrush is oral candidiasis. _____

_____

Choose the best answer for each question.

1. A crack at the end of the rectum is called a _____.

A. Halitosis

B. Pica

C. Peristalsis

D. Fissure

2. Intestinal gas is called _____.

A. GERD

B. Halitosis

C. *Helicobacter pylori*

D. Flatulence

3. Which of the following is NOT a type of antiemetic?

A. Phenothiazines

B. Antihistamines

C. Prostaglandins

D. Cannabinoids

4. Which medication is used to treat GERD?

A. Laxatives

B. Proton pump inhibitors

C. Antiemetics

D. Emetics

5. Which medication causes a reduction in spasms associated with GI disorders?

A. Anticholinergics

B. Laxatives

C. Antiemetics

D. Prostaglandins

6. Inflamed varicose veins located in the rectum are called _____.

A. Pica

B. Peristalsis

C. Hemorrhoids

D. Fissures

7. The medication prescribed for oral thrush is _____.

A. Nystatin

B. Simethicone

C. Amoxicillin

D. Activated charcoal

8. The medication prescribed for *H. pylori* is _____.
   A. Nystatin
   B. Simethicone
   C. Amoxicillin
   D. Activated charcoal

9. The medication taken for flatulence is _____.
   A. Nystatin
   B. Simethicone
   C. Amoxicillin
   D. Activated charcoal

10. A medication administered to treat a drug overdose is _____.
   A. Nystatin
   B. Simethicone
   C. Amoxicillin
   D. Activated charcoal

Application Exercises
Respond to the following situations.

1. Butler is having gastric bypass surgery, and the surgeon is removing most of Butler's stomach. How will that affect the absorption of drugs he takes?_____
   _____
   _____

2. Cliff wants to lose weight. He wants to be put on Xenical but continue his lifestyle. What would you teach him? _____
   _____
   _____

3. Marilyn takes Dulcolax every night to a have bowel movement. Is this a good practice? Why or why not? _____
   _____
   _____

4. Joyce says that her mother always drank milk to treat her stomach ulcer. She does not understand why she is taking antibiotics and told not to use milk to treat the ulcer. What would you say? _____
   _____
   _____

For further study and practice with drug classifications learned in this chapter, complete the following table to the best of your ability. Use resources such as the *PDR,* the Internet, or printed drug guides for help.

Trade Name	Generic Name	Classification	Purpose	Side Effects	Contraindications and Precautions	Examples	Patient Education
Maalox							
Imodium							
Mycostatin							
Ipecac							
Reglan							
Biaxin							
Pepcid							
Cytotec							
Prilosec							

Internet Research

Using your favorite search engine:

1. Find an article on obesity, and download it. Share and discuss this article with your class.

2. Find a body mass index calculator, and figure out yours.

3. Download some weight-loss tips to help make a teaching plan for your patients.

20

Reproductive and Urinary System Medications

The reproductive system is responsible for the procreation of our species, whereas the urinary system's main function is to remove toxins from our body while conserving electrolytes. Reproductive disorders can cause pain, infertility, and sometimes death if they are not treated. Most medications used in the reproductive system are hormone based. A prime example is birth control pills, which can not only prevent pregnancy, but also help to manage painful menstruation. Urinary system disorders can cause discomfort and pain, and untreated urinary system failure can lead to death. One of the most common groups of medications used for the urinary system consists of diuretics, which increase the excretion of water and waste products. Another common group of medications comprises those used for benign prostatic hypertrophy (BPH). These medications decrease the size of the prostate gland and allow urine to flow more freely.

LEARNING OUTCOMES

At the end of this chapter, you should be able to:

20.1   Define all key terms.

20.2   List actions of the reproductive hormones FSH, LH, and ICSH.

20.3   Describe how contraceptives work.

20.4   Describe the effects of estrogens, progestins, agents for cervical ripening, oxytocin, tocolytics, ovulation stimulants, androgens, diuretics, and BPH medications.

20.5   Discuss the relation of diuretics to electrolyte imbalances.

KEY TERMS

Androgen
Benign prostatic
    hypertrophy (BPH)
Enuresis
Estrogen
Follicle-stimulating
    hormone (FSH)

Hormone replacement
    therapy (HRT)
Interstitial cell–stimulating
    hormone (ICSH)
Luteinizing hormone (LH)
Progestin

Sexually transmitted
    disease (STD)
Tocolytic

HORMONES OF THE REPRODUCTIVE SYSTEM

Several hormones, known as gonadotropic hormones, and their interactions are responsible for optimal functioning of the testes and ovaries. These hormones are secreted by the pituitary gland and include **follicle-stimulating hormone (FSH), luteinizing hormone (LH),** and **interstitial cell–stimulating hormone (ICSH).** These hormones are responsible for the production of the female hormones estrogen and progestin and the male hormone androgen (testosterone). Testosterone, estrogen, and progesterone are hormones that promote the health, growth, and function of the reproductive system. The testes in the male (testicles) produce testosterone (Fig. 20-1A). The ovaries in the female secrete female sex hormones (estrogen and progesterone) (Fig. 20-1B).

As discussed in Chapter 15, FSH regulates sperm and egg production. LH triggers the release of the egg in women and promotes secretion of estrogen and progesterone. In men, LH is called ICSH and regulates testosterone production. Table 20-1 summarizes the reproductive hormones.

MEDICATIONS FOR DISORDERS RELATED TO FEMALE HORMONES

If the hormone levels are either too high or too low in women, fertility can be affected. Too little progesterone will not sustain a pregnancy, and too much FSH or LH may lead to multiple births. The classifications of medications used include contraceptives such as medroxyprogesterone (Provera), used to prevent pregnancy and stabilize menstrual cycles, and hormone replacement medications such as testosterone (AndroGel) or estrogen (Premarin), used when a normally occurring hormone is lacking as a result of disease or the aging process (see the Master the Essentials table for a more comprehensive list of medications used in treatment of reproductive health and illness).

Contraceptive Medications

Some of the most common drugs used for contraception are based on hormones that a woman naturally produces. When administered as a drug, they prevent pregnancy by overriding the body's own mechanism to make **estrogens** and **progestins** (the two main hormones secreted by the ovaries). The body, while receiving hormones from an outside source regularly, stops producing its own estrogens and progestins. Contraceptives contain such low doses of the hormones that they usually inhibit the body's ability to conceive by inhibiting ovulation (release of an egg from the ovary), inhibiting fertilization (joining of the egg and sperm to form an embryo), preventing implantation (embedding of the embryo into the uterine wall), or preventing growth of the fetus.

One of the most common forms of birth control is the "pill." It is available in formulations that provide differing amounts of estrogen and progestin during the menstrual cycle. Monophasic pills, such as ethinyl estradiol and norgestrel (Cryselle 28, Lo/Ovral 28, Ogestrel-28) or ethinyl estradiol and norethindrone (Aranelle, Modicon, Ortho-Novum), deliver a constant amount of hormone during the first 21 days of the cycle. Biphasic birth control pills, such as ethinyl estradiol and norethindrone (Jenest-28) and ethinyl estradiol and desogestrel (Apri, Desogen, Mircette, Ortho-Cept), contain a constant dose of estrogen but two different doses of progestin in the monthly cycle dosage. This allows

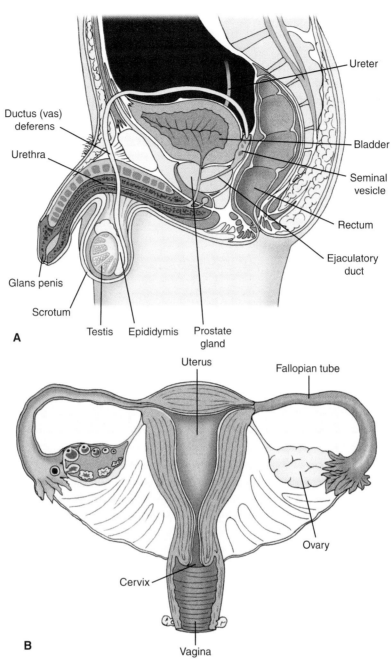

FIGURE 20-1: Male and female reproductive systems. A, Male reproductive system. Internal and external male reproductive system. B, Female reproductive system. Internal female reproductive system.

the lining of the uterus to develop normally during the menstrual cycle. These differing doses are reflected by pills of different colors. Triphasic birth control pills, such as ethinyl estradiol and norethindrone (Aranelle, Junel FE 1/20, Ortho-Novum 7/7/7) and ethinyl estradiol and levonorgestrel (Alesse, Levlite, Lutera, Portia, Tri-Levlen), contain a varying amount of both estrogen and progestin with three different strengths during the monthly cycle dosage, each denoted with a pill of a different color.

In addition, there is the minipill progestin (Errin, Ovrette, Provera), which contains only progestin and therefore is slightly less effective. Evidence proving that any of the three foregoing types of birth control is superior to the others is lacking. A multitude of manufactured variations exists, and it may take experimentation to determine the best birth control method for an individual woman.

TABLE 20.1 Reproductive Hormones

Hormone	Action	Too Much Causes....	Too Little Causes...
Prolactin	Stimulates milk production in the mammary gland	Overproduction of breast milk in women Milk production in non-nursing patient a possible sign of a pituitary tumor Parlodel used to suppress lactation in women who choose not to breastfeed, but side effect is increased fertility	Underproduction of milk in women; baby has difficulty nursing
Follicle-stimulating hormone (FSH)	Stimulates sperm production in men and egg production in women	Increased fertility	Men: sterility Women: irregular or absent menses
Luteinizing hormone (LH)	Stimulates release of a ripened egg in women (ovulation); also helps in the production of female hormones (estrogens and progestins)	Multiple gestations (e.g., twins, triplets)	Infertility (woman cannot ovulate, so cannot conceive)
Interstitial cell–stimulating hormone (ICSH)	Stimulates production of androgens (male hormone testosterone)	Aggressiveness, excessive hair	Feminine attributes in men (e.g., high voice, small muscles)

Sometimes patients experience symptoms of pregnancy while taking contraceptive pills or tablets because normal reproductive functioning shuts down, so the body behaves as though it is pregnant (e.g., weight gain, mood swings, and breast tenderness).

If contraception fails or fails to be used properly, a woman can use postcoital high-dose estrogen to prevent pregnancy. The medications prescribed for this postcoital contraception are levonorgestrel emergency contraceptive (Plan B) and ethinyl estradiol and levonorgestrel (Preven EC).

Contraceptive hormones are also commonly delivered via vaginal ring ethinyl estradiol and etonogestrel (NuvaRing), implants, intrauterine devices (IUDs), and transdermal patches. NuvaRing is a flexible ring containing estrogen and progestin that is inserted into the vagina every month. This prevents ovulation, fertilization, and implantation. This ring is removed after 3 weeks, to allow normal menstruation to occur. A new ring is placed 7 days after removal of the previous ring.

The only available implant currently is etonogestrel (Implanon, Nexplanon), which contains a hormone that prevents ovulation, makes it more difficult for sperm to reach the uterus, and prevents implantation of a fertilized egg. The implant is a small plastic rod containing the medication and is placed in the upper arm. This method provides contraception for up to 3 years.

The levonorgestrel intrauterine system Mirena contains the hormone progestin and is placed in the uterus by a physician. This device makes the uterus a very unwelcoming place for sperm, and the lining of the uterus becomes a difficult place in which to implant a fertilized egg. The hormone-based IUD may be left in place for 5 years. Another type of IUD that does not contain hormones is the copper IUD. Copper is naturally toxic to sperm, and the fluids produced in response by the uterus and fallopian tubes are also deadly to sperm. These copper IUDs may be left in place for 10 years.

Transdermal patches such as the Ortho Evra patch contain ethinyl estradiol and norelgestromin, which are forms of estrogen and progestin, to prevent ovulation. A new patch is applied weekly for 3 weeks, and no patch is used for the fourth week, to allow a normal menstrual period to occur.

All of these hormone-based contraceptive medications must be taken with care. They have a risk for serious side effects, such as the formation of blood clots, especially in women older than 35 years of age. Smoking increases the risk for blood clots. Women with a history of blood clots or diseases involving the vascular system should not be prescribed these medications.

Another common method of birth control is the use of barrier devices such as condoms or diaphragms in combination with spermicides containing nonoxynol-9 such as Encare and Conceptrol. The barrier devices are the only contraceptives effective against sexually transmitted diseases (STDs), as well as preventing pregnancy.

The medication mifepristone (Mifeprex), originally known as RU-486, is used to stop a pregnancy. This medication blocks the hormone progesterone, which is necessary for pregnancy to be successful. The medication is only used during the first 7 weeks since the last menstrual period. Because this medication causes cramping and bleeding, it is not advised in patients taking blood thinners such as Coumadin. This medication is given in an oral form and is taken in the physician's office. If, on rechecking, the patient is still pregnant after 3 days, she will be administered an additional oral dose of mifepristone and rechecked in 2 weeks.

Table 20-2 summarizes the information on contraceptive medications.

Hormone Replacement Therapy

Women experiencing menopause (permanent cessation of menses) may choose to take **hormone replacement therapy (HRT).** This term refers to the administration of hormones to replace those that are no

TABLE 20.2   Examples of Contraceptive Medications

Type	Action	Examples
Monophasic tablets	Prevent ovulation	Ethinyl estradiol and norgestrel (Cryselle 28, Lo/Ovral 28, Ogestrel-28), ethinyl estradiol and norethindrone (Aranelle, Modicon, Ortho-Novum)
Biphasic tablets	Prevent ovulation	Ethinyl estradiol and norethindrone (Jenest-28), ethinyl estradiol and desogestrel (Apri, Desogen, Mircette, Ortho-Cept)
Triphasic tablets	Prevent ovulation	Ethinyl estradiol and norethindrone (Aranelle, Junel FE 1/20, Ortho-Novum 7/7/7), ethinyl estradiol and levonorgestrel (Alesse, Levlite, Lutera, Portia, Tri-Levlen)
Vaginal ring	Inhibits reproductive function	Ethinyl estradiol and etonogestrel (NuvaRing)
Implants	Prevent ovulation, fertilization, and implantation	Etonogestrel (Implanon, Nexplanon)
Transdermal patches	Prevent ovulation	Ethinyl estradiol and norelgestromin (Ortho Evra patch)
IUDs	Prevent implantation, kill sperm	Levonorgestrel intrauterine system (Mirena), copper IUD
Spermicides	Kill sperm	Nonoxynol-9 (Encare and Conceptrol) Diaphragm, male condom, female condom
Barrier devices	Prevent fertilization	Levonorgestrel emergency contraceptive (Plan B), ethinyl estradiol and levonorgestrel (Preven)
Postcoital contraception	Prevents ovulation, fertilization, and implantation	Mifepristone (Mifeprex)
Abortifacient	Kills fetus within 49 days from menstrual period	Ethinyl estradiol and norgestrel (Cryselle 28, Lo/Ovral 28, Ogestrel-28), ethinyl estradiol and norethindrone (Aranelle, Modicon, Ortho-Novum)

IUD, intrauterine device.

longer being naturally produced during and after menopause. If a woman no longer has a uterus, her own estrogen is replaced because there is no buildup of the lining of the uterus. If the woman still has a uterus, estrogen is usually combined with a progestin in this therapy, so the endometrial lining is shed in the same way it would be in the presence of natural hormones. If estrogen is taken without the addition of progesterone in these women, the risk for endometrial cancer is higher. Estrogen therapy is taken as a pill such as Estrace or Premarin, a cream such as Estrace or Dienestrol, or a patch such as Estraderm, Alora, or Vivelle. Combination estrogen-progesterone therapy is prescribed as an oral pill (Prempro) or a patch (Climara-Pro).

Women also produce small amounts of testosterone, and when these levels begin to decline, replacing testosterone may help relieve the symptoms of menopause, such as hot flashes and vaginal dryness. A combination of estrogen and testosterone is administered as a tablet in medications such as Covaryx and Estratest. HRT has been shown to decrease bone loss and cardiovascular dysfunction. However, studies have shown that using HRT increases the risk for breast cancer, stroke, and blood clots. Therefore, HRT is an individual decision. If a woman does not elect HRT, alternative treatments to relieve menopausal symptoms should be discussed, and treatment should be reevaluated on an annual basis.

HRT can also be used to treat prostate cancer in men because estrogen decreases testosterone levels. In addition, men are believed to endure their own form of menopause in which their testosterone levels diminish. Studies are showing a possible decrease in heart disease, diabetes, and death when androgen replacement therapy is administered. The most common method of administering the androgen testosterone in these patients is through a gel (AndroGel) that is rubbed into the skin on a daily basis.

Medications for Abnormal Uterine Bleeding

Abnormal uterine bleeding is a condition in which vaginal bleeding occurs irregularly or too heavily. Correcting the hormonal imbalance that typically causes this condition is often indicated. Combination therapy of estrogen and progesterone, as oral contraceptives, can be prescribed. Progestins (progesterone) alone can also be prescribed to regulate the rhythm and amount of menstruation.

The medications leuprolide (Eligard, Lupron) and goserelin (Zoladex) are gonadotropin-releasing hormone agonists. They are frequently used to suppress buildup of the endometrial lining in patients with endometriosis by reducing estrogen levels in women and thus creating an artificial menopause-like condition that allows the endometrial lining to heal. These medications are injected approximately once a month; treatment is short term, lasting no more than 6 months. In some patients, the side effects are temporary; in others, long-term side effects last 6 months to longer than 5 years. Because of this risk for long-term, sometimes serious side effects, the benefits versus risks must be carefully evaluated. Side effects mimic those of menopause: hot flashes, bone loss, lack of menstrual periods, mood swings, insomnia, headaches, vaginal dryness, and increased cholesterol levels.

■ LABOR MEDICATIONS

Labor needs to occur when the baby is fully developed and able to survive outside the mother's womb. Unfortunately, because of unforeseen circumstances, the baby may be in danger of being born too early to survive. In other cases, the baby does not seem in any hurry to be born but is developmentally ready. In these instances, medications used for labor include those to hasten labor, which include cervical ripening agents and oxytocin, and those to slow or stop labor, such as tocolytics.

Cervical ripening agents are those that are applied topically to the cervix of the uterus to prepare it for labor. The agents soften the cervix in the hopes of initiating dilation. Dinoprostone (Cervidil, Prepidil) is a prostaglandin used for cervical ripening. The gel form is inserted into the cervix; the vaginal insert is placed in the posterior fornix of the vagina. The cervix is then allowed time to soften gently. If labor does not begin in approximately 6 hours, a second dose may be administered, or the patient may be started on oxytocin (Pitocin, Syntocinon), which is the pituitary hormone that causes the uterus to contract. Both medications should not be used simultaneously because this may cause a much stronger effect than with either drug alone. If labor fails to progress, synthetic oxytocin (Pitocin) can be given by the intravenous (IV) route over time to encourage the uterus gently to contract (however, women in labor may argue that there is nothing gentle about this drug) (Fig. 20-2). This medication is administered only in a controlled setting in which the mother is closely monitored for complications such as developing hypertension. It may also be given after the baby is born to contract the uterus and thus help control postpartum bleeding.

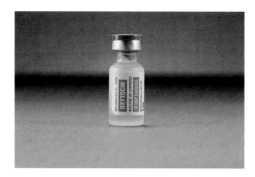

FIGURE 20-2: Oxytocin

Labor **tocolytics** have an effect opposite that of oxytocin. They slow or stop uterine contractions and are indicated to prevent premature birth and allow the baby to mature, especially its lungs. Magnesium sulfate, indomethacin, and nifedipine are agents used as tocolytics. These medications are labeled for other uses, but they are commonly used to stop labor.

Magnesium sulfate is not proven to stop preterm labor, but it is commonly used to treat preeclampsia (a pregnancy-related condition) and premature labor. It may be given by the IV route for a short time (24 to 48 hours) and is thought to act as a calcium channel blocker, by keeping the calcium from the muscles, where it is needed for the uterus to contract. There is some belief that if other tocolytics are ineffective and premature birth is imminent, magnesium sulfate may reduce the possibility of cerebral palsy in the preterm infant. Side effects include hypotension, cardiac arrhythmias, and weakness.

A medication that can be taken orally for preterm labor is nifedipine (Adalat CC, Procardia). This medication is a calcium channel blocker, which relaxes smooth muscles such as the uterus. This medication is used when the cervix is minimally dilated, the amniotic sac remains intact, and other tocolytic medications have not been successful. Again, this medication is preferably used on a short-term basis (for 24 to 48 hours).

Indomethacin (Indocin, Tivorbex) is a strong NSAID that is administered by the IV route, orally, or as a rectal suppository. This drug is commonly used as an anti-inflammatory drug for joint conditions. Indocin has a strong antiprostaglandin effect, which is necessary for uterine contractions. Use should be limited to less than 7 days, to minimize effects on the developing fetus. This medication should not be used during the last 2 months of pregnancy because of the effects on fetal cardiac development.

■ INFERTILITY MEDICATIONS

Medications can also help women increase their fertility. Some medications are used to help ovaries release multiple eggs, to increase the chance that one will be fertilized and grow into a fetus. These drugs are referred to as ovulation stimulants. Clomiphene (Clomid, Serophene) is an example of a drug that increases the hormones FSH and LH, which initiate ovulation. This is the drug of choice when infertility has no obvious cause, and the medication is taken orally with minimal side effects. Menotropins (Humegon, Menopur, Pergonal, Repronex) are given as an injection that stimulates follicle ripening and release. This treatment is indicated in women who have functional ovaries but in whom hormonal stimulation is lacking. Chorionic gonadotropin (Ovidrel, Pregnyl) is given as an injection in combination with clomiphene to stimulate the release of a mature egg. The patient should be prepared for the possibility of not becoming pregnant or becoming pregnant with multiple fetuses when fertility drugs are used.

■ MEDICATIONS FOR OTHER FEMALE REPRODUCTIVE DISORDERS

Premenstrual dysphoric disorder (formerly premenstrual syndrome or PMS) is frequently treated with selective serotonin reuptake inhibitors (SSRIs). Serotonin levels are increased with the use of SSRIs, and this leads to alleviation of many symptoms of PMS such as hot flashes, depression, anxiety, and pain.

Medications are also used to treat infections of the female reproductive tract. Some infections are caused by **sexually transmitted diseases (STDs)** such as syphilis. Among the more popular drugs for vaginal infections are the following: antibacterials such as metronidazole (Flagyl), used orally or by the IV route to treat trichomonas infections; antivirals such as acyclovir (Zovirax), used orally and intravenously to treat herpes infections; and antifungals such as miconazole (Monistat), used topically or orally to treat vaginal yeast infections (see Chapter 17 for a review of immune system medications such as antibacterials, antivirals, and antifungals).

■ MEDICATIONS FOR MALE REPRODUCTIVE DISORDERS

Androgens are male sex hormones that promote maturation of the male sexual organs and male sexual characteristics. Men who have low androgen levels may need testosterone to increase their masculine traits. Testosterone can also be used to lower estrogen levels in women with breast cancer, just as estrogen is used to lower testosterone levels in men who have prostate cancer.

Erectile dysfunction, or impotence, is a fairly common disorder, frequently related to atherosclerosis, diabetes, stroke, and hypertension. This disorder may also have psychological roots, such as guilt, fatigue, depression, and fear of failure to perform adequately.

Erectile dysfunction drugs such as phosphodiesterase type 5 inhibitors usually work by dilating the arteries leading to the penis and constricting the veins and thereby holding the blood in the penis and sustaining an erection. If erectile dysfunction is associated with physiological decline, it is vitally important that the patient give a complete history to the prescriber. Medications such as sildenafil (Revatio, Viagra), vardenafil (Levitra, Staxyn), and tadalafil (Adcirca, Cialis) can be dangerous for patients with a history of cardiovascular disease, stroke, and sickle cell anemia or eye problems. Sildenafil, vardenafil, and tadalafil are taken orally approximately 30 minutes to 1 hour before sexual activity and no more often than one dose per day. Cialis may also be prescribed to be taken orally on a daily basis to provide more flexibility in sexual readiness.

Another medication for erectile dysfunction is alprostadil (Caverject, Edex), which is either injected into the penis or inserted as a urethral pellet. This medication begins to work within 5 to 20 minutes and lasts approximately 1 hour. It should be administered no more than once a day and three times a week. The most common side effects are minor and include mild pain at the site of administration.

 CRITICAL THINKING

Why may erectile dysfunction drugs affect the entire cardiovascular system and not just the penis?

Reduced libido can occur in both men and women as a result of either emotional or physiological changes, such as depression, or the physical changes of aging, which include gaining or losing weight and the development of wrinkled and sagging skin, thus leading to a general feeling of decreased attractiveness. Many medications decrease libido in men and women. Among them are Benadryl, Aldactone, Aldomet, Catapres, Chlor-Trimeton, Valium, alcohol, Zantac, Tagamet, Dopar, and Inderal. Amphetamines increase libido.

A variety of drugs can be used to treat male infertility, including human chorionic gonadotropin (hCG), a substance naturally present in pregnant women. When hCG is administered as an injection in a male patient, it increases testosterone levels, which, in turn, increases sperm production.

■ THE URINARY SYSTEM

The urinary system's main functions are filtration of the blood and removal of the waste products that the kidneys have filtered out as unnecessary or dangerous (Fig. 20-3). This system consists of the kidneys, ureters, bladder, and urethra. The kidneys act as the filters for our blood. The ureters transfer the filtered waste products in water to the bladder, where they are stored until removal from the body

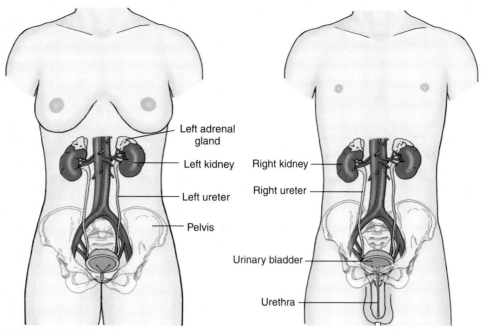

FIGURE 20-3: The urinary system.

via the urethra. This system is closely linked to the reproductive system, especially in men, because the urethra is encased in the penis and acts as a conduit to transfer sperm from the man to the woman during sexual intercourse. The most commonly used medications for treatment of disorders and diseases of the urinary system are diuretics.

Diuretics

Diuretics, commonly referred to as water pills, increase excretion of body fluids from the kidneys. This is necessary in certain medical conditions. The most common conditions for which diuretics are used are hypertension (high blood pressure) and heart failure. If the circulating pressure is too high and/or the heart muscle is not pumping with adequate strength, consequences will include lack of adequate blood flow, damage to tissue, and possible death if these situations remain untreated. Decreasing the amount of circulating volume lessens pressure on the blood vessels. Think of a garden hose. When there is a rapid flow of water (high volume), the pressure is high, but if you turn the hose down (lower the volume), the pressure is reduced to a gentle stream. In addition, if the heart is not pumping adequately, lowering the amount of liquid that it is required to push throughout the body will decrease the effort the heart must exert.

Other medical conditions requiring diuretics include kidney failure when hypertension and edema are present. Kidney stones can be minimized or prevented through the use of diuretics, which limit the amount of calcium excreted in the urine. In addition, glaucoma treatment may include diuretics to decrease the circulating fluid in the body, including the eyes. Diuretics can be categorized into four main areas: loop, thiazide, potassium-sparing, and osmotic. As might be inferred from the name of one of the previous types of diuretics, potassium loss is a serious side-effect of diuretic use and must be considered when prescribing these medications.

Loop Diuretics

The most effective diuretics work in the loop of Henle, located in the nephron (see A Closer Look: The Nephron…Building Block of the Kidney). Not surprisingly, they are called loop diuretics. They mainly are used to treat congestive heart failure by decreasing the volume of blood that the heart must circulate through the body. This effect also decreases the amount of fluid in the lungs and makes breathing easier. In renal insufficiency, it helps the kidneys to produce more urine and thus rids the body of toxins. Examples of loop diuretic drugs include furosemide (Lasix), ethacrynic acid (Edecrin), torsemide (Demadex), and bumetanide (Bumex). These medications are commonly taken orally, but they are also administered by the IV route. Furosemide and bumetanide may be given as an IM injection.

Thiazide Diuretics

Thiazides, which block sodium reabsorption and increase water excretion, are used to treat moderate hypertension. They are less effective than loop diuretics. Examples of thiazides are as follows: chlorothiazide (Diuril); chlorthalidone (Hygroton, Thalitone); indapamide (Lozol); hydrochlorothiazide, also known as HCTZ (Aquazide, HydroDIURIL, Microzide); and metolazone (Mykrox, Zaroxolyn). These medications are all taken orally. Chlorothiazide may also be administered by the IV route.

A CLOSER LOOK: The Nephron...Building Block of the Kidney

The kidneys regulate volume and content of urine. In doing so, they also affect blood pressure. Each kidney is made up of approximately 1 million nephrons. Structures within the nephron form urine by filtration. Each nephron determines which electrolytes are retained and which are disposed of outside the body. Thus, the kidneys have a large role in maintaining the acid-base balance in the body.

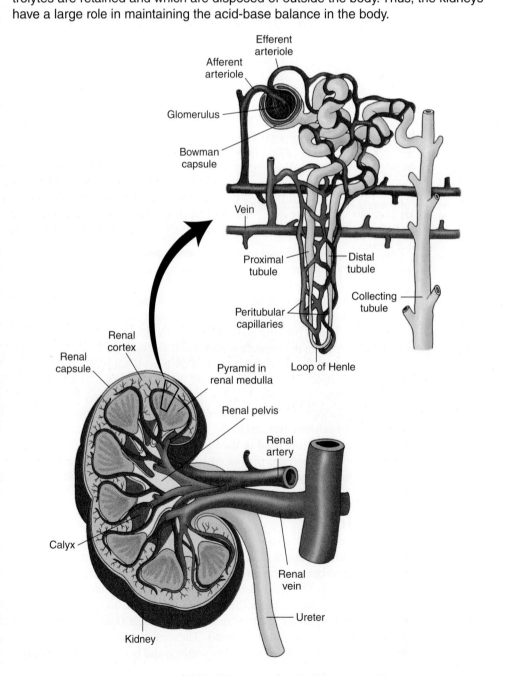

Electrolyte Imbalances and Diuretics

Although diuretics may relieve congestion by removing excess fluid from the body, they can have a devastating effect on the patient's electrolyte balance. To function properly, the body needs electrolytes: sodium (Na), potassium (K), calcium (Ca), and magnesium (Mg). Potassium, for example, is a vital electrolyte and plays a major role in maintaining a proper heart rhythm. With thiazides and loop diuretics, potassium is lost along with the sodium and water. Any time a diuretic is prescribed, the patient must be monitored to make sure that it is not adversely affecting the electrolyte levels. IV infusion therapy may be needed to replenish lost electrolytes; alternatively, electrolytes can be taken orally in supplements or through dietary changes to prevent imbalances. Patients with moderate hypertension may be prescribed a potassium-sparing diuretic instead of thiazides or loop diuretics.

Potassium-Sparing Diuretics

Potassium-sparing diuretics are frequently prescribed instead of or in combination with loop or thiazide diuretics to minimize the risk for potassium imbalances. These drugs block the reabsorption of water and sodium back into the bloodstream, but they allow potassium to be reabsorbed. Examples include amiloride hydrochloride, spironolactone (Aldactone), and triamterene (Dyrenium), which are all given orally.

Osmotic Diuretics

Osmotic diuretics such as mannitol are used for patients who have increased intracranial pressure as a result of head trauma, a brain tumor, or other illness affecting the brain. These diuretics help to lower the pressure exerted on the brain by swelling. In addition, osmotic diuretics may be given to those patients suffering from high intraocular pressure and those who are in the anuric (no urine output) stage of acute renal failure, to lower the amount of edema. These diuretics may also be administered in cases of toxic overdose, to flush the toxins from the body more rapidly. Osmotic diuretics function by pulling more fluid out of the body tissues and into the circulation, where it is then filtered through the kidneys and excreted. Osmotic diuretics such as mannitol (Osmitrol) are given by the IV route only in a controlled setting because the patient must be closely monitored during the administration. Side effects include dizziness, eye pain, anorexia, confusion, and dehydration.

Other Medications for Urinary Disorders

Other common disorders of the urinary system include infection, gout, urinary incontinence, and benign prostatic hypertrophy.

Many older men suffer from **benign prostatic hypertrophy (BPH),** a nonmalignant growth of the prostate gland that constricts the urethra and impedes the outflow of urine (Fig. 20-4). During its early stages, BPH can be treated with alpha-adrenergic blockers, such as alfuzosin (Uroxatral), doxazosin (Cardura, Carduran, Cascor, Doxadura), dutasteride (Avodart), finasteride (Propecia, Proscar), tamsulosin (Flomax), or terazosin (Hytrin). These drugs relax smooth muscle in the prostate gland and decrease blockage of the urethra, thus allowing urination to occur. For a close look at Avodart, see Drug Spotlight 20.1.

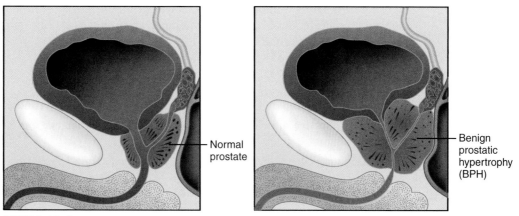

Normal prostate

Benign prostatic hypertrophy (BPH)

FIGURE 20-4: Benign prostatic hypertrophy.

Drug Spotlight 20-1 *Dutasteride (Avodart)*

Classification	Benign prostatic hyperplasia agent
Availability	Capsules
Indications	Treatment of the symptoms of benign prostatic hypertrophy
Mechanism of Action	Prevents conversion of testosterone to DHT, which leads to enlargement of the prostate gland
Adverse Reactions/ Side Effects	Reduced libido, impotence, breast tenderness and enlargement, reduced sperm count
Contraindications/ Precautions	Must be taken for 6 months before determining effectiveness of treatment. Pregnant women should avoid handling drug because of potential birth defects; for the same reason, men should wait 6 months after treatment ends to donate blood, to prevent exposing women to drug

DHT, dihydrotestosterone

Urinary tract infections can cause frequency, urgency, pain, and blood in the urine. They are usually treated with broad-spectrum antibiotics (Bactrim, Augmentin), analgesics (Pyridium), and antispasmodics (methenamine, flavoxate).

Although gout affects the musculoskeletal system, it is caused by the inability of the kidneys to clear uric acid from the bloodstream. Antigout medications can cause rashes in hypersensitive individuals (see Chapter 12 for further information on medications to treat gout).

Certain antispasmodics such as darifenacin (Enablex), fesoterodine (Toviaz), oxybutynin (Ditropan, Urotrol), solifenacin (VESIcare), tolterodine (Detrol), or trospium (Regurin, Sanctura) can effectively treat urinary incontinence by decreasing the contractions of the bladder and thus eliminating urgency symptoms that lead to wetting accidents. These medications are taken orally, and a few are additionally available as a transdermal patch.

Enuresis (bedwetting) can be treated effectively with desmopressin (DDAVP) (nasally or orally) and oral imipramine (Tofranil). DDAVP is a manufactured form of the naturally occurring hormone vasopressin found in the pituitary gland that helps the body control its water volume. You should also advise patients not to drink caffeinated drinks after 6 P.M. because these drinks can irritate the bladder and cause enuresis.

Effects of Medications on Color of the Urine

One side effect of many medications is a change in the color of urine to dark brown or yellow, blue green, orange yellow, or red pink. Usually, this discoloration has no effect on the kidneys, but it may frighten the unprepared patient. Preparing the patient may prevent panicked calls in the middle of the night or during a busy workday. Agents that change the color of urine include some anticoagulants, antibiotics, antidepressants, laxatives, barbiturates, and iron salts. Always check your drug handbook for information on urine color changes.

●●○ SUMMARY

■ Reproductive and urinary system disorders can cause pain, infertility, and sometimes death.

■ Many reproductive disorders result from a hormonal imbalance and are treated with hormones.

■ The gonadotropic hormones follicle-stimulating hormone (FSH), luteinizing hormone (LH), and interstitial cell–stimulating hormone (ICSH) are responsible for the production of the female hormones estrogen and progestin and the male hormone androgen (testosterone).

■ Contraceptives are hormones in low doses that, when used regularly, cause the body to stop producing the hormones that occur naturally to enable fertilization to occur.

■ Hormonal replacement therapy (HRT) and estrogen replacement therapy (ERT) can be used to help women through the symptoms of menopause, but they may also carry the risk for breast cancer, as certain studies have indicated.

■ Medications also exist to treat profuse or irregular bleeding and to encourage the onset of labor by thinning the cervix or by causing the uterus to contract.

■ Infertility medications can facilitate and/or maintain a pregnancy.

■ Other reproductive disorders that require treatment include STDs of the female and male reproductive tracts, yeast infections, and erectile dysfunction in men, as well as libido disorders.

■ The urinary system eliminates wastes and toxic substances and regulates the volume of body fluids.

■ Diuretics are the main treatment for many urinary system disorders.

■ Both loop and thiazide diuretics deplete electrolytes from the body, and this can cause serious adverse effects such as cardiac problems. In these instances, a potassium-sparing diuretic is often prescribed instead.

■ Other disorders and conditions of the urinary system include urinary tract infections, gout, BPH, and enuresis.

Master the Essentials: Reproductive and Urinary Medications

This table shows the various classes of reproductive and urinary medications and key side effects, contraindications and precautions, interactions, and examples for each class.

Class	Indications for Use	Side Effects	Contraindications and Precautions	Interactions	Examples
Androgens	Low testosterone levels, certain breast cancers	Headache, increased or decreased libido, anxiety, depression, acne, hirsutism, nausea, gynecomastia; amenorrhea or virilization in women	Serious heart, kidney, or liver disease; hypersensitivity, pregnancy, male with breast or prostate cancer	Anticoagulants, insulin, propranolol, corticosteroids, cyclosporine	Testosterone (AndroGel)
Antispasmodics	Incontinence resulting from overactive bladder	Dry mouth and eyes, blurred vision, constipation, nausea, dizziness, fatigue, flulike symptoms	Known sensitivity, glaucoma, stomach disorders, difficulty urinating, liver or kidney disease, history of long QT syndrome, myasthenia gravis	Arsenic trioxide, chloroquine, halofantrine, droperidol, HIV/AIDS medications, antibiotics, narcotics, psychiatric medications, cardiac medications, alcohol	Darifenacin (Enablex), fesoterodine (Toviaz), oxybutynin (Ditropan, Urotrol), solifenacin (VESIcare), tolterodine (Detrol), trospium (Regurin, Sanctura)

Continued

Master the Essentials: Reproductive and Urinary Medications—cont'd

Class	Indications for Use	Side Effects	Contraindications and Precautions	Interactions	Examples
BPH medications	Enlarged prostate gland	Decreased libido, mild impotence, palpitations, dizziness, somnolence, asthenia, nausea	Hypersensitivity, liver impairment	Alcohol, beta blockers, verapamil	Alfuzosin (Uroxatral), doxazosin (Cardura, Carduran, Cascor, Doxadura), dutasteride (Avodart), finasteride (Propecia, Proscar), tamsulosin (Flomax), terazosin (Hytrin)
Cervical ripening agents	Inducement of labor	Uterine hyperstimulation, GI effects, back pain, fetal bradycardia	Prior cesarean section, cephalopelvic disproportion, prior traumatic delivery, ruptured membranes, hypersensitivity, placenta previa	Oxytocin, misoprostol, mifepristone, ergonovine, mifepristone, methylergonovine, ureaphil	Dinoprostone (Cervidil, Prepidil)
Erectile dysfunction drugs	Erectile dysfunction (impotence)	Fatal cardiovascular events, flushing, headache, abnormal vision, dyspepsia, back pain	Hypersensitivity, heart disease, kidney or liver impairment	Erythromycin, grapefruit, nitrates, alcohol, alpha blockers, amlodipine, angiotensin II receptor blockers, beta blockers, diuretics, enalapril, metoprolol, protease inhibitors	Alprostadil (Caverject, Edex), sildenafil (Revatio, Viagra), vardenafil (Levitra, Staxyn), tadalafil (Adcirca, Cialis)
Estrogens	Estrogen replacement	Breast enlargement and tenderness, cardiovascular risk, decreased folic acid, edema, gallbladder disease, GI upset, headache, increased triglycerides, irregular menstrual bleeding, visual disturbances, DVT, PE	Asthma, diabetes, heart problems, lactation, liver dysfunction pregnancy, stroke, seizures, smoking, breast cancer, abnormal uterine bleeding, DVT, PE, MI, hypersensitivity	Anticoagulants, anti-infectives, corticosteroids, oral hypoglycemics, tricyclic antidepressants, thyroid hormones, hydantoins, topiramate	Oral: Estrace or Premarin Cream: Estrace, Dienestrol Patch: Alora, Estraderm Vivelle Vaginal: Estring, Vagifem
Loop diuretics	Congestive heart failure, renal insufficiency	Hyperglycemia, fluid and electrolyte loss, GI problems, headache, hypotension, hearing loss	Children, cirrhosis, diabetes, kidney disease, lactation, pregnancy, anuria, hypersensitivity	Blood pressure medications, corticosteroids, lithium, digoxin, aminoglycosides, anticoagulants	Furosemide (Lasix), ethacrynic acid (Edecrin), torsemide (Demadex), bumetanide (Bumex)

Master the Essentials: Reproductive and Urinary Medications—cont'd

Class	Indications for Use	Side Effects	Contraindications and Precautions	Interactions	Examples
Osmotic diuretics	Increased intracranial pressure, increased intraocular pressure	CNS effects, fluid and electrolyte imbalances, hypotension or hypertension, tachycardia, edema, headache, nausea, vomiting, diarrhea	Cardiovascular or kidney failure; pulmonary edema; active intracranial bleeding	Lithium	Mannitol (Osmitrol)
Ovulation stimulants	Female infertility	Ovarian hyperstimulation, headache, gynecomastia, injection site pain, vasomotor flushes	Liver disease, pregnancy, uncontrolled thyroid or adrenal disease, ovarian cyst, abnormal uterine bleeding, hypersensitivity	None reported	Clomiphene (Clomid, Serophene), menotropins (Humegon, Menopur, Pergonal, Repronex), chorionic gonadotropin (Ovidrel, Pregnyl)
Oxytocin	Induction of labor	Uterine rupture, embolism, fetal trauma and death, forceful contractions, hemorrhage, tachycardia, nausea, vomiting	Cephalopelvic disproportion, fetal distress, placenta previa, scarred uterus, unfavorable fetal positions, prolonged use in severe toxemia, hypersensitivity	Cyclopropane anesthesia, sympathomimetics, vasoconstrictors	Oxytocin (Pitocin, Syntocinon)
Potassium-sparing diuretics	Congestive heart failure, polycystic ovary syndrome	GI distress, high blood potassium, hypotension, headache, drowsiness	Cirrhosis, lactation, pregnancy, renal impairment, hypersensitivity, serum potassium <5.5 mEq/L	ACE inhibitors, lithium, NSAIDs, potassium supplements, digoxin	Amiloride hydrochloride, spironolactone (Aldactone), triamterene (Dyrenium)
Progestins	Birth control	Breast tenderness, decreased bone density, headache, irregular menses, swelling, insomnia, depression, nausea, weight changes	Cardiovascular disease, depression, edema, pregnancy, hypersensitivity, thrombophlebitis, thromboembolic disorder, breast cancer, undiagnosed vaginal bleeding, missed abortion	Aminoglutethimide, rifampin	Errin, Ovrette, Provera

Continued

Master the Essentials: Reproductive and Urinary Medications—cont'd

Class	Indications for Use	Side Effects	Contraindications and Precautions	Interactions	Examples
Thiazide diuretics	Hypertension, edema	Hyperglycemia; low chloride, potassium, and blood pressure	Anuria, hypersensitivity, renal decompensation, hepatic coma	Antidiabetic medications, corticosteroids, lithium, NSAIDs, digoxin, anesthetics, anticoagulants, antigout medications	Chlorothiazide (Diuril); chlorthalidone (Hygroton, Thalitone); indapamide (Lozol); hydrochlorothiazide, also known as HCTZ (Aquazide, HydroDIURIL, Microzide); metolazone (Mykrox, Zaroxolyn)

ACE, angiotensin-converting enzyme; BPH, benign prostatic hypertrophy; CNS, central nervous system; DVT, deep vein thrombosis; GI, gastrointestinal; MI, myocardial infarction; NSAID, nonsteroidal anti-inflammatory drug; PE, pulmonary embolism.

Activities

To make sure that you have learned the key points covered in this chapter, complete the following activities.

True or False

Write true if the statement is true. Beside the false statements, write false, and correct the statement to make it true.

1. Testosterone is used to treat breast cancer. _____

_____

2. Luteinizing hormone regulates testosterone production. _____

_____

3. Birth control pills can cause women to experience the symptoms of pregnancy. _____

_____

4. Human chorionic gonadotropin is used to treat male infertility. _____

_____

5. Diuretics cause the retention of potassium. _____

_____

6. The minipill contains both estrogen and progestin. _____

_____

7. BPH is a disease that is usually terminal. _____

_____

8. Reduced libido may occur as a result of daily medication taken by both men and women.

_____

_____

9. One risk associated with fertility drugs is multiple births. _____

_____

10. Cervical ripening refers to the ability of the uterus to accept a fertilized egg. _____

_____

Multiple Choice

Choose the best answer for each question.

1. Which of the following is NOT a type of diuretic?
   A. Loop
   B. Potassium-sparing
   C. Tocolytic
   D. Thiazide

2. **Which drug is used to treat vaginal herpes?**

   A. Zovirax

   B. Pitocin

   C. MetroGel

   D. Monistat

3. **Which drug induces uterine contractions?**

   A. Tocolytics

   B. Pitocin

   C. Dinoprostone

   D. B and C

4. **Which is a medication that can lead to decreased libido?**

   A. Benadryl

   B. Penicillin

   C. Vitamin C

   D. None of the above

5. **Which type of diuretic is used to treat moderate hypertension?**

   A. Loop

   B. Potassium-sparing

   C. Tocolytic

   D. Thiazide

   E. Osmotic

6. **Which of the following hormones are part of the reproductive system?**

   A. Luteinizing hormone (LH)

   B. Interstitial cell–stimulating hormone (ICSH)

   C. Follicle-stimulating hormone (FSH)

   D. All of the above

7. **Which of the following birth control pills contains a consistent amount of both progestin and estrogen in every pill for a period of 3 weeks?**

   A. Monophasic

   B. Biphasic

   C. Triphasic

   D. Minipill

8. **Which of the following medications is used as birth control?**

   A. Lupron

   B. Pitocin

   C. Terbutaline

   D. Implanon

9. What hormone may be given to treat male infertility?

    A. Thyroid

    B. Parathyroid

    C. Human chorionic gonadotropin

    D. Pituitary

10. DDAVP is used to treat which disorder?

    A. Infertility

    B. Enuresis

    C. Benign prostatic hypertrophy

    D. None of the above

Application Exercises

Respond to the following situations.

1. Martin calls the office to state that ever since he started taking Rocephin, his urine is orange. He is worried that his kidneys are being damaged. Explain to Martin why this is happening and what he should do. _____

_____

_____

2. Charlotte is going through menopause. She is concerned about HRT and wants to know why she needs this and whether there is anything else she can do to alleviate the symptoms. Explain the risks and benefits of HRT to her, as well as potential alternative therapies available. _____

_____

_____

3. Mr. Stephens faithfully donated blood every 8 weeks at his local blood bank. He began taking Avodart recently, and now he has been denied as a donor. He is upset and wants to know why this is happening. Explain to Mr. Stephens why taking Avodart makes him ineligible to donate blood. _____

_____

_____

Essentials Review

For further study and practice with drug classifications learned in this chapter, complete the following table to the best of your ability. Use resources such as the *PDR,* the Internet, or printed drug guides for help.

Trade Name	Generic Name	Classification	Purpose	Side Effects	Contraindications and Precautions	Patient Education
Proscar						
Cialis						
Premarin						
Pitocin						
Megace						
Diuril						

Internet Research

Using your favorite search engine, research one drug from each category of contraceptives in Table 20-2 (monophasics through abortifacients). Create a poster to help teach teenagers about contraceptive options.

Vitamins, Minerals, Herbs, and Complementary and Alternative Medicine

Vitamins and minerals are vital to survival and maintaining good health. A well-balanced diet consisting of proteins, fats, carbohydrates, vitamins, and minerals ensures the body's nutritional needs are met to maintain overall energy, health, and vitality. Amino acids and lipids also contribute to overall nutritional health. A healthy diet should provide a patient with sufficient quantities of these substances. If a patient does not or cannot maintain a healthy diet, supplements may be prescribed. They come in powders, capsules, liquids, and tablets.

Herbal supplements have become popular treatments for many conditions and to enhance overall health. Health-care professionals should always inquire whether their patients are taking herbal or vitamin and mineral supplements, and which ones, because many of these over-the-counter formulations have actions that will either increase or inhibit the treatment the physician initiates.

During the last few decades, the health-care community has gradually accepted that complimentary medicines and treatments that were previously used instead of traditional medicine can be a valuable aid to traditional treatment. As treatments such as acupuncture and acupressure gain more credibility, they are used in combination, or as a complement to medication to help patients manage stress, pain, and hypertension. Initially, medication may be prescribed to deal with an acute issue, and complementary therapies may work toward a more long-term goal. As these alternative therapies are used, the medication may be changed, the dosage may be decreased, or the medication may be discontinued altogether. For example, acupuncture is a Chinese art in which thin needles are inserted at certain points of the body to treat pain.

KEY TERMS

Complementary and alternative medicine (CAM)	Homeopathy Inorganic Megadoses	Organic Recommended daily allowance (RDA)

■ VITAMINS

Vitamins are **organic** (containing carbon) nutrients that are essential to regulate the chemical processes in the body. These nutrients work to maintain strong bones, release energy from food, and control hormonal activity.

The FDA has established **recommended daily allowances (RDAs)** for vitamins and minerals. Vitamin and mineral deficiencies can lead to illness. The RDA for each vitamin varies for women, men, pregnant women, infants, children, and adolescents. **Megadoses** (larger than the FDA recommendations) usually are not better and can also cause illness or death. If the doses are too large for long periods, serious health issues may arise, such as the following: kidney, liver, and heart and nerve damage; kidney and bladder stones; and an increased risk for diabetes and gout.

It is common to see changes in the urine with vitamin supplements. The urine may become bright yellow and have a strong odor. If the supplement doses are within the recommended range, it is usually not a concern.

■ **Fat-soluble vitamins:** Fat-soluble vitamins are not excreted from the body. They are stored when they are not currently needed and can build up to toxic levels if more than the recommended intake is ingested. Vitamins A, D, E, and K are fat-soluble vitamins (Table 21-1). Vitamins A, D, and K are stored in the liver, and vitamin E is spread throughout the fatty tissue of the body. Vitamin A is a requirement for healthy skin, teeth, bone, and soft tissue such as mucous membranes. It also is essential for vision, reproductive health, and immune system health. Vitamin D plays a key role in the healthy development of bone and the retention and absorption of calcium and phosphorus in the body. Vitamin E is thought to have a role in the formation of red blood cells and muscles, as well as the support of the immune system. Vitamin K is important in the clotting processes of the human body, and without it, bleeding abnormalities may occur.

■ **Water-soluble vitamins:** Water-soluble vitamins are not stored and are excreted by the body. These vitamins include vitamins B and C and must be ingested daily (Table 21-2). Vitamin B includes B_1 (thiamine), B_2 (riboflavin), B_3 (niacin), B_5 (pantothenic acid),

TABLE 21.1 Fat-Soluble Vitamins

Vitamin	Function	Deficiency	Excess
Vitamin A	Important for: • growth and development • immune function • reproduction • red blood cell formation • skin and bone formation • vision	Susceptibility to vision problems Immunodeficiency	Birth defects Death
Vitamin D	Important for: • blood pressure regulation • bone growth • calcium balance • hormone production • immune and nervous system functions	Tooth and bone deformation and fractures Rickets (children) Osteomalacia Osteoporosis Tetany	Nausea, vomiting, diarrhea Kidney stones Dizziness Redness of skin Muscle and bone pain Cardiac arrhythmias Vertigo Tinnitus
Vitamin E	Important for: • formation of blood vessels • immune function • acts as an antioxidant	Rare because most adults have large vitamin E stores in adipose tissue; may contribute to retinopathy in prematurity and early childhood	Muscle weakness Fatigue Nausea Abnormal blood cell count In large doses significantly decreases clotting time
Vitamin K	Important for: • clotting blood • forming strong bones	Increased clotting time Blood in urine Petechiae Bruising Blood in stool	No known reaction

TABLE 21.2 Water-Soluble Vitamins

Vitamin	Function	Deficiency	Excess
Vitamin B$_1$ (thiamine)	Important for: • conversion of sugar into energy • nervous system function	Emaciation Constipation Anorexia Nausea, GI upset Neuritis Pain, tingling in the extremities Loss of reflexes Muscle weakness Fatigue Ataxia Confusion, memory loss	Rare except when given by IV route: • feeling of warmth • sweating • weakness • nausea • restlessness • symptoms of anaphylactic shock
Vitamin B$_2$ (riboflavin)	Important for: • conversion of food into energy • growth and development • red blood cell formation	Glossitis Cheilosis Dermatitis	Rare: • burning or prickling sensation • hypersensitivity reaction

Continued

TABLE 21.2 Water-Soluble Vitamins—cont'd

Vitamin	Function	Deficiency	Excess
Vitamin B₃ (niacin)	Important for: • cholesterol production • conversion of food into energy • digestion • nervous system function	Peripheral vascular damage Dermatitis Diarrhea	Headache Flushing Burning sensation Postural hypotension Jaundice
Vitamin B₅ (pantothenic acid)	Important for: • conversion of food into energy • fat metabolism • hormone production • nervous system function • red blood cell formation	Extremely rare because available in diet and also produced by intestinal bacteria Fatigue	None reported
Vitamin B₆ (pyridoxine)	Important for: • immune and nervous system functions • protein, carbohydrate, and fat metabolism • red blood cell formation	Dermatitis Glossitis Depression Confusion Anemia Convulsions	Nerve damage to the arms and legs
Vitamin B₇ (biotin, also known as vitamin H)	Important for: • energy storage • protein, carbohydrate, and fat metabolism	Hair loss Rash around face and genitals Neurological symptoms	None reported
Vitamin B₉ (folic acid)	Important for: • birth defect prevention • protein metabolism • red blood cell formation	Anorexia Diarrhea Decreased weight Weakness Sore mouth Irritability	Hypersensitivity reaction
Vitamin B₁₂ (cobalamin)	Important for: • conversion of food into energy • nervous system function • red blood cell formation	Anemia Ataxia Numbness Irritability	Numbness Decreased muscle coordination Irritability Confusion
Vitamin C (ascorbic acid)	Important for: • collagen and connective tissue formation • immune function • wound healing • acts as an antioxidant	Fragility of capillaries Poor wound healing Degenerative bone disease	Diarrhea Stomach pain

GI, gastrointestinal; PMS, premenstrual syndrome.

B_6 (pyridoxine), B_7 (biotin), B_9 (folic acid), and B_{12} (cobalamin). These B vitamins work to support the immune and nervous systems, as well as improve metabolism and maintain healthy skin and muscles. They also help with stress, depression, and cardiac disease. Vitamin C (ascorbic acid) is needed for the production and maintenance of connective tissue, bones, and teeth.

MINERALS, LIPIDS, AND AMINO ACIDS

Minerals are **inorganic** (lack carbon) chemical elements that are necessary to the health and maintenance of the body's many biological processes. Minerals are required for almost every single function in the body. They act as catalysts for many essential vitamins. One example is magnesium, which allows calcium and vitamin C to be metabolized and helps to convert blood sugar into energy. Without magnesium, these nutrients would be excreted from the body without ever being used. Another example is iron. Iron is one key to hemoglobin production, which is necessary to transport oxygen throughout the body.

Minerals can be major or trace. Major minerals are those that the body needs in large amounts such as calcium, magnesium, phosphorus, potassium, sodium, and chloride, and trace minerals are those the body needs in minute amounts. Trace minerals include chromium, cobalt, copper, iron, iodine, manganese, molybdenum, selenium, silica, and zinc. Table 21-3 lists both major and trace minerals and their functions.

TABLE 21.3 Minerals

Vitamin	Function	Deficiency	Excess
Major Minerals			
Calcium	Important for: • blood clotting • bone and teeth formation • constriction and relaxation of blood vessels • hormone secretion • muscle contraction • nervous system function	Bone deformities and fractures Leg cramps Tetany Heart dysrhythmias	Constipation Irritation of tissue if IV infiltrates
Magnesium	Important for: • blood pressure and blood sugar regulation • bone formation • energy production • hormone secretion • immune function • muscle contraction • nervous system function • normal heart rhythm • protein formation	Kidney stones and gallstones Endocrine disorders Nerve numbness	None reported
Phosphorus	Important for: • acid-base balance • bone formation • energy production and storage • hormone activation	Malformed bones and teeth Poor growth and healing Fatigue Malabsorption	None reported
Potassium	Important for: • blood pressure regulation • cardiac function • carbohydrate metabolism • fluid balance • growth and development • muscle contraction • nervous system function • protein formation	Confusion Muscular weakness Paralysis Arrhythmias Lethargy Fatigue	Hypotension Listlessness Paralysis Confusion Arrhythmias

Continued

TABLE 21.3 Minerals—cont'd

Vitamin	Function	Deficiency	Excess
Sodium and chloride	Important for: • acid-base balance • blood pressure regulation • conversion of food into energy • digestion • fluid balance • muscle contraction • nervous system function	Nausea, vomiting Dizziness Headache Muscle cramps	Hypertension Malfunction in cells

Trace Minerals

Vitamin	Function	Deficiency	Excess
Chromium	Important for: • insulin production • protein, carbohydrate, and fat metabolism	Rare: • Diabetes mellitus symptoms: impairs ability to use glucose for energy	None reported
Copper	Important for: • bone, collagen, and connective tissue formation • energy production • iron metabolism • nervous system function • acts as an antioxidant	Infection CV disease	Anxiety Insomnia Poor concentration Depression Tinnitus Headache Rash
Fluoride	Important for health of teeth	Dental caries Kidney stones	Mottling of teeth, possible brain underdevelopment in children
Iron (ferrous)	Important for: • energy production • growth and development • immune function • red blood cell production • reproduction • wound healing	Fatigue Anemia Pallor Pica (craving to eat nonfoods such as clay and laundry starch) Lethargy Weakness Vertigo Air hunger Confusion Irregular heartbeat Learning disabilities in children Insomnia	Constipation GI bleeding
Iodine	Important for: • growth and development • metabolism • reproduction • thyroid hormone production	Goiter Thyroid disease	Thyroid underactivity
Manganese	Important for: • blood pressure and blood sugar regulation • bone formation	Hearing loss Dizziness Ataxia Fainting	Decreased iron absorption leading to iron-deficiency anemia

TABLE 21.3 Minerals—cont'd

Vitamin	Function	Deficiency	Excess
	• energy production • hormone secretion • immune function • muscle contraction • nervous system function • heart function • protein formation	Weakness in joints; linked to myasthenia gravis Impaired glucose metabolism Reduced insulin production	
Molybdenum	Important for: • enzyme production	Cavities Anemia Impotence Gout Malabsorption	Weight loss Stunted growth Anemia Diarrhea Swollen joints
Selenium	Important for: • immune function • reproduction • thyroid function • acts as an antioxidant	Immune, CV, liver, and sexual disorders	Nausea, vomiting, diarrhea Hair loss Rash Brittle nails Fatigue Nerve damage Garlic odor to breath
Silica	Important for: • connective tissue and skeletal tissue functioning	Hair Skin, CV, and bone disorders	None reported
Zinc	Important for: • growth and development • immune and nervous system functions • protein formation • reproduction • taste and smell • wound healing	Alcohol tolerance Anemia Poor wound healing Decreased taste Hair loss Dermatitis Immune deficiency Growth retardation	Nausea and vomiting, diarrhea Headache

CV, cardiovascular; GI, gastrointestinal.

Amino acids are compounds that contain an amino group and have an acidic function. They are considered the building blocks of protein. The eight "essential" amino acids include alanine, valine, tryptophan, isoleucine, methionine, lysine, threonine, and leucine (Table 21-4). They are called essential because the body can only obtain them through diet and does not store them for future use. In addition, there are 12 "nonessential" amino acids; nonessential means that they can usually be made from other substances in the body if needed.

Lipids (fats) are necessary for life in that they store energy, insulate body tissues from heat and cold, and cushion and protect our internal organs. Saturated fats are obtained from animals and are solid at room temperature. Unsaturated fats originate from plant sources and are liquid at room temperature. Cholesterol is used to synthesize hormones, vitamin D, and bile. It also serves to stabilize cell membranes throughout the body. Fatty acids found in fish are available as fish oil and are considered helpful in patients with high triglycerides or familial history of heart disease, and they may also lower blood pressure. For patients who are receiving all their nutrients through IV therapy, an IV form of lipids (Intralipid 20%) is available to provide essential fatty acids and calories. Lipids are available as oral supplements and are used to lower harmful types of cholesterol, treat poor blood flow, lower the body's production of triglycerides, and treat wrinkles (Table 21-5).

TABLE 21.4 Key Amino Acids

Amino Acid	Purpose
Alanine	Removal of waste products from the body
Glycine	Wound healing
Arginine	Protein synthesis
Aspartic acid	Synthesis of other amino acids
Cysteine	Immune system function
Glutamine	Synthesis of RNA and DNA
Histidine	Production and synthesis of red blood cells (RBCs) and white blood cells (WBCs)
Lysine	Synthesis of enzymes and other hormones
Methionine	Healthy skin
Phenylalanine	Immune system function
Tryptophan	Appetite
Tyrosine	Production of thyroid hormones

TABLE 21.5 Examples of Lipid Supplements

Supplement	Purpose
Fish oils	Lower triglycerides in the blood
Inositol	Reduces bad cholesterol, and increases good cholesterol in the blood

CRITICAL THINKING

If an athlete takes excessive amounts of vitamins and complains that his urine has changed color and has a strong odor, what is the likely cause?

■ HERBAL MEDICINES

Herbs have been used as medications for centuries. Today, the value of the active agents in plant sources as an addition to or instead of artificial sources is gaining wider acceptance. In Chapter 1, the foxglove plant was described as a potent treatment for heart disease that has been in use for hundreds of years. Many people use herbs to self-medicate, such as by drinking chamomile tea for relaxation and insomnia or using aloe vera plants to treat burns. Herbal remedies are not harmful in most cases; however, some herbs can be dangerous if taken in the wrong quantities or when they interact with certain medications. For example, St. John's wort affects the way the liver metabolizes many medications. St. John's wort can make hormonal birth control much less effective, thus leading to unplanned pregnancy.

For the foregoing reasons, it is essential that patients discuss with their physician the herbal remedies they are using, to avoid any detrimental effects from interactions. In addition, because self-medication occurs routinely, patients may fail to seek a physician's assistance for many serious health issues. An open, accepting attitude by the office staff is critical in successful discussions of these treatments.

If you visit any herbal store, you may be surprised to see the variety of herbal and/or natural products and the routes by which they can be administered. Most are swallowed as tablets, but others can be brewed as teas, chewed on as a root, or rubbed on the skin. Furthermore, some herbs (e.g., eucalyptus for asthma) are used as aromatherapy, in which they are burned and their aroma inhaled. Herbs are also just one type of plant substance used in homeopathy.

Some sources of information on commercially available herbal remedies may not contain data about safety, efficacy, and dosing. Furthermore, because herbs are not regulated as strictly as most pharmaceutical preparations by the Food and Drug Administration (FDA), there might be inconsistent amounts of an herb in different manufacturers' products or hidden ingredients. As a result, herbal remedies are often considered complementary and alternative medicine. See Appendix G for a comprehensive list of plants, vitamins, minerals, amino acids, and lipids and their use as complimentary or alternative treatments.

■ COMPLEMENTARY AND ALTERNATIVE MEDICINE

Complementary and alternative medicine (CAM) therapies include treatments such as massage therapy, aromatherapy, acupuncture, acupressure, and medications such as herbs, minerals, and vitamins used to complement or as an alternative to conventional medical therapy. Sometimes the patient believes that conventional treatment does not or cannot eliminate the disease. Other patients may consider modern medical treatment dangerous.

Aromatherapy involves the use of fragrant oils in baths, as inhalants, or during massage to relieve stress and to treat skin conditions. Acupressure originates from an ancient Chinese treatment in which the application of pressure at certain points of the body is used to promote healing. Likewise, acupuncture is a Chinese practice in which thin needles are inserted at certain points of the body to treat pain or illness (Fast Tip 21.1).

 Fast Tip 21.1   Acupuncture

Advise patients who are interested in trying acupuncture to seek certified professionals who use sterile or disposable needles.

With the exception of acupuncture, most of these therapies have had less, if any, scientific testing than modern treatments and drugs. This is the main reason that insurance companies refuse to pay for many alternative therapies, including herbal remedies. These companies believe that the evidence supporting CAM effectiveness is insufficient. For example, therapeutic touch involves the use of hand movements to stimulate circulation and healing; however, there is no rigorous scientific basis for its efficacy.

A CLOSER LOOK: **Homeopathy**

Homeopathy is a type of complementary and alternative medicine based on the principle that "like cures like" with highly diluted preparations. The idea is that a patient takes a small amount of a substance similar to the one that is harming his or her body, thereby training the body to fight the dangerous substance. For example, a patient who experiences allergy symptoms to cat dander would be exposed to an extremely dilute (1:1,000) mixture of water and cat dander.

Continued

A CLOSER LOOK: Homeopathy—cont'd

A German physician, Samuel Hahnemann (1755–1843), developed homeopathy and homeopathic remedies. In the 1800s, physicians would often cut people open to bleed them because they believed that bleeding purged the body of evil disease. Physicians also administered harsh enemas to force the body to purge disease. Not surprisingly, these drastic measures failed to work and often, in fact, killed patients, so Dr. Hahnemann developed homeopathy.

Three premises support homeopathy and how it should work:

- A remedy starts healing from the top of the body and works downward.
- A remedy starts from within the body, working outward, and from major to minor organs.
- Symptoms clear in reverse order to their manner of appearance.

More than 2,000 homeopathic remedies are available from animal, vegetable, and mineral sources. Homeopaths are practitioners who are skilled in homeopathy and who advise patients on the selection and dosing of homeopathic preparations. Homeopaths are usually not regulated by any medical board or governmental agency.

It is important to understand the different philosophies that patients and health-care providers may have toward healing. If, for example, a patient who values Eastern philosophy visits a provider who values Western philosophy, conflicts in the choice of treatment may result.

Many CAM therapies emphasize an Eastern philosophy rather than a Western philosophy of healing. Eastern philosophy focuses on the body's ability to heal itself and uses herbs to promote self-healing. Practitioners of Eastern medicine believe that disease is a result of imbalance within the body and that health returns once balance is restored. Some examples of CAM include acupuncture, acupressure, and reflexology. Practitioners of Western medicine believe that disease is caused by physiological disorders and that health is the absence of disease. Western medicine uses medications to target specific problems.

Many practitioners are combining Eastern and Western philosophies, conventional medical treatment and CAM therapies, as integrative therapy.

 CRITICAL THINKING

If a placebo (inactive medication) works almost 60% of the time, what does this say about the role of faith in healing?

SUMMARY

- Vitamins and minerals are vital to survival and maintaining good health.
- Vitamins are organic (containing carbon) nutrients.
- Fat-soluble vitamins (A, D, E, and K) are stored in the body and can build up to toxic levels if more than the recommended intake is ingested.
- Water-soluble vitamins (B and C) are excreted by the body and must be replenished.
- Major and trace minerals are inorganic (lack carbon) chemical elements that are necessary to the health and maintenance of the body's many biological processes.
- People often use herbal remedies to supplement health or medications. Herbal remedies are considered complementary and alternative medicine. An awareness of their effects and interactions with other herbs or medications is important.

■ Packaging on commercially available herbal remedies may not contain data about ingredients, safety, efficacy, and dosing.

■ CAM therapies include treatments such as massage therapy, aromatherapy, acupuncture, and acupressure.

■ Complementary medicine is used in addition to conventional treatment. Alternative medicine is used as a substitute for conventional treatment.

■ Insurance companies will not pay for many CAM treatments because the evidence supporting effectiveness of CAM is insufficient.

■ Practitioners of Eastern medicine believe that disease is a result of imbalance within the body and that health returns once balance is restored. Practitioners of Western medicine believe that disease is caused by physiological disorders and that health is the absence of disease.

■ Always ask your patients about the type, if any, of CAM therapies they may be using, so you can be aware of any potential interactions with prescribed medications.

Activities

To make sure that you have learned the key points covered in this chapter, complete the following activities.

True or False

Write true if the statement is true. Beside the false statements, write false, and correct the statement to make it true.

1. Vitamin B is a water-soluble vitamin. _____

    _____

2. Vitamin A is stored in the liver. _____

    _____

3. Chamomile tea helps to keep someone alert. _____

    _____

4. Lipids are the building blocks of protein. _____

    _____

5. Niacin is a form of vitamin B. _____

    _____

6. Vitamins and minerals are regulated by the FDA as medications. _____

    _____

7. St. John's wort should not be taken by patients using hormonal birth control. _____

    _____

8. Commercially available herbal remedies might include inconsistent amounts of an herb or hidden ingredients. _____

    _____

9. Insurance companies routinely pay for CAM and herbal remedies. _____

    _____

10. CAM therapies are rooted in Eastern philosophy. _____

    _____

Choose the best answer for each question.

1. **CAM therapies include all of the following EXCEPT** _____.

    A. Acupuncture

    B. Acupressure

    C. Reflexology

    D. Oncology

    E. Aromatherapy

2. **Which of the following is a substance closely regulated by the FDA?**

    A. Antibiotics

    B. Herbs

    C. Vitamins

    D. Minerals

3. **Which vitamin is important to blood clotting?**

    A. A

    B. D

    C. E

    D. K

4. **Herbal medicine forms include which of the following?**

    A. Tablets

    B. Teas

    C. Roots

    D. Topical preparations

    E. All of the above

5. **The basis for Eastern philosophy is** _____.

    A. The body's ability to heal itself

    B. Medications to target specific problems

    C. Disease is caused by physiological disorders

    D. None of the above

6. **Western philosophy focuses on** _____.

    A. The body's ability to heal itself

    B. Medications to target specific problems

    C. Disease is caused by physiological disorders

    D. B and C

7. B vitamins include which of the following?

   A. Niacin

   B. Riboflavin

   C. Folic acid

   D. All of the above

8. Which of the following vitamins must be taken on a daily basis?

   A. A

   B. C

   C. D

   D. K

9. Amino acids are the building blocks of which substance?

   A. Protein

   B. Carbohydrate

   C. Fat

   D. None of the above

10. RDA stands for _____.

   A. Ratio of daily allowance

   B. Required daily allowance

   C. Recommended daily allowance

   D. None of the above

Application Exercises

Respond to the following situations.

1. Patrick tells you that he is treating his depression with phenylalanine but still has very little energy and has no interest in his children's activities. What would you tell him? _____

_____

_____

2. Ryan is undergoing chemotherapy for lung cancer. He is losing weight and has a very poor appetite. How will this affect his health? What would you suggest? _____

_____

_____

For further study and practice with drug classifications learned in this chapter, complete the following table to the best of your ability. Use resources such as the *PDR,* the Internet, or printed drug guides for help.

Classification	Purpose	Side Effects	Contraindications and Precautions	Examples	Patient Education
Vitamin A					
Vitamin B					
B_1					
B_2					
B_3					
B_5					
B_6					
B_7					
B_9					
B_{12}					
Vitamin C					
Vitamin D					
Vitamin E					
Vitamin K					
Calcium					
Chromium					
Cobalt					
Copper					

Internet Research

1. Using your favorite search engine, research one form of alternative medicine. Find a few specific herbs that are used in that therapy, and share this information with the class.

2. Using your preferred search engine, go the FDA website to find information to help you make a brochure on safe herbal medication use for patients.

Glossary

A

Absorption—passage of a substance through some surface of the body into body fluids and tissues

a.c.—before meals

ACE inhibitor—drug that inhibits the action of angiotensin-converting enzyme

Acne—inflammatory disease of the sebaceous glands of the skin

Acromegaly—chronic syndrome of growth hormone excess, most often caused by a pituitary macroadenoma, and characterized by gradual coarsening and enlargement of bones and facial features

ACTH—adrenocorticotropic hormone

Active artificial immunity—immunity obtained through the administration of a vaccine that allows the patient to form antibodies to a virus, toxin, or bacterium

Active natural immunity—immunity obtained through a microorganism's entry into the body and the body's learning to fight it

Acupressure—traditional Chinese medicine's use of pressure on certain points on the body to promote healing

Acupuncture—traditional Chinese medicine's use of needles at certain points on the body to promote healing

a.d.—right ear

Addiction—the abnormal psychological and/or physical dependence on a drug

Addison disease—gradual, progressive failure of the adrenal glands and insufficient production of steroid hormones

Addition—to combine two or more numbers together

Additive—effect that one drug or substance contributes to the action of another drug or substance

ADH—antidiuretic hormone

Adrenergic—relating to nerve fibers that release norepinephrine or epinephrine at the synapses

Adverse reaction—undesired side effects or toxicity caused by a treatment

Aerobic—taking place in the presence of oxygen

Agonist—drug that binds to the receptor and stimulates the receptor's function

Al-Hawi—large 20-volume Arabian medical book written by a single author Al-Razi and having a significant influence on medicine in medieval Europe

Alimentary canal—another name for the gastrointestinal tract

Alopecia—absence or loss of hair

Alternative medicine—the practice of using natural healing in conjunction with mainstream medicine. Some examples are acupuncture, massage therapy, and aromatherapy.

Alveoli—plural of alveolus; an air sac in the lungs

Ampule—small glass container that can be sealed and its contents sterilized

Anaerobic—taking place in the absence of oxygen

Analgesic—medication that relieves pain

Anaphylaxis—hypersensitivity reaction between an allergenic antigen and immunoglobulin E bound to mast cells; stimulates the sudden release of immunologic mediators locally or throughout the body

Androgen—substance producing or stimulating the development of male characteristics, such as the hormones testosterone and androsterone

Angina pectoris—oppressive pain or pressure in the chest caused by inadequate blood flow and oxygenation to heart muscle

Anoxia—absence of oxygen

Antagonist—that which counteracts the action of something else, such as a muscle or drug

Antibody—substance produced by lymphocytes in response to a unique antigen to fight against it

Antigen—any substance capable of eliciting an immune response (foreign invader)

Antihistamine—drug that opposes the action of histamine

Antihypertensive—drug used to treat hypertension

Antineoplastic—drug used to destroy neoplasms

Antispasmodic—drug that prevents or relieves spasm

Antitussive—drug that prevents or relieves coughing

Anxiolytic—medication that reduces anxiety

Apnea—cessation of breathing

Apothecary—druggist or pharmacist

Aqueous humor—thin, watery fluid contained in the anterior chamber of the eye

Aromatherapy—use of fragrant oils in baths, as inhalants, or during massage to relieve stress and to treat skin conditions

a.s.—left ear

Atherosclerosis—the most common form of arteriosclerosis, marked by cholesterol-lipid-calcium deposits in the walls of the arteries

Attenuate—to render weak or make less virulent

a.u.—both ears

Aura—subjective, but recognizable sensation that precedes and signals the onset of a convulsion or migraine headache

Automatic stop order—an order that discontinues a medication at a certain time

Autoimmune disorder—condition in which the immune system attacks tissue normally present in the body (attacks itself)

Autoimmunity—the body's tolerance of the antigens on its own cells

Autonomic—self-controlling, functioning independently

Available dose—amount of medication on hand to administer to a patient

Avoirdupois—system of weighing or measuring articles in which 7,000 grains equal 1 pound

B

Bactericidal—capable of killing bacteria

Bacteriostatic—inhibits the growth of bacteria

Barrel—part of the syringe through which the plunger passes

Benign—not recurrent or progressive, not malignant

Beta-adrenergic agent—synthetic or natural drug that stimulates beta receptors

bid—two times per day

Bioavailability—the amount of a drug that the body can absorb and use

Biotransformation—chemical alteration that a substance undergoes in the body

Bisphosphonates—any of a class of medications that inhibit the resorption of bones by osteoclasts

Blister pack—method of delivering medications; usually contains one dose in each small sac

Blood-borne pathogens—microorganisms capable of producing disease, transmitted by body fluids

Blood-brain barrier—densely packed cells that allow nutrients and certain other chemicals, but no others, to pass into the central nervous system

Blood-placental barrier—densely packed cells that allow nutrients and certain other chemicals, but not others, to pass through the placenta

Blood-testicular barrier—densely packed cells that allow nutrients and certain other chemicals, but not others, to pass into the testicles

Booster—additional dose of an immunizing agent to increase the protection afforded by the original series of injections

Bovine—refers to products produced from cows

BPH—benign prostatic hypertrophy

Brand name—drug name given by the drug manufacturer

Broad spectrum—in reference to antibiotics; ones that combat a wide variety of microorganisms

BSA—body surface area (computed using height and weight)

Buccal—route in which a medication is administered into the buccal pouch (cheek)

Buffered—treated in such a way to offset the reaction of an agent administered in conjunction with it

Bulk—mass; in reference to medication, a container holding multiple doses

BUN—blood urea nitrogen

C

c̄—with

cc—unit of measure in which one cubic centimeter of space will hold 1 mL of fluid

C & S—see *Culture and sensitivity*

Calcitonin—hormone produced by the human thyroid gland that is important for maintaining a dense, strong bone matrix and regulating the blood calcium level

Calculus—stone commonly formed from calcium found in the gallbladder or kidneys

Calibrated—determined as accurate

CAM—see *Complementary and alternative medicine*

Cannula—tube used to deliver oxygen or through which a trocar is withdrawn after insertion

Cap—abbreviation for capsule

Caplet—delivery mode for medication that is similar to both capsules and tablets

Capsule—delivery mode for medication that holds a measured drug inside a substance that dissolves

Carcinogen—any substance or agent that produces cancer or increases the risk for developing cancer in humans or animals

Cathartic—purging the body quickly; example, cleaning the bowels of stool

Centi—prefix used in the metric system to denote one-hundredth (1/100)

Cerumen—earwax; secreted by the glands at the outer third of the ear canal

Chemotherapy—also known as antineoplastic medications; those used to fight cancer cells or neoplasms

Chemical name—drug name that reflects the chemical makeup of the drug

CHF—congestive heart failure

Cholinergic—agent that produces the effect of acetylcholine

Chyme—mixture of food and stomach acid passing into the small intestine

Clinical trials—scientific tests that research the efficacy and safety of a medication

CNS—central nervous system

CO_2—carbon dioxide

Comedo—small skin lesion of acne vulgaris and seborrheic dermatitis

Compassionate use—the use of an investigational new drug (IND) in patients who are suffering greatly and may die without the drug

Complementary and alternative medicine (CAM)—treatments, such as massage therapy or acupuncture, and remedies, such as herbs. Complementary medicine is used in addition to conventional treatment, and alternative medicine is used as a substitute.

Compound—mix

Condyloma—wart, found on the genitals or near the anus, with a textured surface that may resemble coral, cauliflower, or cobblestone

Constipation—stool with lowered liquid content and less frequent defecation

Contractility—having the ability to contract or shorten

Contraindications—symptoms or circumstances that make treatment with a drug or device unsafe or inappropriate

Control group—group of people in clinical trials who receive the placebo or usual treatment, in contrast to the group given the treatment or medication being studied

Controlled substances—substances monitored under the Comprehensive Drug Abuse Prevention and Control Act, a law enacted in 1971 to control the distribution and use of all depressant and stimulant drugs and other drugs of abuse or potential abuse as may be designated by the Drug Enforcement Administration of the U.S. Department of Justice

Conversion factor—number used to change a mathematical number from one condition to another

COPD—chronic obstructive pulmonary disease

CPAP—continuous positive airway pressure

Cream—semisolid delivery system for medications

Cretinism—congenital condition caused by a lack of thyroid hormones and characterized by arrested physical and mental development, myxedema, dystrophy of the bones and soft tissues, and lowered basal metabolism

Crystalloid—substance capable of crystallization, which in solution can be diffused through animal membranes

CSF—cerebrospinal fluid

Culture and sensitivity (C&S)—identification of microorganisms in a specimen and the determination of the appropriate drug needed to kill them

Cumulation—increasing in effect by successive additions

Curative—having healing or remedial properties

Cushing disease—caused by excessive production of adrenocorticotropic hormone (ACTH) in the body

CVA—cerebrovascular accident

Cyanosis—blue, gray, slate, or dark purple discoloration of the skin or mucous membranes caused by deoxygenated or reduced hemoglobin in the blood

D

d/c—discontinue(d)

DEA—Drug Enforcement Administration of the U.S. Department of Justice

Débride—to perform the action of débridement, the removal of foreign material and dead or damaged tissue, especially in a wound

Deci—prefix used in the metric system to denote one-tenth (1/10)

Decimal—numeric system using numbers from 0 to 9

Decongestant—agent that reduces congestion, especially nasal

Deep vein thrombosis (DVT)—a blood clot within the deep veins of the legs or, less often, the arms or pelvis

Delayed action—action occurring a considerable time after a stimulus

Deltoid—triangular muscle on the upper arm

Delusion—false belief brought about without appropriate external stimulation and inconsistent with the individual's own knowledge and experience

Dementia—progressive, irreversible decline in mental function, marked by memory impairment and, often, deficits in reasoning, judgment, abstract thought, registration, comprehension, learning, task execution, and use of language

Denominator—number on lower part of a fraction; used to divide into the numerator

Dependent—supported by, nurtured by, or relying on another person or variable

Depression—mood disorder marked by loss of interest or pleasure in living

Desired dose—dose of medication ordered by the prescriber (also known as ordered dose)

Destructive—causing injury or death

Dextrose—glucose, sugar

Diabetes insipidus—excessive urination caused by inadequate amounts of antidiuretic hormone (ADH) in the body or by failure of the kidney to respond to ADH

Diabetes mellitus—chronic metabolic disorder marked by hyperglycemia

Diagnostic—pertaining to the disease or syndrome a person has or is believed to have

Dialysis—passage of a solute through a membrane

Diarrhea—increased frequency of stool and higher fluid content

Digestion—the process of converting food into chemical substances that can be used in the body

Diluent—fluid used to reconstitute a powdered medication

Dimensional analysis—calculating dosages using the measurement, such as milligrams or milliliters, to set up the calculation

Distribution—dividing and spreading of a medication to a target organ

Dividend—number being divided in a division problem

Division—to separate into smaller parts

Divisor—number doing the division in a division problem

DMARD—disease-modifying antirheumatic drug

Dorsogluteal—injection site in the gluteus maximus on the dorsal (back) side

Double-blind—neither the patient nor the researcher in the clinical trial knows who has the placebo and who has the drug being tested

Drip chamber—part of an intravenous line where the medication drips into the chamber at a regulated rate

Droog—Dutch word meaning "dry," as in dried herbs used for healing; source of the word *drug*

Drug—substance that can change a function in a living being

Drug cycle—absorption, distribution in the body, metabolism, and excretion of medications

Drug holiday—period in which a patient with Parkinson's disease stops taking medications for a period of time to allow the medications to be resumed at much lower doses while still obtaining desired benefits

Drug Information for Health Providers—the first of this two-volume set published by the United States Pharmacopeial Convention, Inc., in Rockville, Maryland. *Drug Information for Health Providers* is written primarily for prescribers; the other volume, *Advice for the Patient,* is written in language that is easy for patients to understand, with tips for proper use of drugs and a pronunciation key.

DVT—see *Deep vein thrombosis*

Dwarfism—condition of being abnormally small

Dyspnea—difficult breathing

Dysrhythmias—abnormal heart rhythms

Dystonia—prolonged involuntary muscular contractions that may cause twisting of body parts, repetitive movements, and increased muscular tone

E

Ebers Papyrus—preserved medical document listing some 700 recipes to remedy a wide range of illnesses; written in approximately 1550 BC in Egypt

Eczema—general term for an itchy red rash that initially weeps or oozes serum and may become crusted, thickened, and scaly

EEG—see *Electroencephalogram*

Effervescent—bubbling; rising in little bubbles of gas

Efficacy—ability to produce a desired effect

Electroencephalogram—recording of the electrical activity of the brain

Electrolytes—substances that, in solution, conduct an electric current and are decomposed by its passage

Electronic prescription (e-prescription)—an order for medication created electronically (online) by the prescriber and sent directly to the patient's pharmacy

Elix—abbreviation for elixir

Elixir—sweetened, aromatic, hydroalcoholic liquid used when compounding oral medication

Embolus—mass of undissolved matter present in a blood or lymphatic vessel and brought there by the blood or lymph

Emesis—evacuation of stomach contents

Emulsions—mixtures of two liquids not mutually soluble

Endogenous—produced or originating from within a cell or organism

Enema—introduction of a solution into the rectum and colon to stimulate bowel activity and cause emptying of the lower intestine for feeding or therapeutic purposes; sometimes used to give anesthesia or to aid in radiographic studies

Enteric-coated—coated with a substance so the drug is dissolved and absorbed only in the small intestine

Enuresis—bedwetting

Equivalent—equal in power or force or value

ERT—estrogen replacement therapy

Estrogen—any natural or artificial substance that induces estrus and the development of female sex characteristics; more specifically, an estrogenic hormone produced by the ovaries

EtOH—ethyl alcohol

Excretion—elimination of waste products from the body

Expectorant—agent, such as guaifenesin, that promotes clearance of mucus from the respiratory tract

Expiration—death or end of usefulness; relaxation of lungs causing the exhalation of waste in the form of CO_2

Extremes—numbers on the far ends (front and back) of a ratio and proportion problem

F

Factor—the number that divides another number

FDA—see *Food and Drug Administration*

Fight or flight—body's natural response to prepare to flee or defend itself from attack

Filter—to pass a liquid through any porous substance that prevents particles larger than a certain size from passing through

Fissure—cracks in the anus

Flatulence—air in the gastrointestinal system

Flow regulator—piece of equipment on the intravenous line that regulates the rate of passage of fluid; can be used to stop or start the flow

Food and Drug Administration (FDA)—the U.S. government agency responsible for regulation and supervision of food and medication to ensure the safety of the public's health

Formula—rule prescribing how to calculate a dosage; for example, D/H × Q = answer

Fraction—ratio of a numerator to a denominator

FSH—follicle-stimulating hormone

G

g—abbreviation for gram

GABA—gamma-aminobutyric acid

Gastroesophageal reflux disease (GERD)—the condition of acid regurgitating from the stomach up into the esophagus causing irritation and erosion

Gauge—measurement representing the circumference of the inner opening of an object such as a needle

Gel—semisolid condition of a precipitated or coagulated colloid, jelly, or jelly-like colloid

Generic name—official name of the drug; nonproprietary

GERD—see *Gastroesophageal reflux disease*

Geriatrics—branch of health care concerned with care of the aged

GH—growth hormone

Gigantism—excessive development of a body or body part

Glucocorticoids—general classification of adrenal cortical hormones primarily active in protecting against stress and affecting protein and carbohydrate metabolism

Goiter—enlarged thyroid

Gout—form of arthritis marked by the deposition of monosodium urate crystals in joints and other tissues

gr—abbreviation for grain

Gram negative—bacterial microorganism that is unable to retain the color applied in a Gram stain test

Gram positive—bacterial microorganism that is able to retain the color applied in a Gram stain test

Graves' disease—distinct type of hyperthyroidism caused by an autoimmune attack on the thyroid gland

gtt—abbreviation for drop

H

Habituated—process of becoming accustomed to a stimulus

Halitosis—bad breath

Half-life—the length of time required for the concentration of a drug to decrease by one-half in the plasma

Hallucination—false perception having no relation to reality and not accounted for by any exterior stimulus

HCl—hydrochloric acid

HDL—high-density lipoprotein

Health Insurance Portability and Accountability Act (HIPPA)—a group of federal laws that, in part, establishes patients' rights, including their rights to privacy of their medical information

Heartburn—pain in the area of the heart caused by irritation of refluxed acid into the esophagus

Hemorrhoid—varicose veins found in the anus

Hemostasis—arrest of bleeding or of circulation

HIPAA—see *Health Insurance Portability and Accountability Act*

HMO—health maintenance organization

Homeopathy—school of American healing, founded by Dr. Samuel Hahnemann, based on the idea that very dilute doses of medicines that produce symptoms of a disease in healthy people can cure that disease in affected patients

Host—human, animal, or thing that harbors a potentially infectious microorganism

Household—measuring system used by laypersons, not apothecaries, in their home

Helicobacter pylori—bacterium responsible for the majority of ulcers

HPV—human papillomavirus

HRT—hormone replacement therapy

HTN—see *Hypertension*

Hub—part of the needle where the syringe attaches

Hydantoins—colorless bases; glycolyl urea; derived from urea and allantoin

Hyperglycemia—abnormally high blood glucose levels, as are found in people with diabetes mellitus or people treated with some drugs

Hyperlipidemia—abnormally high lipids in the blood

Hypertension—high blood pressure (higher than 140 mm Hg systolic or 90 mm Hg diastolic)

Hypocalcemia—abnormally low calcium in the blood

Hypodermic—under or inserted under the skin

Hypoglycemia—abnormally low glucose levels in the blood

Hypoxia—oxygen deficiency in body tissues

I

ICSH—interstitial cell–stimulating hormone

ID—intradermal

IDDM—insulin-dependent diabetes mellitus

Idiosyncratic—relating to idiosyncrasy; how a person differs from another

IM—intramuscular

Impaired provider—professional caregiver who is under the influence of a drug or disease and thus is not as competent

Impetigo—a bacterial infection of the skin

Implanted device—object inserted into the body

Improper—referring to a fraction, one in which the numerator is larger than the denominator

IND—see *Investigational new drug*

Induration—area of hardened tissue

Inert—having little or no tendency or ability to react with other chemicals; not active

Infarction—area of tissue in an organ or part that undergoes necrosis following cessation of blood supply

Infiltration—deposition and accumulation of an external substance (infiltrate) in a cell, tissue, or organ, such as fat deposition in a damaged liver

Inflammation—the body's natural response (redness, swelling, heat, and pain) against any microbial invasion to help limit the spread of microbes or injury

Infusion—any liquid substance (other than blood) introduced into the body for therapeutic purposes

Inhalation—introduction of dry or moist air or vapor into the lungs for therapeutic purposes, such as by metered-dose bronchodilators in the treatment of asthma

Inhaler—device for administering medications by inhalation

Inorganic—not containing carbon; not derived from animal or vegetable matter

Inscription—body of the prescription, which gives the names of the drug prescribed and the dosage

Insert—implanting something inside something else

Insomnia—inability to sleep

Inspiration—inhalation, breathing in

Intradermal—within the dermis, intracutaneous

Intramuscular—within a muscle

Invert—to turn inside out or upside down

Investigational new drug—a drug under development and in the first three phases of clinical trials

IOP—intraocular pressure

Ischemia—temporary deficiency of blood flow to an organ or tissue

IUD—intrauterine device, usually for contraception

IV—intravenous

IV push (IVP)—inject quickly, not drip, a small amount of medication into an intravenous line

J

Jelly—thick, semisolid, gelatinous mass

K

Keratinization—process of keratin formation that takes place in keratocytes as they progress upward through the layers of the epidermis of skin to the stratum corneum

Ketoacidosis—faulty fat metabolism

Kilo—prefix used in the metric system to denote 1,000

L

Lactated Ringer's solution—intravenous medication containing fluid, dextrose, and electrolytes in a healthy combination, developed by Sydney Ringer

Latent TB—harboring of the tuberculosis tubercle, but without active infection

Lavage—irrigation of a cavity

LDL—low-density lipoprotein

Least common denominator—number on the bottom of a fraction that is common to the multiples of another number but is the least denominator those numbers have in common

LH—luteinizing hormone

Liniment—liquid vehicle (usually water, oil, or alcohol) containing a medication to be rubbed on or applied to the skin

Lipid—fat

Lotion—liquid medicinal preparation for local application to, or bathing, a part

Lozenge—small, dry, medicinal solid to be held in the mouth until it dissolves

Lumen—space within a tube

Lymphatic—pertaining to the lymph system

M

Magma—mass left after extraction of principal; salve or paste; suspension of finely divided material in a small amount of water

Malignant—growing worse; resisting treatment; said of cancerous growth; tending or threatening to produce death; harmful

Mania—mental disorder characterized by excessive excitement

MAO inhibitor—medication that affects the action of monoamine oxidase at the synapse; used to treat depression and Parkinson's disease

Mast cell stabilizer—stabilizes large tissue cells; resembles a basophil; essential for inflammatory reactions; does not circulate in the blood

mcg—microgram; one-millionth part of a gram

Means—numbers in the center of a ratio and proportion problem, not those at the ends

Megadose—overly large dosage

Melanocyte—cell that forms melanin; found in the lower epidermis of the skin

Melatonin—peptide hormone produced by the pineal gland; influences sleep-wake cycles and other circadian rhythms

Meniscus—curved upper surface of a liquid in a container

mEq—milliequivalent; one-thousandth of a chemical equivalent

Metabolism—breaking down into its constituents

Metastasis—change in location of a disease

Metastasize—to invade a distant body structure

Metric—measurement system based on grams for weight, liters for liquid, and meters for distance

mg—milligram, one-thousandth of a gram

MI—myocardial infarction; heart attack

Micro—small

Migraine headache—familiar disorder marked by periodic, usually unilateral, pulsatile headaches that begin during childhood or early adult life and tend to recur with diminishing frequency in later life

Milli—prefix used in the metric system to denote one-thousandth (1/1,000)

Mixed—when referring to numbers, a fraction that contains a whole number and a fractional part

mL—milliliter, one-thousandth of a liter

Monoamine oxidase inhibitor (MAOI)—medication that affects the action of monoamine oxidase at the synapse; used to treat depression and Parkinson's disease

Morbidly obese—weight 20% or more above the recommended ideal weight; usually associated with increased health risks

Mortar—vessel with a smooth interior in which crude drugs are crushed or ground with a pestle

Mucolytic—medication that breaks down mucus and improves breathing

Multiplication—adding repetitively

Myxedema—clinical and metabolic manifestations of hypothyroidism in adults, adolescents, and children

N

Narcotic—strong painkiller, generally made from opium, or synthetically made; may be addictive both psychologically and physically

Nausea—feeling of impending vomiting

NDA—new drug application

Nebulizer—apparatus for producing a fine spray or mist

Negative feedback system—result of a process that reverses or shuts off a stimulus

Nephrotoxic—substance with the potential to damage the kidney

Neuroleptic—medication used to treat psychoses

Neurotransmitter—substance released when the axon terminal of a presynaptic neuron is excited and acts by inhibiting or exciting a target cell

Nevus (nevi)—congenital discoloration of a circumscribed area of the skin resulting from pigmentation; a mole

NIDDM—non–insulin-dependent diabetes mellitus

Nit—egg of a louse or any other parasitic insect

Nodule—a small node or cluster of cells

Normal flora—normally occurring microorganisms on the human body; nonpathogenic with normal immune system

Nosocomial—infection contracted in a health-care facility

NPO—nothing by mouth

NSS—normal saline solution; isotonic solution

Numerator—number on the top of a fraction

O

O$_2$—oxygen

o.d.—right eye

Occupational Safety and Health Administration (OSHA)—the U.S. government agency that establishes and enforces the standards for safe and healthful working conditions

Ointment—viscous, semisolid vehicle to apply medication to the skin

Ophthalmic—pertaining to the eye

Oral—concerning the mouth; taking medications by mouth

Ordered dose—dose ordered by the prescriber (also known as desired dose)

Organic—containing carbon; composed of animal or vegetable matter

o.s.—left eye

OSHA—see *Occupational Safety and Health Administration*

Osmosis—passage of a solvent through a semipermeable membrane that separates solutions of different concentrations

Osteoarthritis—inflammation of bone and joints

Osteomalacia—softening of bone (an adult form of rickets)

Osteoporosis—loss of bone mass that occurs throughout the skeleton and predisposes patients to fractures

OTC—see *Over-the-counter*

Otic—pertaining to the ear

Ototoxicity—having a detrimental effect on the eighth nerve or organs of hearing

o.u.—both eyes

Over-the-counter (OTC)—in reference to medications and health-care products that can be purchased without a prescription

Oxytocin—pituitary hormone that stimulates the uterus to contract and thus induces parturition

oz—abbreviation for ounce

P

Package insert—information included with the product and written by the manufacturer

Packed cells—red blood cells that have been separated from plasma; used in treating conditions that require red blood cells but not liquid components of whole blood

Palliative—relieving or alleviating without curing

Papules—small lump or pimple, typically larger than a grain of salt but smaller than a peppercorn, that rises above the surface of the neighboring skin

Paranoia—condition in which patients show persistent persecutory delusions or delusional jealousy

Parasympathetic—of or pertaining to the craniosacral division of the autonomic nervous system

Parasympathomimetic—medication that stimulates the parasympathetic nervous system

Parathormone—hormone produced by the parathyroid; increases blood calcium

Parenteral—denoting any medication route other than the alimentary canal, such as intravenous, subcutaneous, intramuscular, or mucosal

Particulate—made up of particles

Passive artificial immunity—immunity obtained when patient is given antibodies from a donor to provide immunity

Passive natural immunity—the transfer of antibodies from one person to a nonimmune person (e.g., from mother to the newborn) that is temporary

Patch—drug delivery system that enhances uptake of a medicine through the skin

Patent medicine—remedy of questionable value that may harm the patient

Pathogenic—disease-causing microorganism

p.c.—after meals, on a full stomach

PCA—patient-controlled analgesia; delivery of pain medication that is controlled by the patient

PDR—*Physician's Desk Reference*

Pediatric—concerning the treatment of children

Percent—number divided by 100

Peripheral—located at, or pertaining to, the periphery; occurring away from the center

Peristalsis—movement of food and stool through the gastrointestinal tract

Pernicious anemia—chronic, macrocytic anemia; an autoimmune disease marked by a reduction in the mass of circulating red blood cells

Pestle—device for macerating drugs in a mortar

Pharmacodynamics—a drug's negative and positive biochemical or physiological changes to the body

Pharmacokinetics—study of metabolism and action of drugs with particular emphasis on the time required for absorption, duration of action, distribution in the body, and method of excretion

Pharmacology—study of drugs and their origin, nature, properties, and effects on living organisms

Pharmakon—from ancient Greek meaning "medicine"; also means poison or remedy

Phlebitis—inflammation of the vein

PICC (catheter)—peripherally inserted central catheter; ends in a large vein close to the heart, but is inserted from a peripheral site such as the lower arm

Piggyback—when medication is hung above another intravenous line and delivered before the main line is allowed to drip in

Placebo—inactive substance or treatment used as a nonspecific or inactive control in a test of a therapy that is suspected of being useful for a particular disease or condition; also, given to satisfy a patient's demand for medicine

Plasma—liquid part of blood or lymph

Plaster—topical preparation in which the constituents are formed into a tenacious mass of substance harder than an ointment and spread on muslin, linen, skin, or paper

Platelet—round or oval disk found in the blood of vertebrates; fragments of megakaryocytes that contribute to forming a clot

Plunger—part of a syringe that pushes the medication out of the syringe

PO—by mouth

Polymerized hemoglobin—hemoglobin that has been chemically changed; when added to solutions, polymerized hemoglobin gives concentrated hemoglobin; used only when other blood products are not available

Polypharmacy—concurrent use of a large number of drugs, a condition that increases the likelihood of unwanted side effects and adverse drug-drug interactions

Porcine—indicates substance is derived from pigs

Port—site of entry into the intravenous system of tubing allowing a health-care professional to insert medication

Potency—a drug's strength or ability to provide the desired effect

Potentiate—strengthen

Powder—an aggregation of fine particles of one or more substances that may be passed through fine meshes; a dose of such a powder, contained in a paper

PPD—see *Purified protein derivative*

Priming—removing air from an intravenous line by allowing fluid to flow through it

Productive cough—cough producing and expectorating mucus

prn—as needed

Progestin—corpus luteum hormone that prepares the endometrium for implantation of the fertilized ovum; a term used to cover a large group of synthetic drugs that have a progesterone-like effect on the uterus

Prolactin—hormone produced by the anterior pituitary gland; in humans, in association with estrogen and progesterone, stimulates breast development and the formation of milk during pregnancy

Proper—in mathematics, a fraction in which the numerator is smaller than the denominator

Prophylactic—pertaining to prevention

Proportion—in mathematics, a comparison or relationship of numbers

Proprietary name—name given to a medication by the pharmaceutical company that developed it; trade name

Prostaglandins—any of a large group of biologically active, carbon-20, unsaturated fatty acids produced by the metabolism of arachidonic acid through the cyclooxygenase pathway

Protective cap—top devised to maintain sterility or to prevent accidental injury

Psoriasis—chronic skin disorder in which red, scaly plaques with sharply defined borders appear on the body surface

Psychotropic—affecting the mind, emotions, or behaviors

Purified protein derivative (PPD)—substance used in an intradermal test for tuberculosis

Q

qd—every day

qid—four times per day

Quotient—answer in a division problem

R

Random—in research, a method used to assign subjects to experimental groups without introducing bias into a study

Ratio—relation in degree or number between two things

RDA—recommended daily allowance for vitamins and minerals

Receipts—recipes for preparation and administration of a treatment

Receptors—structures in the cell that enable the attachment of a drug, hormone, or infectious agent, which affects the functioning of the cell

Reconstitute—return a substance previously altered for preservation or storage to its original state

Reflux—regurgitation of acid up into the esophagus from the stomach

Releasing factor—chemical that triggers the release of hormones

Remainder—in mathematics, the amount left after subtracting two numbers

Replacement—restoration of something depleted or missing

Respiration—interchange of gases (CO_2 and O_2)

Rheumatoid arthritis—acute and chronic conditions marked by inflammation, muscle soreness and stiffness, and pain in joints and associated structures

Rickets—disease of bone formation in children, most commonly the result of vitamin D deficiency and marked by inadequate mineralization of developing cartilage and newly formed bone; causes abnormalities in the shape, structure, and strength of the skeleton

Rosacea—chronic eruption, usually localized in the middle of the face, in which papules and pustules appear on a flushed or red background

RSV—respiratory syncytial virus

Rx—means take; prescription; therapy

S

s̄ —without

Saline—sodium chloride solution

Salve—ointment; viscous, semisolid vehicle for applying medications to the skin

SC—under the skin, subcutaneous

Schlemm canal—drainage tube in the eye that drains aqueous humor

Scored—marked with a line to facilitate taking one-half of a tablet

Seborrhea—disease of the sebaceous glands marked by an increase in the amount and often an alteration of the quality, of the fats secreted by the sebaceous glands

Selective serotonin reuptake inhibitor (SSRI)—drug used to treat depression related to low amounts of the neurotransmitter serotonin

Seven rights of medication administration—seven rules to follow to administer medication safely

Shock—clinical syndrome marked by inadequate perfusion and oxygenation of cells, tissues, and organs; usually a result of marginal or markedly lowered blood pressure

SIADH—syndrome of inappropriate antidiuretic hormone

Side effect—any action or effect other than that intended

Signature—part of the prescription; giving instructions to the patient

Smoking cessation—stopping smoking

Solution—liquid containing dissolved substances

Somatic—pertaining to the body

Somatotropin—human growth hormone

Spacer—attachment to inhalers that promotes easier hand-holding; saves the medication in a chamber for entry during the next inhalation

Spastic—afflicted with spasms

Spike—in relation to intravenous (IV) therapy, opening an IV bag with a sharp device (spike) to allow fluid to flow out of the bag

ss—one-half

SSRI—see *Selective serotonin reuptake inhibitor*

Standing orders—orders that a prescriber leaves to administer certain medications automatically, usually in the prescriber's absence

Stat orders—orders to be executed immediately

Status asthmaticus—persistent and intractable asthma

Status epilepticus—continuous seizure activity without a pause

STD—sexually transmitted disease

Stomatitis—inflammation of the mouth including the gums, lips, and tongue

Street name—slang name for a drug; drug name used on the "street"

Subcutaneous—under the skin

Sublingual—under the tongue

Subscription—the part of a prescription that contains directions for compounding ingredients

Substance abuse—misuse or improper use of medications

Subtraction—removing one amount from another

Succinimides—class of antiseizure drugs that delay calcium moving over the neurons

Sum—answer to an addition problem

Superinfection—new infection caused by an organism different from that which caused the initial infection

Superscription—beginning of the prescription, denoted by the symbol R_x, meaning "take"

Suppository—semisolid substance for introduction into the rectum, vagina, or urethra, where it dissolves

Suspension—state of a solid when its particles are mixed with, but not dissolved in, a fluid or another solid

Sympathetic—division of the autonomic nervous system that produces a general rather than a specific effect and prepares the body to cope with stressful circumstances

Sympathomimetic—medication that stimulates the sympathetic nervous system

Synapse—space at the junction of two neurons

Synergism—action of two or more agents or organs working with each other

Synthetic—related to or made by synthesis; artificially prepared

Syrup—concentrated solution of sugar in water to which specific medicinal substances are usually added

Systemic—concerning a system or organized according to a system, pertaining to the whole body rather than one of its parts

T

t—teaspoon

T—tablespoon

T_3—triiodothyronine, a thyroid hormone

T_4—thyroxine, a thyroid hormone

Tab—abbreviation for tablet

Tablet—a small, disklike mass of medicinal powder

Telephone orders—orders received from a prescriber over the telephone

Tension headache—head pain that feels like pressure on the skull

Teratogenic—literally, creating a monster; anything that adversely affects normal cellular development in the embryo or fetus

Therapeutic level—refers to the point at which the blood value of the drug has the optimum desired effect

Therapeutic range—the range of blood levels from low to high in which the medication will work as desired

Therapeutic touch—the use of hand movements to stimulate circulation and healing

Thrombolytic—substance that breaks apart clots

Thrombus—blood clot that adheres to the wall of a blood vessel or organ

Thrush—candidal (yeast) infection of the mouth where white patches are noted

Thyroid storm—life-threatening situation resulting from untreated hyperthyroidism and characterized by hyperthermia, tachycardia, chest pain, sweating, weakness, heart failure, anxiety, shortness of breath, and disorientation

Thyroxine (T_4)—one of the thyroid hormones

tid—three times per day

Timed-release—medication that is released over a period of time to allow continuous treatment

Tinnitus—subjective ringing, buzzing, tinkling, or hissing sound in the ear

Tip—part of the syringe where the needle is attached

Titer—level of a specific item in the blood

TNF—tumor necrosis factor

Tocolytic—capable of relieving uterine contraction by reducing the excitability of myometrial muscle

Tolerance—capability to endure a large amount of a substance without an adverse effect and show decreased sensitivity to subsequent doses of the same substance

Tonometer—instrument for measuring tension or pressure

Topical—pertaining to a definite surface area; local

Total parenteral nutrition (TPN)—the patient receives nutrition only through this parenteral route; also known as hyperalimentation

Toxic—pertaining to, resembling, or caused by poison

Toxin—poisonous substance

TPN—see *total parenteral nutrition*

Trade name—name given to a drug by the pharmaceutical company that developed it; brand name

Transdermal—method of delivering medicine by placing it in a special gel-like matrix that is applied to the skin

Triiodothyronine (T_3)— one of the thyroid hormones

Troche—solid, discoid, or cylindrical mass consisting of chiefly medicinal powder, sugar, and mucilage

TSH—thyroid-stimulating hormone

Tuberculin—solution of purified protein derivative of tuberculosis that is injected intradermally to determine the presence of a tuberculosis infection

U

Ulcer—lesion of the skin or mucous membranes

Unit—a determined amount; insulin, vitamins, and some antibiotics are usually measured in units

United States Pharmacopeia/National Formulary (USP/NF)—a comprehensive listing of all FDA-approved drugs in the United States

Urticaria—multiple swollen, raised areas on the skin that are intensely itchy and last up to 24 hours

USP/DI—see *Drug Information for Health Providers*

USP/NF—see *United States Pharmacopeia/National Formulary*

V

Vasopressin—causes contraction of smooth muscle, including blood vessels

Vastus lateralis—muscle on the side of the thigh; usual site for injecting medication in infants

Ventrogluteal—site for injecting medication wherein the patient is lying on the side and the gluteus maximus muscle is accessed

Verbal orders—orders given by a prescriber that are not written

Verruca(e)—wart(s)

Vertigo—sensation of moving around in space or having objects move about the person

Vial—small glass or plastic bottle for medicine or chemicals

Viscous—sticky, gummy, gelatinous

Vitamin—accessory, but vital, nutrient that serves as a coenzyme or cofactor in an essential metabolic process

Vitreous humor—thick liquid found in the posterior chamber of the eye

VLDL—very low-density lipoprotein

W

Wheal—more or less round, temporary elevation of the skin, white in the center with a pale red periphery, accompanied by itching

Whole blood—all blood components, including plasma

Whole numbers—numbers that have no fractional component, except to be placed over 1

Withdrawal—cessation of administration of a drug, especially a narcotic; cessation of ingesting alcohol to which the individual has become either physiologically or psychologically addicted

Z

Z-track—intramuscular injection route that displaces the skin before entry to decrease skin staining

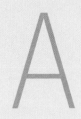

Drug Classifications

Drugs are classified according to what they do in the body. They may be used to treat specific illnesses or symptoms and to diagnose diseases. It is important to understand the general effects of drugs in these classifications. You can then learn about drugs more easily because those in the same class share many of the same purposes and effects. This is an extensive, but not complete, list of all drug classes.

A

Analgesics—reduce pain. Nonopioid analgesics are used for mild pain. Opioid analgesics are used to treat moderate to severe pain.

Anesthetics—remove sensation to the desired area to allow for medical procedures. General anesthesia renders the patient unconscious, and local anesthesia allows the patient to remain conscious, but removes sensation from the desired area of the body.

Anorexiants—used in the management of obesity. This therapy should be combined with a reduced-calorie diet and exercise.

Antacids—neutralize stomach acids to treat symptoms of acid reflux, heartburn, and indigestion.

Anti-Alzheimer's agents—work to manage the dementia that occurs with Alzheimer's disease. They attempt to prevent further deterioration of reasoning and memory. They are not curative.

Antianemics—prevent and treat anemias, which are most commonly caused by low iron levels in the blood.

Antianginals—treat and prevent angina, or chest pain.

Antianxiety medications—used to treat anxiety, such as generalized anxiety disorder (GAD) or post-traumatic stress disorder (PTSD).

Antiarrhythmics—suppress cardiac arrhythmias, or irregular heartbeats.

Antiasthmatics—manage both acute and chronic attacks of bronchospasm or asthma.

Antibiotics—treat bacterial infections. They may be used for a current infection or to prevent infection (prophylaxis). For example, antibiotics can be given before surgery to prevent infections that could result from opening the patient's body during surgery.

Anticholinergics—have many uses, including slowing a fast heart rate and relieving spasms of the respiratory system and nasal discharge. They may also be used to treat nausea and vomiting, motion sickness, and dizziness; some decrease gastric secretions and increase esophageal sphincter muscle tone. Finally, anticholinergics can be used to treat eye and urinary tract disorders, as well as neurological disorders.

Anticoagulants—prevent blood from clotting. They can cause a prolonged bleeding time (a laboratory test).

Anticonvulsants—decrease the incidence and severity of seizures. Sometimes they are used for immediate relief of symptoms (usually given intramuscularly, intravenously, or via endotracheal tube for this purpose). Blood levels may be measured to evaluate the effectiveness of the therapy.

Antidepressants—treat depression and elevate mood, usually in conjunction with psychotherapy. They are also used for the following: to treat anxiety, bedwetting, and chronic pain syndromes; for smoking cessation and eating disorders; and for obsessive-compulsive and generalized anxiety disorders.

Antidiabetics—manage diabetes mellitus. In some cases, injecting insulin is necessary. In others, tablets can be given to stimulate the body to release its own insulin.

Antidiarrheals—control and give symptomatic relief for both acute and chronic diarrhea.

Antiemetics/antivertigo agents—manage nausea, vomiting, and motion sickness.

Antifungal agents—treat fungal infections. Usually, they are rubbed on the skin or mucosa. Severe cases may require systemic treatment with an oral or intravenous form.

Antihistamines—relieve symptoms associated with allergies, including nasal inflammation, itching, and vessel swelling. They are used to treat anaphylaxis, a life-threatening allergic reaction.

Antihypertensives—decrease blood pressure. They are usually taken orally to reduce chronic hypertension, although some may be given intravenously in an emergency.

Anti-inflammatories—decrease swelling.

Antineoplastics—fight new growths caused by cancer. They are also used against autoimmune diseases, such as rheumatoid arthritis.

Antiparkinsonian agents—treat Parkinson's disease, a neurological disorder caused by low levels of dopamine, a chemical substance that transmits nerve impulses in the body.

Antiplatelet agents—prevent thromboembolic (clots that move) events, such as a stroke (cerebrovascular accident [CVA]) or heart attack. They are frequently used after cardiac surgery and can be combined with anticoagulants and thrombolytic (clot-busting) drugs.

Antipsychotic drugs—treat both acute and chronic psychoses, such as schizophrenia. They are also used to suppress tics that originate in the brain, such as in Tourette's syndrome.

Antipyretics—lower fevers resulting from infection, inflammation, or cancer.

Antiretrovirals—manage human immunodeficiency virus (HIV) infections. They increase the CD4 cell count and decrease the viral load.

Antirheumatics—manage symptoms of rheumatoid arthritis (pain and swelling), slow joint destruction, and preserve joint function.

Antituberculars—prevent and treat tuberculosis. They are also used to prevent meningitis and influenza.

Antiulcer agents—prevent or treat stomach ulcers. They are also used in the management of gastroesophageal reflux disease (GERD).

Antiviral medications—manage viral infections, such as herpes, chickenpox, influenza A, and cytomegalovirus (CMV) infection.

B

Beta blockers—help to manage blood pressure, chest pain, fast heart rates, vessel narrowing, migraine headaches, glaucoma, and heart failure. They can also prevent heart attacks and manage symptoms of low thyroid function.

Biologicals—antivenins and antitoxins used to treat poisonings or snakebites.

Bone resorption inhibitors—primarily used to treat and prevent osteoporosis in postmenopausal women. They are also used to manage high blood calcium and Paget's disease.

Bronchodilators—treat reversible airway obstruction resulting from asthma or chronic obstructive pulmonary disease (COPD).

C

Calcium channel blockers—treat high blood pressure, chest pain, and coronary artery spasm. They act to control the rhythm of the heart and to prevent neurological damage.

Central nervous system stimulants—treat narcolepsy, attention deficit disorder (ADD), and attention deficit–hyperactivity disorder (ADHD).

Corticosteroids—correct adrenocortical insufficiency. In large dosages, corticosteroids are used for anti-inflammatory, immunosuppressive, and antineoplastic activity. They can be used to reduce blood calcium and to treat autoimmune diseases. Topically, they are used to decrease inflammation and allergic conditions. Inhaled corticosteroids are used for asthma and vasoconstriction. They are also used for eye disorders.

D

Diuretics—used alone or in combination to reduce high blood pressure and swelling resulting from congestive heart failure (CHF) and other disorders. Potassium-sparing diuretics conserve potassium while decreasing fluid.

H

H$_2$ antagonists—used to decrease the production of acid in the stomach by blocking histamine-induced gastric acid secretion in the treatment of GERD, gastric ulcers, and other hypersecretory illnesses.

Hormones—used to treat deficiencies in disorders such as diabetes and thyroid disease.

I

Immunosuppressants—prevent transplant rejection. However, they also suppress the body's own immune system. For this reason, they may be used to treat some autoimmune disorders.

L

Laxatives—treat and prevent constipation. They are also used to cleanse the bowel in preparation for radiological or endoscopic procedures.

Lipid-lowering agents—used in conjunction with diet and exercise to lower blood lipid levels in an effort to decrease the morbidity associated with cardiovascular disease.

M

Minerals/electrolytes/pH modifiers—treat deficiencies or excesses of electrolytes to maintain correct acid-base balance.

N

Natural/herbal products—used for a wide variety of disorders. As discussed in the text, the Food and Drug Administration (FDA) does not regulate all herbal remedies as stringently as more accepted over-the-counter (OTC) and prescription medications, so the quality and effectiveness of herbal remedies can vary. Herbs are used extensively to treat menopausal symptoms, improve mood, reduce nausea, prevent motion sickness, boost the immune system, strengthen muscles, and improve gastric and urinary functioning.

Nonsteroidal anti-inflammatory drugs (NSAIDs)—control mild to moderate pain, fever, and inflammatory symptoms resulting from conditions such as rheumatoid arthritis and osteoarthritis. Ophthalmic NSAIDs decrease inflammation after eye surgery.

P

Proton pump inhibitors—decrease the production of stomach acid, which allows gastric ulcers to heal and prevents new ulcers from forming.

S

Sedative-hypnotics—provide sedation. They are frequently given before procedures or to induce sleep.

Skeletal muscle relaxants—reduce spasticity associated with neurological disorders or for symptomatic relief of musculoskeletal conditions.

T

Thrombolytic agents—dissolve clots and prevent heart attacks. As their name suggests, they are "clot-busters."

V

Vaccines/immunizing agents—prevent infectious diseases by promoting the body's own production of antibodies against diseases.

Vascular headache suppressants—change vascular tension to decrease pain.

Vitamins—prevent and treat vitamin deficiencies. They are also used as supplements in metabolic disorders.

Drug Classification Index by Generic Name

Generic Name	Trade Names	Classification
acetaminophen	Acephen, Infant's Feverall, Tylenol, Ofirmev (IV)	Antipyretics, nonopioid analgesics
acyclovir	Sitavig, Zovirax	Antivirals
adenosine	Adenocard, Adenoscan	Antiarrhythmics
albiglutide	Tanzeum	Antidiabetics
albuterol	Accuneb, ProAir HFA, ProAir Respiclick, Proventil HFA, Ventolin HFA, VoSpire ER	Bronchodilators
alendronate	Binosto, Fosamax	Bone resorption inhibitors
alfuzosin	Uroxatral	Urinary tract antispasmotics
allopurinol	Alloprim, Lopurin, Zyloprim	Antigout agents, antihyperuricemics
almotriptan	Axert	Vascular headache suppressants
alogliptin	Nesina	Antidiabetics
alprazolam	Xanax, Xanax XR	Antianxiety agents
aluminum hydroxide	AlternaGel, Alu-Cap, Aluminet, Alu-Tab, Amphojel, Basalgel, Dialume	Antiulcer agents, hypophosphatemics
alteplase	Activase, Cathflo Activase, tissue plasminogen activator (t-PA)	Thrombolytics
aminocaproic acid	Amicar	Hemostatic agents
amiodarone	Nexterone, Pacerone	Antiarrhythmics (class III)
amitriptyline	Elavil	Antidepressants
amlodipine	Norvasc	Antihypertensives
amoxicillin	Moxatag	Anti-infectives, antiulcer agents
amoxicillin/clavulanate	Augmentin, Augmentin ES, Augmentin XR	Anti-infectives
amphetamine mixtures	Adderall XR, Amphetamine Salt	Central nervous system stimulants
amphotericin B liposome	AmBisome	Antifungals
ampicillin	None listed	Anti-infectives
anidulafungin	Eraxis	Antifungals
apixaban	Eliquis	Anticoagulants
aprepitant	Emend	Antiemetics
aripiprazole	Abilify, Abilify Maintena	Antipsychotics, mood stabilizers
asparaginase	Erwinaze	Antineoplastics
atazanavir	Reyataz	Antiretrovirals
atenolol	Tenormin	Antianginals, antihypertensives
atorvastatin	Lipitor	Lipid-lowering agents
atropine	AtroPen	Antiarrhythmics
avanafil	Stendra	Erectile dysfunction agents
azathioprine	Azasan, Imuran	Immunosuppressants

Continued

Generic Name	Trade Names	Classification
azithromycin	Zithromax, Zmax	Agents for atypical mycobacterium, anti-infectives
aztreonam	Azactam, Cayston	Anti-infectives
baclofen	Gablofen, Lioresal	Antispasticity agents, skeletal muscle relaxants (centrally acting)
basiliximab	Simulect	Immunosuppressants
becaplermin	Regranex	Wound/ulcer/decubiti healing agent
beclomethasone (nasal)	QVAR	Antiasthmatics, Anti-inflammatories (steroidal)
benazepril	Lotensin	Antihypertensives
benztropine	Cogentin	Antiparkinsonian agents
bicalutamide	Casodex	Antineoplastics
bisacodyl	Bisac-Evac, Biscolax, Correctol, Dacodyl, Doxidan, Dulcolax, Ex-Lax Ultra, Femilax, Fleet Laxative	Laxatives
bismuth subsalicylate	Bismatrol, Kaopectate, Kao-Tin, Kapectolin, Peptic Relief, Pepto-Bismol	Antidiarrheals, antiulcer agents
bisoprolol	Zebeta	Antihypertensives
bivalirudin	Angiomax	Anticoagulants
bleomycin	Blenoxane	Antineoplastics
bortezomib	Velcade	Antineoplastics
bumetanide	None listed	Diuretics
bupivacaine liposome	Exparel	Anesthetics (topical/local)
buprenorphine	Buprenex, Subutex	Opioid analgesics
bupropion	Aplenzin, Forfivo XL, Wellbutrin, Wellbutrin SR, Wellbutrin XL, Zyban	Antidepressants, smoking deterrents
bupropion/naltrexone	Contrive	Weight-control agents
buspirone	BuSpar	Antianxiety agents
busulfan	Busulfex, Myleran	Antineoplastics
butalbital, acetaminophen	Axocet, Bucet, Bupap, Butex Forte, Dolgic, Marten-Tab, Phrenilin, Phrenilin Forte, Repap CF, Sedapap, Tencon, Triapin	Nonopioid analgesics (combination with barbiturate)
butalbital, acetaminophen, and caffeine	Endolor, Esgic, Esgic-Plus, Fioricet, Margesic, Medigesic, Repan, Triad	Nonopioid analgesics (combination with barbiturate)
butalbital, aspirin, and caffeine	Fiorinal, Fiortal	Nonopioid analgesics (combination with barbiturate)
butorphanol	Stadol, Stadol NS	Opioid analgesics
caffeine citrate	Cafcit	Central nervous system stimulants
canagliflozin	Invokana	antidiabetics
candesartan	Atacand	Antihypertensives
cangrelor	Kengreal	Antiplatelet agents
capsaicin	Capsin HP, Capzasin-P, DiabetAid Pain and Tingling Relief, Qutenza, Solonpas Hot, Zostrix, Zotrix Diabetic Foot Pain, Zostrix-HP	Nonopioid analgesics (topical)
captopril	None listed	Antihypertensives
carbamazepine	Carbatrol, Epitol, Equetro, Tegretol, Tegretol-XR, Teril	Anticonvulsants, mood stabilizers
carbidopa-levodopa	Duopa, Rytary, Sinemet, Sinemet CR	Antiparkinsonian agents
carboplatin	None listed	Antineoplastics
carisoprodol	Soma	Skeletal muscle relaxants (centrally acting)
carvedilol	Coreg, Coreg CR	Antihypertensives
caspofungin	Cancidas	Antifungals (systemic)
cefdinir	None listed	Anti-infectives
cefepime	Maxipime	Anti-infectives

Generic Name	Trade Names	Classification
cefprozil	Cefzil	Anti-infectives
ceftriaxone	Rocephin	Anti-infectives
cefuroxime	Ceftin, Zinacef	Anti-infectives
celecoxib	Celebrex	Antirheumatics, nonsteroidal anti-inflammatory agents
cephalexin	Keflex	Anti-infectives
certolizumab pegol	Cimzia	Gastrointestinal anti-inflammatories, antirheumatics
cetirizine	Zyrtec	Allergy, cold, and cough remedies; antihistamines
cetuximab	Erbitux	Antineoplastics
chlorpheniramine	Aller-Chlor, Allergy, Chlo-Amine, Chlorate, Chlor-Trimeton, Chlor-Trimeton Allergy 4 Hour, Chlor-Trimeton Allergy 8 Hour, Chlor-Trimeton Allergy 12 Hour, PediaCare Allergy Formula, Phenetron, Telachlor, Teldrin	Allergy, cold, and cough remedies; antihistamines
cholestyramine	LoCHOLEST, LoCHOLEST Light, Prevalite, Questran, Questran Light	Lipid-lowering agents
cidofovir	Vistide	Antivirals
cilostazol	Pletal	Antiplatelet agents
cimetidine	Tagamet, Tagamet HB	Antiulcer agents
ciprofloxacin	Cipro, Cipro XR	Anti-infectives
cisplatin	Platinol-AQ	Antineoplastics
citalopram	Celexa	Antidepressants
cladribine	Leustatin	Antineoplastics
clarithromycin	Biaxin, Biaxin XL	Agents for atypical mycobacteria, anti-infectives, antiulcer agents
clevidipine	Cleviprex	Antihypertensives
clindamycin	Cleocin, Cleocin T, Clinda-Derm, Clindagel, Clindesse, Clindets, Evoclin	Anti-infectives
clofarabine	Clolar	Antineoplastics
clonazepam	Klonopin	Anticonvulsants
clonidine	Catapres, Catapres-TTS, Duraclon, Kapvay	Antihypertensives
clopidogrel	Plavix	Antiplatelet agents
clorazepate	Tranxene T-Tab, Tranxene-SD	Anticonvulsants, sedative-hypnotics
clozapine	Clozaril, FazaClo, Versacloz	Antipsychotics
codeine	None listed	Allergy, cold, and cough remedies; antitussives; opioid analgesics
colchicine	Colcrys, Mitigare	Antigout agents
colesevelam	Welchol	Lipid-lowering agents
colestipol	Colestid	Lipid-lowering agents
crofelemer	Fulyzaq	Antidiarrheals
cyclobenzaprine	Amrix, Flexeril	Skeletal muscle relaxants (centrally acting)
cyclosporine	Gengraf, Neoral, Sandimmune	Immunosuppressants, antirheumatics (DMARDs)
cyproheptadine	Periactin	Allergy, cold, and cough remedies; antihistamines
cytarabine	Cytosar, Cytosar-U, Tarabine PFS	Antineoplastics
dabigatran	Pradaxa	Anticoagulants
dacarbazine	DTIC-Dome	Antineoplastics
dalfampridine	Ampyra	Anti–multiple sclerosis agents
dantrolene	Dantrium, Ryanodex	Skeletal muscle relaxants (direct acting)
daptomycin	Cubicin	Anti-infectives

Continued

Generic Name	Trade Names	Classification
darbepoetin	Aranesp	Antianemics
darifenacin	Enablex	Urinary tract antispasmodics
darunavir	Prezista	Antiretrovirals
daunorubicin hydrochloride	Cerubidine	Antineoplastics
decitabine	Dacogen	Antineoplastics
deferoxamine	Desferal	Antidotes
denosumab	Prolia, Xgeva	Bone resorption inhibitors
desipramine	Norpramin	Antidepressants
desirudin	Iprivask	Anticoagulants
desloratadine	Clarinex, Clarinex Reditabs	Allergy, cold, and cough remedies; antihistamines
desmopressin	DDAVP, DDAVP Rhinal Tube, DDAVP Rhinyle Drops, Stimate	Hormones
desvenlafaxine	Khedezla, Pristiq	Antidepressants
dexlansoprazole	Dexilant	Antiulcer agents
dexmedetomidine	Precedex	Sedative-hypnotics
dexmethylphenidate	Focalin, Focalin XR	Central nervous system stimulants
dexrazoxane	Totect, Zinecard	Cardioprotective agents
dextroamphetamine	Dexedrine Spansule, ProCentra, Zenzedi	Central nervous system stimulants
dextromethorphan	Creo-Terpin, Creomulsion Adult Formula, Creomulsion for Children, Delsym, PediaCare Children's Long Acting Cough, Robafin Cough, Robitussin, Scot-Tussin Diabetes, Triaminic Thin Strips Long Acting Cough, Vicks 44 Cough Relief, Vicks DayQuil Cough	Allergy, cold, and cough remedies; antitussives
diazepam	Diastat, Valium	Antianxiety agents, anticonvulsants, sedative-hypnotics, skeletal muscle relaxants (centrally acting)
diclofenac sodium	Voltaren XR	Nonopioid analgesics, nonsteroidal anti-inflammatory agents
dicyclomine	Bentyl	Antispasmodics
digoxin	Lanoxicaps, Lanoxin	Antiarrhythmics, inotropics
diltiazem	Cardizem, Cardizem CD, Cardizem LA, Cartia XT, Taztia XT, Tiazac	Antianginals, antiarrhythmics (class IV), antihypertensives
dimenhydrinate	Calm X, Dramamine, Dramanate, Triptone Caplets	Antiemetics, antihistamines
dimethyl fumarate	Tecfidera	Anti–multiple sclerosis agents
dinoprostone	Cervidil Vaginal Insert, Prepidil Endocervical Gel, Prostin E Vaginal Suppository	Cervical ripening agents
diphenhydramine (oral, parenteral)	Banophen, Benadryl, Benadryl Dye-Free Allergy, Compoz, Compoz Nighttime Sleep Aid, Diphen AF, Diphen Cough, Genahist, 40 Winks, Hyrexin-50, Maximum Strength Nytol, Maximum Strength Sleepinal, Midol PM, Miles Nervine, Nighttime Sleep Aid, Nytol, Scot-Tussin Allergy DM, Siladryl, Silphen, Sleep-Eze 3, Sleepwell 2-night, Snooze Fast, Sominex, Tusstat, Twilite, Unisom Nighttime Sleep-Aid	Allergy, cold, and cough remedies; antihistamines; antitussives
diphenoxylate-atropine	Logen, Lomate, Lomotil, Lonox	Antidiarrheals
dipyridamole	Persantine, Persantine IV	Antiplatelet agents, diagnostic agents (coronary vasodilators)
dobutamine	Dobutrex	Inotropics
docetaxel	Docefrez, Taxotere	Antineoplastics
docosanol	Abreva	Antivirals

Generic Name	Trade Names	Classification
docusate sodium	Colace, Correctol, Diocto, Docu-Soft, Ducosoft S, DOK, DSS, Dulcolax, Dulcolax Stool Softener, Enemeeez, Fleet Pedia-Lax, Fleet Sof-Lax, Phillips Liqui-Gels	Laxatives
dofetilide	Tikosyn	Antiarrhythmics (class III)
dolasetron	Anzemet	Antiemetics
dolutegravir	Tivicay	Antiretrovirals
donepezil	Aricept	Anti-Alzheimer's agents
dopamine	Intropin	Inotropics, vasopressors
doripenem	Doribax	Anti-infectives
doxazosin	Cardura, Cardura XL	Antihypertensives
doxepin	Silenor, Zonalon	Antianxiety agents, antidepressants, antihistamines (topical), sedative/hypnotics
doxorubicin	None listed	Antineoplastics
dronedarone	Multaq	Antiarrhythmics
droperidol	Inapsine	Sedative-hypnotics
dulaglutide	Trulicity	Antidiabetics
duloxetine	Cymbalta	Antidepressants
dutasteride	Avodart	Benign prostatic hyperplasia (BPH) agents
edoxaban	Svaysa	Anticoagulants
efavirenz	Sustiva	Antiretrovirals
eletriptan	Relpax	Vascular headache suppressants
elvitegravir	Vitekta	Antiretrovirals
empagliflozin	Jardiance	Antidiabetics
emtricitabine	Emtriva	Antiretrovirals
enalapril, enalaprilat	Epaned, Vasotec	Antihypertensives
enoxaparin	Lovenox	Anticoagulants
entacapone	Comtan	Antiparkinsonian agents
entecavir	Baraclude	Antivirals
epinephrine	Adrenaclick, Adrenalin, Auvi-Q, EpiPen, Micronefrin, Nephron, Twin-Ject	Antiasthmatics, bronchodilators, vasopressors
epirubicin	Ellence	Antineoplastics
eplerenone	Inspra	Antihypertensives
epoetin	Epogen, Procrit	Antianemics
eprosartan	Teveten	Antihypertensives
eptifibatide	Integrilin	Antiplatelet agents
ergotamine	Ergomar	Vascular headache suppressants
erlotinib	Tarceva	Antineoplastics
ertapenem	Invanz	Anti-infectives
erythromycin base	Eryc, Ery-Tab, PCE	Anti-infectives
erythromycin (topical)	Akne-Mycin, Erygel	Anti-infectives
escitalopram	Lexapro	Antidepressants
esmolol	Brevibloc	Antiarrhythmics (class II)
esomeprazole	Nexium	Antiulcer agents
estradiol	Estrace	Hormones
estrogens, conjugated	Premarin	Hormones
eszopiclone	Lunesta	Sedative-hypnotics
etanercept	Enbrel	Antirheumatics (EMARDs)
ethambutol	Myambutol	Antituberculars
etidronate	Didronel	Bone resorption inhibitors
etodolac	None listed	Antirheumatics, nonopioid analgesics
etravirine	Intelence	Antiretrovirals
evolocumab	Repatha	Lipid-lowering agents
exenatide	Bydureon, Byetta	Antidiabetics
ezetimibe	Zetia	Lipid-lowering agents

Continued

Generic Name	Trade Names	Classification
famciclovir	Famvir	Antivirals
famotidine	Pepcid, Pepcid AC	Antiulcer agents
febuxostat	Uloric	Antigout agents
felodipine	Plendil	Antianginals, antihypertensives
fenofibrate	Antara, Fenoglide, Lipofen, Lofibra, Tricor, Triglide	Lipid-lowering agents
fenofibric acid	Fibricor, Trilipix	Lipid-lowering agents
fenoldopam	Corlopam	Antihypertensives
fentanyl (parenteral)	Sublimaze	Opioid analgesics
fentanyl (transdermal)	Duragesic	Opioid analgesics, analgesic adjuncts
ferumoxytol	Feraheme	Antianemics
fesoterodine	Toviaz	Urinary tract antispasmodics
fexofenadine	Allegra, Mucinex Allergy	Allergy, cold, and cough remedies; antihistamines
fidaxomicin	Dificid	Anti-infectives
filgrastim	Neupogen, Zarxio	Colony-stimulating factors
finasteride	Propecia, Proscar	Hair regrowth stimulants
fingolimod	Gilenya	Anti–multiple sclerosis agents
flecainide	Tambocor	Antiarrhythmics
fluconazole	Diflucan	Antifungals (systemic)
fludarabine	Fludara	Antineoplastics
flumazenil	Romazicon	Antidotes
flunisolide	Aerospan HFA	Antiasthmatics, anti-inflammatories (steroidal)
fluorouracil	Carac, Efudex, Fluoroplex, 5-FU	Antineoplastics
fluoxetine	Prozac, Prozac Weekly, Sarafem, Selfemra	Antidepressants
fluphenazine	Permitil, Prolixin, Prolixin Decanoate, Prolixin Enanthate	Antipsychotics
flurazepam	Dalmane	Sedative-hypnotics
fluticasone (inhaled)	Arnuity Ellipta, Flovent Diskus, Flovent HFA	Antiasthmatics, anti-inflammatories (steroidal)
fluticasone (nasal)	Flonase, Veramyst	Anti-inflammatories (steroidal)
fluvastatin	Lescol, Lescol XL	Lipid-lowering agents
fluvoxamine	Luvox, Luvox CR	Antidepressants, antiobsessive agents
folic acid	folate, Folvite, vitamin B	Antianemics, vitamins
fondaparinux	Arixtra	Anticoagulants
formoterol	Perforomist	Bronchodilators
fosamprenavir	Lexiva, Telzir	Antiretrovirals
foscarnet	None listed	Antivirals
fosinopril	None listed	Antihypertensives
fosphenytoin	Cerebyx	Anticonvulsants
frovatriptan	Frova	Vascular headache suppressants
furosemide	Lasix	Diuretics
gabapentin	Gralise, Horizant, Neurontin	Analgesic adjuncts, therapeutic; anticonvulsants; mood stabilizers
galantamine	Razadyne, Razadyne ER	Anti-Alzheimer's agents
ganciclovir	Cytovene	Antivirals
gatifloxacin	Zymaxid	Anti-infectives (ophthalmic)
gefitinib	Iressa	Antineoplastics
gemcitabine	Gemzar	Antineoplastics
gemfibrozil	Lopid	Lipid-lowering agents
gemifloxacin	Factive	Anti-infectives
gemtuzumab ozogamicin	Mylotarg	Antineoplastics
gentamicin	None listed	Anti-infectives
glimepiride	Amaryl	Antidiabetics
glipizide	Glucotrol, Glucotrol XL	Antidiabetics
glucagon	GlucaGen	Hormones

Generic Name	Trade Names	Classification
glyburide	DiaBeta, Glynase PresTab, Micronase	Antidiabetics
glycopyrrolate	Cuvposa, Robinul, Robinul-Forte	Antispasmodics
golimumab	Simponi, Simponi Aria	Antirheumatics
goserelin	Zoladex	Antineoplastics, hormones
granisetron	Kytril	Antiemetics
guaifenesin	Alfen Jr, Altarussin, Breonesin, Diabetic Tussin, Ganidin NR, Guiatuss, Hytuss, Hytuss-2X, Mucinex, Naldecon Senior EX, Organidin NR, Robitussin, Scot-tussin Expectorant, Siltussin DAS, Siltussin SA	Allergy, cold, and cough remedies; expectorants
guanfacine	Intuniv, Tenex	Antihypertensives
haloperidol	Haldol, Haldol Decanoate	Antipsychotics
heparin	Hep-Lock, Hep-Lock U/P	Anticoagulants
human papillomavirus quadrivalent (types 6, 11, 16, and 18)	Gardasil	Vaccines/immunizing agents
hydralazine	None listed	Antihypertensives
hydrocodone	Hysingla ER, Zohydro ER	Allergy, cold, and cough remedies (antitussive); opioid analgesics
hydrocodone and acetaminophen	Anexsia, Norco	Allergy, cold, and cough remedies (antitussive); Opioid analgesics
hydrocodone and ibuprofen	Reprexain, Vicoprofen	Allergy, cold, and cough remedies (antitussive); Opioid analgesics
hydromorphone	Dilaudid, Dilaudid-HP, Exalgo	Allergy, cold, and cough remedies (antitussives); opioid analgesics
hydroxychloroquine	Plaquenil	Antimalarials, antirheumatics (DMARDs)
hydroxyzine	Vistaril	Antianxiety agents, antihistamines, sedative-hypnotics
hyoscyamine	Anaspaz, A-Spas S/L, Cystospaz, Cystospaz-M, Donnamar, ED-SPAZ, Levbid, Levsin, Levsinex, NuLev	Antispasmodics
ibandronate	Boniva	Bone resorption inhibitors
ibuprofen, oral	Advil, Advil Migraine Liqui-Gels, Children's Advil, Children's Motrin, Excedrin IB, Junior Strength Advil, Medipren, Midol Maximum Strength Cramp Formula, Motrin, Motrin Drops, Motrin IB, Motrin Junior Strength, Motrin Migraine Pain, Nuprin, PediaCare Children's Fever	Antipyretics, antirheumatics, nonopioid analgesics, nonsteroidal anti-inflammatory agents
ibutilide	Corvert	Antiarrhythmics (class III)
idarubicin	Idamycin PFS	Antineoplastics
idarucizumab	Praxbind	Antidotes
ifosfamide	Ifex	Antineoplastics
iloperidone	Fanapt	Antipsychotics
imatinib	Gleevec	Antineoplastics
imipenem/cilastatin	Primaxin	Anti-infectives
imipramine	Tofranil, Tofranil PM	Antidepressants
imiquimod	Aldara	Antivirals, immune modifiers
indacaterol	Aracept Neohaler	Bronchodilators, COPD agents
indomethacin	Indocin, Tivorbex	Antirheumatics, ductus arteriosus patency adjuncts (IV only), nonsteroidal anti-inflammatory agents

Continued

Generic Name	Trade Names	Classification
infliximab	Remicade	Antirheumatics (DMARDs), gastrointestinal anti-inflammatories
insulin, regular (injection, concentrated)	Humulin R, Humulin R Regular U-500 (Concentrated), Novolin R	Antidiabetics, hormones
ipratropium	Atrovent, Atrovent HFA	Allergy, cold, and cough remedies; bronchodilators
irbesartan	Avapro	Antihypertensives
irinotecan	Camptosar	Antineoplastics
isoniazid	INH	Antituberculars
isosorbide	Dilatrate-SR, Isordil	Antianginals
isotretinoin	Absorica, Amnesteem, Claravis, Myorisan, Sotret, Zenatane	Antiacne agents
isradipine	DynaCirc, DynaCirc CR	Antianginals
itraconazole	Onmel, Sporanox, Sporanox PulsePak	Antifungals (systemic)
ivabradine	Corlanor	Heart failure agents
ixabepilone	Ixempra	Antineoplastics
ketoconazole (systemic)	Extina, Nizoral, Nizoral A-D, Xolegel	Antifungals
ketoprophen	None listed	Antipyretics, antirheumatics, nonopioid analgesics, nonsteroidal anti-inflammatory agents
ketorolac	Sprix, Toradol	Nonsteroidal anti-inflammatory agents, nonopioid analgesics
labetalol	None listed	Antianginals, antihypertensives
lacosamide	Vimpat	Anticonvulsants
lactulose	Cholac, Constilac, Constulose, Enulose, Generlac, Kristalose	Laxatives
lamivudine	Epivir, Epivir-HBV	Antiretrovirals, antivirals
lamotrigine	Lamictal, Lamictal CD, Lamictal ODT, Lamictal XR	Anticonvulsants
lansoprazole	Prevacid, Prevacid 24 HR	Antiulcer agents
lapatinib	Tykerb	Antineoplastics
leflunomide	Arava	Antirheumatics (DMARDs)
letrozole	Femara	Antineoplastics
leucovorin	None listed	Antidotes (for methotrexate), vitamins
leuprolide	Eligard, Lupron Depot, Lupron Depot-Ped	Antineoplastics
levalbuterol	Xopenex, Xopenex HFA	Bronchodilators
levetiracetam	Keppra, Keppra XR	Anticonvulsants
levofloxacin	Levaquin	Anti-infectives
levomilnacipran	Fetzima	Antidepressants
levothyroxine	Levo-T, Levoxyl, Synthroid, T4, Tirosint, Unithroid	Hormones
lidocaine (parenteral)	Xylocaine	Anesthetics (topical/local), antiarrhythmics (class IB)
linagliptin	Trajenta	Antidiabetics
lindane	gamma-benzene hexachloride	Pediculicides, scabicides
linezolid	Zyvox	Anti-infectives
liraglutide	Saxenda, Victoza	Antidiabetics
lisinopril	Prinivil, Zestril	Antihypertensives
lithium	Lithobid	Mood stabilizers
loperamide	Imodium, Imodium A-D, Neo-Diaral	Antidiarrheals
lopinavir/ritonavir	Kaletra	Antiretrovirals
loratadine	Alavert Allergy 24 Hour, Alavert Children's Allergy, Claritin 24-Hour Allergy, Claritin Children's Allergy, Claritin Liqui-Gels 24-Hour Allergy, Claritin Reditabs 24 Hour Allergy, Lordamed, Tavist ND Allergy	Antihistamines
lorazepam	Ativan	Analgesic adjuncts, antianxiety agents, sedative-hypnotics

Generic Name	Trade Names	Classification
lorcaserin	Belviq	Weight-control agents
losartan	Cozaar	Antihypertensives
lovastatin	Altoprev	Lipid-lowering agents
lurasidone	Latuda	Antipsychotics
magaldrate and simethicone	Riopan Plus	Antiulcer agents
magnesium oxide (60.3% Mg; 49.6 mEq Mg/g)	Mag-Ox 400, Uro-Mag	Mineral and electrolyte replacements/supplements
mannitol	Osmitrol, Resectisol	Diuretics
maraviroc	Selzentry	Antiretrovirals
meclizine	Antivert, Bonine, Dramamine Less Drowsy Formula	Antiemetics, antihistamines
medroxyprogesterone	Depo-Provera, Depo-Sub Q Provera 104, Provera	Antineoplastics, contraceptive hormones
megestrol	Megace, Megace OS	Antineoplastics, hormones
meloxicam	Mobic	Nonsteroidal anti-inflammatory agents
melphalan	Alkeran	Antineoplastics
memantine	Namenda	Anti-Alzheimer's agents
meperidine	Demerol	Opioid analgesics
meropenem	Merrem	Anti-infectives
mesalamine	Apriso, Asacol HD, Canasa, Delsicol, Lialda, Pentasa, Rowasa	Gastrointestinal anti-inflammatories
mesna	Mesnex	Antidotes
metaxalone	Skelaxin	Skeletal muscle relaxants (centrally acting)
metformin	Fortamet, Glucophage, Glucophage XR, Glumetza, Riomet	Antidiabetics
methadone	Methadose	Opioid analgesics
methocarbamol	Robaxin	Skeletal muscle relaxants (centrally acting)
methotrexate	Otrexup, Rasuvo, Rheumatrex, Trexall	Antineoplastics, antirheumatics (DMARDs), immunosuppressants
methyldopa	None listed	Antihypertensives
methylergonovine	Methergine	Oxytocic agents
methylnaltrexone	Relistor	Laxatives
methylphenidate	Aptensio XR, Concerta, Metadate CD, Metadate ER, Methylin, Methylin ER, Quillivant XR, Ritalin, Ritalin LA, Ritalin-SR	Central nervous system stimulants
methylprednisolone	A-Methapred, Depo-Medrol, Medrol, Solu-Medrol	Therapeutic antiasthmatics, corticosteroids
metoclopramide	Metozolv ODT, Reglan	Antiemetics
metolazone	Zaroxolyn	Antihypertensives, diuretics
metoprolol	Lopressor, Toprol-XL	Antianginals, antihypertensives
metronidazole	Flagyl, Flagyl ER, MetroCream, MetroGel, MetroGel-Vaginal, Metro IV, MetroLotion, Noritate, Nuvessa, Vandazole	Anti-infectives, antiprotozoals, antiulcer agents
micafungin	Mycamine	Antifungals
midazolam	None listed	Antianxiety agents, sedative-hypnotics
mifepristone	Korlym, Mifeprex	Abortifacients, antidiabetics
miglitol	Glyset	Antidiabetics
milnacipran	Savella	Antifibromyalgia agents
milrinone	None listed	Inotropics
mirabegron	Myrbetriq	Urinary tract antispasmotics
mirtazapine	Remeron RD, Remeron SolTab	Antidepressants
misoprostol	Cytotec	Antiulcer agents, cytoprotective agents
mitomycin	None listed	Antineoplastics

Continued

Generic Name	Trade Names	Classification
mitoxantrone	Novantrone	Antineoplastics, immune modifiers
modafinil	Provigil	Central nervous system stimulants
moexipril	Univasc	Antihypertensives
mometasone	Asmanex HFA, Asthmanex Twisthaler (inhaled), Nasonex (nasal)	Anti-inflammatories (steroidal)
montelukast	Singulair	Allergy, cold, and cough remedies; bronchodilators
morphine	Astramorph, Duramorph, Embeda, Infumorph, Kadian, MS Contin	Opioid analgesics
moxifloxacin	Avelox	Anti-infectives
mupirocin	Bactroban, Bactroban Nasal, Centany	Anti-infectives
muromonab-CD3	Orthoclone OKT3	Immunosuppressants
mycophenolate mofetil	CellCept	Immunosuppressants
nabumetone	Relafen	Antirheumatics, nonsteroidal anti-inflammatory agents
nadolol	Corgard	Antianginals, antihypertensives
nafarelin	Synarel	Hormones
nalbuphine	None listed	Opioid analgesics
naloxegol	Movantik	Laxatives
naloxone	Evzio	Antidotes (for opioids)
naproxen	Aleve, Anaprox, Anaprox DS, EC-Naprosyn, Naprelan, Naprosyn	Nonopioid analgesics, nonsteroidal anti-inflammatory agents, antipyretics
naratriptan	Amerge	Vascular headache suppressants
nateglinide	Starlix	Antidiabetics
nebivolol	Bystolic	Antihypertensives
nefazodone	None listed	Antidepressants
neostigmine	Prostigmin	Antimyasthenics
nesiritide	Natrecor	Vasodilators
nevirapine	Viramune, Viramune XR	Antivirals
niacin	Niacor, Niaspan, Nicobid, Nicolar, Nicotinex, Nicotinic acid, Slo-Niacin, Vitamin B_3	Lipid-lowering agents, vitamins
niacinamide	Edur-Acin, Nia-Bid, Niac, Niacels, Niacor, Niaspan, Nicobid, Nico-400, Nicolar, Nicotinex, nicotinic acid, Slo-Niacin, vitamin B	Lipid-lowering agents, vitamins
nicardipine	Cardene, Cardene IV	Antianginals, antihypertensives
nicotine	Gum: Nicorette, Thrive Inhaler: Nicotrol inhaler Lozenge: Commit, Nicorette Nasal spray: Nicotrol NS Transdermal: NicoDerm CQ	Smoking deterrents
nifedipine	Adalat CC, Afeditab CR, Procardia, Procardia XL	Antianginals, antihypertensives
nilotinib	Tasigna	Antineoplastics
nimodipine	Nymalize	Subarachnoid hemorrhage therapy agents
nisoldipine	Sular	Antihypertensives
nitrofurantoin	Furadantin, Macrobid, Macrodantin	Anti-infectives
nitroglycerin	Capsules: Nitro-Time IV: none listed Translingual spray: Nitrolingual, NitroMist Ointment: Nitro-Bid Sublingual: Nitrostat Transdermal: Minitran, Nitro-Dur	Antianginals
nitroprusside	Nitropress	Antihypertensives
nizatidine	Axid, Axid AR	Antiulcer agents
norepinephrine	Levophed	Vasopressors

Generic Name	Trade Names	Classification
nortriptyline	Pamelor	Antidepressants
NPH insulin (isophane insulin suspension)	Humulin N, Novolin N	Antidiabetics, hormones
nystatin	Mycostatin, Nilstat	Antifungals (topical/local)
octreotide	Sandostatin, Sandostatin LAR	Antidiarrheals, hormones
ofloxacin	None listed	Anti-infectives
olanzapine	Zyprexa, Zyprexa Relprevv, Zyprexa Zydis	Antipsychotics, mood stabilizers
olmesartan	Benicar	Antihypertensives
olodaterol	Striverdi	Bronchodilators
olsalazine	Dipentum	Gastrointestinal anti-inflammatories
omalizumab	Xolair	Antiasthmatics
omega-3 acid ethyl esters	Lovaza, Omtryg	Lipid-lowering agents
omeprazole	Prilosec, Prilosec OTC	Antiulcer agents
ondansetron	Zofran, Zofran ODT, Zuplenz	Antiemetics
oprelvekin	Neumega	Colony-stimulating factors
oritavancin	Orbactiv	Anti-infectives
orlistat	Alli, Xenical	Weight-control agents
oseltamivir	Tamiflu	Antivirals
oxaliplatin	Eloxatin	Antineoplastics
oxaprozin	Daypro	Antirheumatics, nonsteroidal anti-inflammatory agents
oxazepam	Serax	Antianxiety agents, sedative-hypnotics
oxcarbazepine	Oxtellar XR, Trileptal	Anticonvulsants
oxybutynin (oral)	Ditropan XL	Urinary tract antispasmodics
oxybutynin (transdermal)	Oxytrol, Oxytrol for Women	Urinary tract antispasmodics
oxycodone	Oxaydo, OxyContin, Roxicodone	Opioid analgesics
oxytocin	Pitocin	Hormones
paclitaxel	Abraxane	Antineoplastics
palifermin	Kepivance	Cytoprotective agents
paliperidone	Invega, Invega Sustenna, Invega Trinza	Antipsychotics
palonosetron	Aloxi	Antiemetics
pamidronate	Aredia	Bone resorption inhibitors
pancrelipase	Creon, Pancreaze, Pertyze, Ultresa, Viokace, Zenpep	Digestive agents
pancuronium	None listed	Neuromuscular blocking agents
panitumumab	Vectibix	Antineoplastics
pantoprazole	Protonix, Protonix IV	Antiulcer agents
paroxetine hydrochloride	Paxil, Paxil CR	Antianxiety agents, antidepressants
pazopanib	Votrient	Antineoplastics
pegaspargase	Oncaspar	Antineoplastics
pegfilgrastim	Neulasta	Colony-stimulating factors
peginterferon beta-1a	Plegridy	Immune modifiers
pegloticase	Krystexxa	Antigout agents
pemetrexed	Alimta	Antineoplastics
penciclovir	Denavir (topical)	Antivirals
penicillin G	None listed	Anti-infectives
pentamidine	NebuPent, Pentam 300	Antiprotozoals
pentazocine	Talvin, Talvin NX	Opioid analgesics
perampanel	Fycompa	Anticonvulsants
perindopril	Aceon	Antihypertensives
permethrin	Elimite	Pediculicides
phenazopyridine	Baridium, Pyridium, Pyridium Plus	Nonopioid analgesics
phenobarbital	None listed	Anticonvulsants, sedative-hypnotics
phentermine and topiramate	Qsymia	Weight-control agents

Continued

Generic Name	Trade Names	Classification
phenytoin	Dilantin, Phenytek	Antiarrhythmics, anticonvulsants
phosphate-biphosphate	Fleet Enema, OsmoPrep	Laxatives
phytonadione	Mephyton, vitamin K	Antidotes, vitamins
pimecrolimus	Elidel	Immunosuppressants (topical)
pioglitazone	Actos	Antidiabetics (oral)
piperacillin-tazobactam	Zosyn	Anti-infectives
piroxicam	Feldene	Antirheumatics, nonsteroidal anti-inflammatory agents
polyethylene glycol	GlycoLax, MiraLax	Laxatives
polyethylene glycol-electrolyte	Colyte, GoLYTELY, MoviPrep, NuLYTELY, Suclear, TriLyte	Laxatives
posaconazole	Noxafil	Antifungals
potassium chloride	Klor-Con, Klor-Con M10, Klor-Con M15, Klor-Con M20, K-Tab, Micro-K, Micro-K10	Mineral and electrolyte replacements/supplements
pramipexole	Mirapex, Mirapex ER	Antiparkinsonian agents
pramlintide	SymlinPen 120, SymlinPen 60, Symlin	Antidiabetics
prasugrel	Effient	Antiplatelet agents
pravastatin	Pravachol	Lipid-lowering agents
prazosin	Minipress	Antihypertensives
prednisolone	Orapred, Orapred ODT, Pediapred, Prelone	Antiasthmatics, corticosteroids
prednisone	None listed	Antiasthmatics, corticosteroids
pregabalin	Lyrica	Analgesics, anticonvulsants
procainamide	None listed	Antiarrhythmics (class IA)
procarbazine	Matulane	Antineoplastics
prochlorperazine	Compro	Antiemetics, antipsychotics
progesterone	Crinone, Endometrin, Prochieve, Prometrium	Hormones
promethazine	None listed	Antiemetics, antihistamines, sedative-hypnotics
propafenone	Rythmol, Rythmol SR	Antiarrhythmics (class IC)
propofol	Diprivan	General anesthetics
propranolol	Hemangeol, Inderal, Inderal LA, InnoPran XL	Antianginals, antiarrhythmics (class II), antihypertensives, vascular headache suppressants
propylthiouracil	None listed	Antithyroid agents
protamine sulfate	None listed	Antidotes (heparin)
pseudoephedrine	Silfedrine Children's, Sudafed 12 Hour, Sudafed 24 Hour, Sudafed Children's, SudoGest, SudoGest 12 Hour	Allergy, cold, and cough remedies; nasal drying agents/decongestants
psyllium	Alramucil, Cillium, Effer-Syllium, Fiberall, Fibrepur, Hydrocil, Konsyl, Metamucil, Modane Bulk, Mylanta Natural Fiber Supplement, Naturacil Caramels, Perdiem, Pro-Lax, Reguloid Natural, Serutan, Siblin, Syllact, Vitalax, V-Lax	Laxatives
pyrazinamide	Tebrazid	Antituberculars
pyridostigmine	Mestinon, Mestinon Timespan, Regonol	Antimyasthenics
pyridoxine	Neuro-K-250 TD, Nuero-K-250 Vitamin B_6, Neuro-K50, Neuro-K-500, Pyri 500, vitamin B_6	Vitamins
pyrimethamine	Daraprim	Antimalarials, antiprotozoals
quetiapine	Seroquel, Seroquel XR	Antipsychotics, mood stabilizers
quinapril	Accupril	Antihypertensives
quinine	Qualaquin, QM-260, Quinamm	Antimalarials
rabeprazole	Aciphex, Aciphex Sprinkle	Antiulcer agents
raloxifene	Evista	Bone resorption inhibitors
raltegravir	Isentress	Antiretrovirals
ramelteon	Rozerem	Sedative-hypnotics
ramipril	Altace	Antihypertensives
ranitidine	Zantac, Zantac EFFERdose, Zantac 75, Zantac 150	Antiulcer agents
ranolazine	Ranexa	Antianginals

Generic Name	Trade Names	Classification
rasagiline	Azilect	Antiparkinsonian agents
rasburicase	Elitek	Antigout agents, antihyper-uricemics
repaglinide	Prandin	Antidiabetics
reteplase	Retavase	Thrombolytics
ribavirin	Copegus, Ribasphere, Virazole	Antivirals
rifabutin	Mycobutin	Agents for atypical mycobacterium
rifampin	Rifadin	Antituberculars
rifaximin	Xifaxan	Anti-infectives
rilpivirine	Edurant	antiretrovirals
risedronate	Actonel, Atelvia	Bone resorption inhibitors
risperidone	Risperdal, Risperdal Consta, Risperdal M-TAB	Antipsychotics, mood stabilizers
ritonavir	Norvir	Antiretrovirals
rituximab	Rituxan	Antineoplastics
rivaroxaban	Xarelto	Anticoagulants
rivastigmine	Exelon	Anti-Alzheimer's agents
rizatriptan	Maxalt, Maxalt-MLT	Vascular headache suppressants
rolapitant	Varubi	Antiemetics
ropinirole	Requip, Requip XL	Antiparkinsonian agents
rosiglitazone	Avandia	Antidiabetics
sacubitril and valsartan	Entresto	Vasodilators, antihypertensives
salmeterol	Serevent Diskus	Bronchodilators
sargramostim	Leukine, rHu GM-CSF (recombinant human granulocyte-macrophage colony-stimulating factor)	Colony-stimulating factors
saxagliptin	Onglyza	Antidiabetics
scopolamine	Transderm-Scōp	Antiemetics
selegiline	Eldepryl, Zelapar	Antiparkinsonian agents
selegiline transdermal	Emsam	Antidepressants
sennosides	Black-Draught, Ex-Lax, Ex-Lax Chocolated, Fletchers' Castoria, Maximum Relief Ex-Lax, Sena-Gen, Senexon, Senokot, SenokotXTRA	Laxatives
sertaconazole	Ertaczo	Antifungals
sertraline	Zoloft	Antidepressants
sevelamer	Renagel, Renvela	Electrolyte modifiers
sildenafil	Revatio, Viagra	Erectile dysfunction agents
silodosin	Rapaflo	Benign prostatic hyperplasia (BPH) agents
simeprevir	Olysio	Antivirals
simethicone	Degas, Extra Strength Gas-X, Flatulex, Gas-X, Genasyme, Maximum Strength Mylanta Gas, Mylanta Gas, Mylicon, Phazyme	Antiflatulents
simvastatin	Zocor	Lipid-lowering agents
sirolimus	Rapamune	Immunosuppressants
sitagliptin	Januvia	Antidiabetics
sodium bicarbonate	Baking soda, Bell-Ans, Citrocarbonate, Neut, Soda Mint	Antiulcer agents
sodium citrate and citric acid	Bicitra, Oracit, Shohl's Solution modified	Antiurolithics, mineral and electrolyte replacements/supplements
sodium polystyrene sulfonate	Kalexate, Kayexalate, Kionex, SPS	Hypokalemics, electrolyte modifiers
solifenacin	Vesicare	Urinary tract antispasmodics
sotalol	Betapace, Betapace AF, Sorine, Sotylize	Antiarrhythmics (class III)
spironolactone	Aldactone	Diuretics
stavudine	Zerit, Zerit XR	Antiretrovirals
streptokinase	Streptase	Thrombolytics

Continued

Generic Name	Trade Names	Classification
streptomycin	None listed	Anti-infectives
sucralfate	Carafate	Antiulcer agents
sulfasalazine	Azulfidine, Azulfidine EN-tabs	Antirheumatics (DMARDs), gastrointestinal anti-inflammatories
sulindac	Clinoril	Antirheumatics, nonsteroidal anti-inflammatory agents
sumatriptan	Alsuma, Imitrex, Imitrex STATdose, Sumavel DosePro, Zecuity	Vascular headache suppressants
sunitinib	Sutent	Antineoplastics
suvorexant	Belsomra	Sedative/hypnotics
tacrolimus	Astragraf XL, Envarsus XR, Prograf	Immunosuppressants
tadalafil	Adcirca, Cialis	Erectile dysfunction agents, vasodilators
tamoxifen	None listed	Antineoplastics
tamsulosin	Flomax	None assigned
tapentadol	Nucynta, Nucynta ER	Analgesic (centrally acting), opioid analgesics
tedizolid	Sivextro	Anti-infectives
telavancin	Vibativ	Anti-infectives
telmisartan	Micardis	Antihypertensives
temazepam	Restoril	Sedative-hypnotics
tenecteplase	TNKase	Thrombolytics
tenofovir	Viread	Antiretrovirals
terazosin	None listed	Antihypertensives
terbinafine	Lamisil	Antifungals (systemic)
terbutaline	None listed	Bronchodilators
teriflunomide	Aubagio	Anti–multiple sclerosis agents
teriparatide	Forteo	Hormones
tetracycline	None listed	Anti-infectives
thalidomide	Thalomid	Immunosuppressants
theophylline	Quibron-T, Slo-Bid Byrocaps, Theobid, Theochron, Theo-24, Uniphyl	Bronchodilators
thiamine	vitamin B_1	Vitamins
thioridazine	Mellaril, Mellaril-S	Antipsychotics
thyroid, desiccated	Armour thyroid, Nature-Throid, NP Thyroid, Westhroid, WP Thyroid	Hormones
tiagabine	Gabitril	Anticonvulsants
ticagrelor	Brillinta	Antiplatelet agents
tigecycline	Tygacil	Anti-infectives
timolol	Blocadren	Antihypertensives, vascular headache suppressants
tinidazole	Fasigyn, Tindamax	Antiprotozoals
tiotropium	Spiriva Handihaler, Spiriva Respimat	Bronchodilators
tirofiban	Aggrastat	Antiplatelet agents
tizanidine	Zanaflex	Antispasticity agents (centrally acting)
tocilizumab	Actemra	Antirheumatics, immunosuppressants
tofacitinib	Xelijanz	Antirheumatics
tolcapone	Tasmar	Antiparkinsonian agents
tolterodine	Detrol, Detrol LA	Urinary tract antispasmodics
tolvaptan	Samsca	Electrolyte modifiers
topiramate	Qudexy XR, Topamax, Topamax Sprinkle, Trokendi XR	Anticonvulsants, mood stabilizers
topotecan	Hycamtin	Antineoplastics
torsemide	Demadex	Antihypertensives
tramadol	ConZip, Ultram, Ultram ER	Analgesics (centrally acting)

Generic Name	Trade Names	Classification
trandolapril	Mavik	Antihypertensives
tranylcypromine	Parnate	Antidepressants
trastuzumab	Herceptin	Antineoplastics
trazodone	None listed	Antidepressants
triazolam	Halcion	Sedative-hypnotics
trimethoprim-sulfamethoxazole	Bactrim, Bactrim DS, Septra, Septra DS, Sulfatrim, TMP/SMX, TMP/SMZ	Anti-infectives, antiprotozoals
trospium	Sanctura, Sanctura XR	Urinary tract antispasmodics
umeclidinium	Incruse Ellipta	Bronchodilators
valacyclovir	Valtrex	Antivirals
valganciclovir	Valcyte	Antivirals
valproate sodium	Depacon	Anticonvulsants, vascular headache suppressants
valproic acid	Depakene	Anticonvulsants, vascular headache suppressants
valsartan	Diovan	Antihypertensives
vancomycin	Vancocin	Anti-infectives
vardenafil	Staxyn, Levitra	Erectile dysfunction agents
varenicline	Chantix	Smoking deterrents
vasopressin	Vasotrict	Hormones
vedolizumab	Entyvio	Gastrointestinal anti-inflammatories
venlafaxine	Effexor XR	Antidepressants, antianxiety agents
verapamil	Calan, Calan SR, Covera-HS, Isoptin SR, Verelan, Verelan PM	Antianginals, antiarrhythmics (class IV), antihypertensives, vascular headache suppressants
vigabatrin	Sabril	Anticonvulsants
vilazodone	Viibryd	Antidepressants
vinblastine	None listed	Antineoplastics
vincristine	None listed	Antineoplastics
vinorelbine	Navelbine	Antineoplastics
vorapaxar	Zontivity	Antiplatelet agents
voriconazole	Vfend	Antifungals
warfarin	Coumadin, Jantoven	Anticoagulants
zafirlukast	Accolate	Antiasthmatics, bronchodilators
zaleplon	Sonata	Sedative-hypnotics
zanamivir	Relenza	Antivirals
ziconotide	Prialt	Analgesics
zidovudine	AZT, Retrovir	Antiretrovirals
zinc sulfate	Orazinc, Verazinc, Zinc 220, Zincate, Zinkaps	Mineral and electrolyte replacements/supplements
ziprasidone	Geodon	Antipsychotics, mood stabilizers
zoledronic acid	Reclast, Zometa	Bone resorption inhibitors, electrolyte modifiers, hypocalcemics
zolmitriptan	Zomig, Zomig-ZMT	Vascular headache suppressants
zolpidem	Ambien, Ambien CR, Edluar, Intermezzo, Zolpimist	Sedative-hypnotics
zonisamide	Zonegran	Anticonvulsants

DMARD, disease-modifying antirheumatic drug.

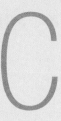

Controlled Substances Schedules

Classes or schedules are determined by the U.S. Drug Enforcement Administration (DEA), an arm of the U.S. Department of Justice, and are based on the potential for abuse and dependence liability (physical and psychological) of the medication. Some states have stricter prescription regulations. Physicians, dentists, podiatrists, and veterinarians may prescribe controlled substances. Nurse practitioners and physician assistants may prescribe controlled substances with certain limitations.

■ SCHEDULE I (C-I)

The potential for abuse is so high as to be unacceptable. These substances may be used for research with appropriate limitations, but otherwise have no acceptable medical use.

The following are examples of Schedule I drugs:

- Heroin
- Lysergic acid diethylamide (LSD)
- Marijuana (cannabis)
- Methaqualone 3,4-methylenedioxymethamphetamine (ecstasy)
- Peyote

■ SCHEDULE II (C-II)

These substances have high potential for abuse and extreme potential for physical and psychological dependence (amphetamines, opioid analgesics, dronabinol, certain barbiturates). Outpatient prescriptions must be in writing. In emergencies, telephone orders may be acceptable if a written prescription is provided within 72 hours. No refills are allowed.

The following are examples of Schedule II drugs:

- Adderall
- Cocaine
- Combination products with less than 15 mg of hydrocodone per dosage unit (Vicodin)
- Dexedrine
- Fentanyl
- Hydromorphone (Dilaudid)
- Meperidine (Demerol)
- Methamphetamine
- Methadone
- Methylphenidate (Ritalin)
- Oxycodone (OxyContin)

■ SCHEDULE III (C-III)

These substances have intermediate potential for abuse (less than C-II) and intermediate liability for physical and psychological dependence (certain nonbarbiturate sedatives, certain nonamphetamine central nervous system stimulants, limited dosages of certain opioid analgesics). Outpatient prescriptions can be refilled five times within 6 months from the date of issue if authorized by the prescriber. Telephone orders are acceptable.

The following are examples of Schedule III drugs:

- Anabolic steroids
- Codeine (less than 90 mg in combination with nonopioid analgesics: solid oral dosage forms such as Tylenol with codeine)
- Ketamine
- Testosterone

■ SCHEDULE IV (C-IV)

These substances have less potential for abuse than Schedule III drugs, with minimal liability for physical or psychological dependence (certain sedative-hypnotics, certain antianxiety agents, some barbiturates, benzodiazepines, chloral hydrate, pentazocaine, propoxyphen). Outpatient prescriptions can be refilled six times within 6 months from the date of issue if authorized by the prescriber. Telephone orders are acceptable.

The following are examples of Schedule IV drugs:

- Alprazolam (Xanax)
- Aspirin and carisoprodol (Soma)
- Darvocet
- Darvon
- Diazepam (Valium)
- Lorazepam (Ativan)
- Petazocine (Talwin)
- Tramadol
- Zolpidem (Ambien)

■ SCHEDULE V (C-V)

These substances have minimal potential for abuse. The number of outpatient refills is determined by the prescriber. Some products (cough suppressants with less than 200 mg of codeine per 100 mL, antidiarrheals containing paregoric) may be available without a prescription to patients older than 18 years of age.

The following are examples of Schedule IV drugs:

- Atropine and diphenoxylate (Lomotil)
- Pregabalin (Lyrica)
- Difenoxin and atropine (Motofen)
- Parepectolin
- Robitussin AC

Source: U.S. Drug Enforcement Administration: Drug Schedules. Available at https://www.dea.gov/druginfo/ds.shtml. Accessed November 23, 2017.

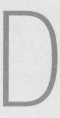
Routine Pediatric and Adult Immunizations

Immunization recommendations change frequently: For the latest recommendations, visit www.cdc.gov.

Routine Pediatric Immunizations (0–18 Years)

Generic Name (Brand Names)	Route and Dosage	Contraindications and Precautions	Adverse Reactions and Side Effects	Notes
Hepatitis B vaccine (HepB, Engerix-B, Recombivax HB)	0.5 mL IM at 0, 1–2, and 6–18 mo; dose is same for patients age 0–19 yr. *Infants born to HBsAg-positive mothers:* Administer 0.5 mL hepatitis B immune globulin IM and first dose of hepatitis B vaccine; give second and third doses of hepatitis B vaccine at 1 mo and 6 mo, respectively.	Serious allergic reaction to this vaccine or any of its components, hypersensitivity to yeast	Local soreness	A two-dose series (separated by ≥4 mo) of the adult formulation. (Recombivax HB) can be used in children 11–15 yr.
Rotavirus vaccine (RV, Rotarix [RV1], RotaTeq [RV5])	*Rotarix:* 1 mL PO at 2 and 4 mo. *RotaTeq:* 2 mL PO at 2, 4, and 6 mo; first dose of either product may be given as early as age 6 wk; final dose should be given no later than age 8 mo.	Serious allergic reaction to this vaccine or any of its components. History of uncorrected congenital malformation of the GI tract (Rotarix); intussusception; severe immunodeficiency	Fever, irritability, diarrhea, vomiting	Series should not be started in infants >15 wk. Complete series with same product if possible.
Diphtheria toxoid, tetanus toxoid, and acellular pertussis vaccine (DTaP, Daptacel, Infanrix)	0.5 mL IM at 2, 4, 6, 15–18 mo, and 4–6 yr (first dose may be given as early as age 6 wk; fourth dose	Serious allergic reaction to this vaccine or any of its components, encephalopathy	Crying, decreased appetite, fever, irritability, malaise, redness or tenderness at site, vomiting	Individual components may be given as separate injections if unusual reactions occur. Do not give *Continued*

Routine Pediatric Immunizations (0–18 Years)—cont'd

Generic Name (Brand Names)	Route and Dosage	Contraindications and Precautions	Adverse Reactions and Side Effects	Notes
	may be given at age 12 mo).	within 7 days of previous dose.		to children >7 yr. Complete series with same product if possible.
Haemophilus b conjugate vaccine (Hib, PedvaxHIB, ActHIB, Hiberix)	*ActHIB:* 0.5 mL IM at 2, 4, and 6 mo, with a booster dose at 12–15 mo. *PedvaxHIB:* 0.5 mL IM at 2 and 4 mo with a booster dose at 12–15 mo (first dose as early as age 6 wk). *Hiberix:* can be used only for the booster dose (any of the products can be used for the booster dose).	Serious allergic reaction to this vaccine or any of its components.	Anorexia, crying, diarrhea, fever, irritability, malaise, tenderness, vomiting, weakness	If different brands are used for first and second dose, administer third dose followed by booster after 12 mo.
Pneumococcal conjugate vaccine (13-valent) (PCV13, Prevnar13)	0.5 mL IM at 2, 4, 6, and 12–15 mo (first dose as early as age 6 wk)	Serious allergic reaction to this vaccine or any of its components.	Arthralgia, chills, anorexia, fatigue, fever, headache, insomnia, irritability, myalgia, pain at injection site, rash	One dose may also be given to previously unvaccinated healthy children age 24–59 mo and for high-risk children (e.g., sickle cell disease; anatomic or functional asplenia; chronic cardiac, pulmonary, or renal disease; diabetes; HIV; immunosuppression; cochlear implant) age 24–71 mo; give two doses (≥8 wk apart, with first dose given >8 wk after most recent dose).
Polio vaccine, inactivated (IPV, IPOL)	0.5 mL IM or SC at 2, 4, and 6–18 mo and at 4–6 yr (first dose may be given as early as age 6 wk)	Serious allergic reaction to this vaccine or any of its components including neomycin, streptomycin, or polymyxin B.	Anorexia, fatigue, irritability, pain at injection site; fever	Oral polio vaccine (OPV) no longer recommended for use in the United States.
Influenza vaccine *injection (inactivated):* (Afluria, Fluarix, FluLaval, Fluvirin,	Injection: *age 6–35 mo:* two doses of 0.25 mL IM given 4 wk apart for first	Hypersensitivity to eggs or egg products; hypersensitivity to thimerosal	*Injection:* local soreness, fever, myalgia, possible neurological toxicity	Immunosuppression may decrease antibody response to injection and

Routine Pediatric Immunizations (0–18 Years)—cont'd

Generic Name (Brand Names)	Route and Dosage	Contraindications and Precautions	Adverse Reactions and Side Effects	Notes
Fluzone); *intranasal (live attenuated):* (FluMist)	season, then one dose annually; *age 3–8 yr:* two doses of 0.5 mL IM given 4 wk apart for first season, then one dose annually; *age ≥9 yr:* 0.5 mL IM single dose annually. Intranasal: *age 2–8 yr:* if not previously vaccinated with influenza vaccine, two doses of 0.2 mL (given as 0.1 mL in each nostril) 4 wk apart, then one dose annually; if previously vaccinated with influenza vaccine, one dose of 0.2 mL (given as 0.1 mL in each nostril) annually; *age ≥9 yr:* one dose of 0.2 mL (given as 0.1 mL in each nostril) annually.	(injection only); avoid use in patients with acute neurological compromise. Fluvirin should only be used in children ≥4 yr. Fluarix should only be used in children ≥3 yr. Serious allergic reaction to this vaccine or any of its components, including eggs and egg products (injection). Avoid in patients with acute neurologic compromise. *FluMist* should be avoided in children <2 yr; pregnancy; chronic pulmonary conditions (including asthma); cardiovascular disorders (not hypertension); renal, hepatic, neurological, hematological, or metabolic (including diabetes) disorders; immunosuppression (including HIV); chronic salicylate therapy (children 6 mo–18 yr); children <5 yr with wheezing in past year; anyone who has taken influenza antiviral medication in previous 48 hr.	*Intranasal:* upper respiratory congestion, malaise	increase risk for viral transmission with intranasal route.
Measles, mumps, and rubella vaccines (MMR, M-M-R II)	0.5 mL SC at 12–15 mo and at 4–6 yr	Serious allergic reaction to this vaccine or any of its components (including eggs, gelatin, or neomycin); active infection; severe immunosuppression (in the absence of	Pain at injection site; arthralgia; fever; encephalitis	If unusual reactions occur, individual components may be given as separate injections; immunosuppression may decrease antibody response to injection and increase *Continued*

Routine Pediatric Immunizations (0–18 Years)—cont'd

Generic Name (Brand Names)	Route and Dosage	Contraindications and Precautions	Adverse Reactions and Side Effects	Notes
		severe immunosuppression, HIV is not a contraindication); pregnancy		risk for viral transmission.
Varicella vaccine (Var, Varivax)	0.5 mL SC at 12–15 mo and at 4–6 yr (second dose may be given earlier if ≥3 mo have elapsed since the first dose); for patients 7–18 yr who have not been vaccinated or without a history of chickenpox, two doses should be given (≥3 mo apart if 7–12 yr or ≥4 wk apart if ≥13 yr).	Serious allergic reaction to this vaccine or any of its components (including gelatin or neomycin); active infection; severe immunosuppression (in the absence of severe immunosuppression, HIV is not a contraindication); pregnancy.	Local soreness, fever, anorexia, chills, diarrhea, fatigue, headache, irritability, nausea, vomiting	Immunosuppression may decrease antibody response to injection and increase risk for viral transmission.
Hepatitis A vaccine (HepA, Havrix, Vaqta)	Should be given to all children age 12–23 mo; give a total of two doses of pediatric formulation (each 0.5 mL) IM at least 6 mo apart.	Serious allergic reaction to this vaccine or any of its components.	Local reactions, headache, anorexia, drowsiness, fever, irritability, weakness	Also recommended in children ≥2 yr who live in areas with high rates of hepatitis A or in other high-risk groups (e.g., chronic liver disease, clotting factor disorders, illicit drug users, close personal contact within first 60 days of arrival of international adoptee from country where hepatitis A is endemic).
Meningococcal conjugate vaccine (MCV4, Menactra, Menveo)	0.5 mL IM single dose at 11–12 yr with a booster at age 16 yr or 13–15 yr with a booster at 16–18 yr at least 8 wk between doses. If first dose given after 16 yr, no booster needed. Single dose should be given to all unvaccinated college freshman (18–21 yr) living in dormitories.	Serious allergic reaction to this vaccine or any of its components.	Fatigue, malaise, anorexia, arthralgia, diarrhea, fever, headache, myalgia, nausea, irritability, pain at injection site, vomiting	Routine vaccination with meningococcal vaccine also recommended for children ≥2 yr who are at high risk (anatomic or functional asplenia, persistent complement component deficiency, travel or residence in areas in which meningococcal disease is hyperendemic or epidemic).

Routine Pediatric Immunizations (0–18 Years)—cont'd

Generic Name (Brand Names)	Route and Dosage	Contraindications and Precautions	Adverse Reactions and Side Effects	Notes
Human papillomavirus vaccine (HPV2, Cervarix)	11–26 yr (may give as early as age 9 yr) females, 0.5 mL IM, repeat at 2 and 6 mo after first dose.	Serious allergic reaction to this vaccine or any of its components (including yeast).	Arthralgia, fatigue, itching, local soreness	Used to prevent cervical cancer caused by HPV types 16 and 18 in females. Complete series with same product if possible.
Human papillomavirus vaccine quadrivalent (HPV4, Gardasil)	0.5 mL IM in males and females age 11–26 yr (first dose may be given as early as age 9 yr); repeat at 1–2 mo, and 6 mo after first dose.	Serious allergic reaction to this vaccine or any of its components (including yeast).	Diarrhea, dizziness, fever, headache, nausea, pain at injection site, syncope	Used to prevent cervical, vulvar, and vaginal cancer caused by HPV types 16 and 18 in females and to prevent genital warts caused by HPV types 6 and 11 and anal cancer caused by HPV types 16 ad 18 in males and females. Complete series with same product if possible.
Human papillomavirus vaccine 9-valent (HPV9, Gardasil 9)	0.5 mL in males and females age 11–26 yr (first dose as early as age 9 yr); repeat at 1–2 mo and 6 mo after first dose.	Serious allergic reaction to this vaccine or any of its components (including yeast).	Dizziness, fever, headache, pain at injection site, syncope	Used to prevent cervical, vulvar, and vaginal cancer caused by HPV types 16, 18, 31, 33, 45, 52, and 58 in females and to prevent genital warts caused by HPV types 6 and 11 and anal cancer caused by HPV types 16, 18, 31, 33, 45, 52, and 58 in males and females. Complete series with same product if possible.

■ NURSING IMPLICATIONS

Assessment
Assess the previous immunization history and history of hypersensitivity.

Assess the patient for a history of asthma or reactive airway disease. Patients with a positive history should not receive FluMist.

Assess for a history of latex allergy. Some prefilled syringes may use latex components and should be avoided in patients with hypersensitivity.

Potential Nursing Diagnoses
Infection, risk for (indications)

Knowledge, deficient, related to medication regimen (patient/family teaching)

Implementation

The following may be given concomitantly: measles, mumps, and rubella (MMR) vaccine; trivalent oral poliovirus vaccine; and diphtheria toxoid, tetanus toxoid, and pertussis vaccine. Live attenuated flu vaccine (LAIV, Nasal Spray) may be given at the same time as other vaccines. Administering vaccines at the same time may increase the risk for seizures resulting from fever, so risks must be evaluated.

Do not administer FluMist concurrently with other vaccines or in patients who have received a live virus vaccine within 1 month or an inactivated vaccine within 2 weeks of vaccination.

Administer each immunization by the appropriate route:

- Oral: Rotavirus vaccine

- Subcutaneous: MMR; Varicella vaccine, IPV

- Intramuscular: Hepatitis B, Diphtheria toxoid; tetanus toxoid, and acellular pertussis; *Haemophilus* b; Pneumococcal; IPV; Influenza vaccine; Hepatitis A; Meningococcal and Human papillomavirus

- Intranasal: FluMist, LAIV

- Intradermal: Fluzone

Patient and Family Teaching

Inform the parent of potential and reportable side effects of the immunization, and provide the appropriate Vaccine Information Statement (VIS) for him or her to read prior to administration of the vaccine. The physician should be notified if the patient develops the following: a fever higher than 39.4°C (103°F); difficulty breathing; hives; itching; swelling of the eyes, face, or inside of the nose; sudden, severe tiredness or weakness; convulsions.

Review the next scheduled immunization with the parent.

Evaluation

Effectiveness of therapy can be demonstrated by prevention of diseases through active immunity.

Routine Adult Immunizations

Generic Name (Brand Names)	Indications	Dosage and Route	Contraindications	Adverse Reactions and Side Effects
Tetanus toxoid, reduced diphtheria toxoid and acellular pertussis vaccine absorbed (Tdap, Adacell, Boostrix)	Single dose should be given instead of Td in adults (19–64 yr) if they received their last dose of Td ≥10 yr ago (and did not previously receive a dose of Tdap). Single dose should also be given to all pregnant women (preferred during 27–36 weeks gestation), close contacts of infants <12 mo, and health-care workers with direct patient contact	0.5 mL IM	Serious allergic reactions to this vaccine or any of its components, encephalopathy within 7 days of previous dose.	Abdominal pain, arthralgia, chills, diarrhea, fatigue, headache, myalgia, nausea, pain at injection site, vomiting

Routine Adult Immunizations—cont'd

Generic Name (Brand Names)	Indications	Dosage and Route	Contraindications	Adverse Reactions and Side Effects
Tetanus-diphtheria (Td, Tenivac)	All adults who lack written documentation of a primary series of tetanus- and diphtheria-toxoid–containing vaccine; booster dose should be given to all adults every 10 yr (see foregoing information on use of Tdap to replace one dose of Td in booster series).	Unimmunized: two doses 0.5 mL IM ≥4 wk apart, then a third dose 6–12 mo later. Immunized: 0.5 mL IM booster every 10 yr.	Severe allergic reaction to this vaccine or any of its components.	Arthralgia, chills, diarrhea, fatigue, headache, myalgia, nausea, local pain and swelling
Human papillomavirus vaccine (HPV2, Cervarix)	All previously unvaccinated women through age 26 yr; Not indicated for males.	0.5 mL IM, repeat at 2 and 6 mo after first dose.	Serious allergic reaction to this vaccine or any of its components, pregnancy.	Arthralgia, fatigue, myalgia, local soreness
Human papillomavirus vaccine, quadrivalent (HPV4m Gardasil)	All previously unvaccinated females and males through age 26 yr.	0.5 mL IM, repeat at 2 and 6 mo after first dose.	Serious allergic reaction to this vaccine or any of its components, pregnancy.	Dizziness, fever, headache, injection site reactions, syncope
Varicella vaccine (Var, Varivax)	Any adult without a history of chickenpox or herpes zoster (shingles), a history of receiving 2 doses of varicella vaccine, or laboratory evidence of immunity. Health-care workers and pregnant women born in the United States before 1980 who do not meet the above criteria should be tested for immunity.	0.5 mL SC; repeat 4–8 wk after first dose.	Previous serious allergic reaction to this vaccine or any of its components (including gelatin or neomycin), active infection, severe immunosuppression (in the absence of severe immunosuppression, HIV is not a contraindication), pregnancy (also avoid becoming pregnant for 4 wk after immunization).	Local soreness, fever. Immunosuppression may decrease antibody response to injection and increase risk for viral transmission.
Zoster vaccine (Zos, Zostavax)	All adults ≥60 yr (regardless of previous history of chickenpox or herpes zoster).	0.65-mL SC, single dose.	Allergy to gelatin or neomycin, active infection, immunosuppression (in the absence of severe immunosuppression, HIV is not a contraindication), pregnancy.	Local soreness, fever. Immunosuppression may decrease antibody response to injection and increase risk for viral transmission.

Continued

Routine Adult Immunizations—cont'd

Generic Name (Brand Names)	Indications	Dosage and Route	Contraindications	Adverse Reactions and Side Effects
Measles, mumps, and rubella vaccine (MMR, M-M-RII)	Adults born in 1957 or later with unreliable documentation of previous vaccination (unless have laboratory evidence of immunity to all three diseases); health-care workers born before 1957 who do not have laboratory evidence of immunity to all measles, mumps, and/or rubella.	0.5 mL SC, one or two doses in adults born in 1957 or later with unreliable history; high-risk groups should receive a total of two doses given 1 mo apart.	Serious allergic reaction to this vaccine or any of its components (including eggs, gelatin, or neomycin); active infection; severe immunosuppression (in the absence of severe immunosuppression, HIV is not a contraindication); pregnancy (also avoid becoming pregnant for 4 wk after immunization).	Burning, stinging pain at injection site; arthritis or arthralgia; fever; encephalitis; allergic reactions; immunosuppression may decrease antibody response to injection and increase risk for viral transmission.
Influenza vaccine *injection (inactivated):* (Afluria, Fluarix, Flublok, Flucelvax, FluLaval, Fluvirin, Fluzone;) *intranasal (live attenuated):* (FluMist)	All adults	Injection: 0.5 mL IM annually. Intranasal (for adults <50 yr): single dose of 0.2 mL (given as 0.1 mL in each nostril) annually.	Previous serious allergic reaction to this vaccine or any of its components including eggs or egg products and thimerosal (injection only); avoid use in patients with acute neurological compromise. FluMist should be avoided in pregnancy; chronic pulmonary conditions (including asthma), cardiovascular (not hypertension), renal, hepatic, neurological, hematological, or metabolic (including diabetes) disorders. Immunosuppression (including HIV); age ≥50 yr.	Injection: local soreness, fever, myalgia; intranasal: abdominal pain, cough, anorexia, headache, irritability, lethargy, nasal congestion, myalgia, rhinorrhea, sore throat; immunosuppression may decrease antibody response to injection and increase risk for viral transmission.
Pneumococcal polysaccharide vaccine (PPSV23, Pneumovax 23)	All adults ≥65 yr; high-risk patients <65 yr (e.g., chronic cardiac or pulmonary disease [including COPD and asthma], chronic liver disease, alcoholism, diabetes, cigarette smoking, anatomic or functional asplenia,	0.5 mL IM or SC; one-time revaccination should also be given ≥5 yr after first dose to those ≥65 yr (if first dose was given before age 65) and to high-risk patients.	Serious allergic reaction to this vaccine or any of its components.	Chills, fever, injection site reactions.

Routine Adult Immunizations—cont'd

Generic Name (Brand Names)	Indications	Dosage and Route	Contraindications	Adverse Reactions and Side Effects
	sickle cell disease, immunosuppression [including HIV], chronic renal failure, cochlear implants, cerebrospinal fluid leaks, residents of long-term care facilities)			
Hepatitis A vaccine (HepA, Havrix, Vaqta)	High-risk groups (e.g., chronic liver disease, clotting factor disorders, illicit drug use, men who have sex with men, working with infected primates or with hepatitis A virus in research laboratory setting), travel to endemic areas, unvaccinated individuals who anticipate close personal contact within first 60 days of arrival of international adoptee from country where hepatitis A is endemic, from a country with intermediate or high endemicity.	1 mL IM, followed by 1 mL IM 6–12 mo (for Havrix) or 6–18 mo later (Vaqta).	Serious allergic reaction to this vaccine or any of its components.	Anorexia, drowsiness, fever, local reactions, headache, irritability.
Hepatitis B vaccine (HepB, Engerix-B, Recombivax HB)	High-risk patients (e.g., household contacts or sex partners of HBsAg-positive persons, IV drug users, sexually active persons not in a monogamous relationship, men who have sex with men, HIV, STDs, hemodialysis, health-care workers, inmates), chronic liver disease, all unvaccinated adolescents	Immunocompetent: 1 mL IM, given at 0, 1, and 6 mo. Immunosuppressed: 1 mL (Recombivax HB) or 2 mL (Engerix-B) IM at 0, 1, and 6 mo. Three doses of 1 mL IM at 0, 1–2, and 4–6 mo.	Serious allergic reaction to this vaccine or any of its components.	Local soreness.

Continued

Routine Adult Immunizations—cont'd

Generic Name (Brand Names)	Indications	Dosage and Route	Contraindications	Adverse Reactions and Side Effects
Meningococcal conjugate vaccine (Menactra [MCV4 or MenACWY-D], Menveo [MenACWY-CRM], *Polysaccaride,* menomune-A/C/Y/W-135 [MPSY4])	College freshmen (up to age 21) living in dormitories who have not previously received a dose on or after their 16th birthday; military recruits, anatomic or functional asplenia, persistent complement component deficiency, travel or residence in areas in which meningococcal disease is hyperendemic or epidemic; persons at risk during an outbreak due to a vaccine serogroup	Age ≤55 yr: 0.5-mL IM single dose; age ≤55 yr with anatomic or functional asplenia, persistent complement component deficiency, or HIV: 0.5 mL IM; repeat at least 2 mo after first dose. Revaccination with MenACWY every 5 yr as indicated in patients previously vaccinated with MenACWY OR MPSV4 and who also remain at increased risk for infection. MenACWY is preferred for adults ≥56 yr who previously received MenACWY and must be revaccinated or for whom multiple doses are needed; MPSV4 is preferred for adults ≥56 yr who have not previously received MenACWY and who only require a single dose.	Serious allergic reaction to this vaccine or any of its components.	Arthralgia, diarrhea, fever, headache, myalgia, nausea, irritability, vomiting, fatigue, malaise, anorexia, pain at injection site.

Source: Adapted from the recommendations of the National Immunization Program. Available at http://www.cdc.gov. *Davis's Drug Guide for Nurses,* ed 15. Philadelphia: FA Davis; 2017.

Administering Medications to Children

GENERAL GUIDELINES

Medication administration to a pediatric patient can be challenging. Prescribers should order dosage forms that are age appropriate for their patients, but they do not always specify beyond the route desired. If a child is unable to take a particular dosage form, ask the pharmacist whether another form is available. If no other form is available, you may need to crush a tablet and mix it with a small amount of food. Always verify that the ordered medication can be crushed.

ORAL LIQUIDS

Pediatric liquid medicines may be given with plastic medicine cups, oral syringes, oral droppers, or cylindrical dosing spoons. Parents should be taught to use these calibrated devices, rather than household utensils, because household teaspoons, tablespoons, and cups have a variety of sizes. For young children, it is best to use an oral syringe to squirt a small amount of the dose at a time into the side of the cheek, away from the bitter taste buds at the back of the tongue. This approach also prevents choking and aspiration because you are not squirting the liquid directly toward the back of the throat.

EYE DROPS AND OINTMENTS

Tilt the child's head back, gently press the skin under the lower eyelid, and pull the lower lid away slightly until a small pouch is visible. Insert the ointment or drop (one drop at a time), and close the eye for a few minutes to keep the medicine in place.

EAR DROPS

Shake the otic suspensions well before administration. For children younger than 3 years of age, pull the outer ear outward and downward before you instill the drops. For children 3 years of age and older, pull the outer ear outward and upward. Keep the child on his or her side (affected side up) for 2 minutes, and place a cotton plug in the ear.

NOSE DROPS

First, clear the child's nose of secretions with a nasal aspirator (bulb syringe), or a cotton swab may be used in infants and young children. Ask older children to blow their nose. Then tilt the child's head back over a pillow, and squeeze the dropper without touching the nostril. Keep the child's head back for 2 minutes.

SUPPOSITORIES

Keep suppositories refrigerated for easier administration. While wearing gloves, moisten the rounded end of the suppository with water or petroleum jelly before insertion. Using your pinky finger for children younger than 3 years of age and your index finger for those 3 years of age and older, insert the suppository into the rectum about 1/2 to 1 inch beyond the sphincter. If the suppository slides out, insert it a little farther than before. Hold the child's buttocks together for a few minutes, and have the child hold the position for about 20 minutes, if possible.

TOPICALS

Clean the affected area and dry it well before topical application. Apply a thin layer of medication to the skin, and rub it in gently. Children absorb medication more rapidly through their skin than do adults, so it is important to keep the layer thin unless otherwise ordered. Do not apply a covering over the area unless instructed to do so by the prescriber.

METERED-DOSE INHALERS

Generally, the same principles apply to children as to adults, except the use of spacers is recommended for young children.

Pediatric Dosage Calculations

Most drugs in children are dosed according to body weight (mg/kg) or body surface area (BSA) (mg/m^2). The health-care professional's role is obtaining extremely accurate height and weight measurements of the patient. Care must be taken to convert body weight from pounds to kilograms (1 kg = 2.2 lb) before calculating doses based on body weight. Doses are often expressed as mg/kg/*day* or mg/kg/*dose*; therefore, orders written "mg/kg/d" are confusing and require clarification from the prescriber.

The calculations are done by the physician and pharmacist. It is a good idea to understand how these calculations are done, to assist in recognizing errors in calculations. Medications are available in multiple concentrations; therefore, orders written in "mL" rather than "mg" are not acceptable and require clarification.

Dosing also varies by indication; therefore, diagnostic information is helpful when calculating doses. The following examples are typically encountered when dosing medication in children.

■ EXAMPLE 1

Calculate the dose of amoxicillin suspension in milliliters for otitis media for a 1-year-old child who weighs 22 lb. The dose required is 40 mg/kg/day divided twice daily (bid), and the suspension comes in a 400 mg/5 mL concentration.

Step 1: Convert pounds to kilograms:	22 lb × 1 kg/2.2 lb = 10 kg
Step 2: Calculate the dose in milligrams:	40 mg × 10 kg = 400 mg/day
Step 3: Divide the dose by the frequency:	400 mg/day ÷ 2 (bid) = 200 mg/dose bid
Step 4: Convert the milligrams dose to milliliters:	200 mg/dose ÷ 400 mg/5 mL = 2.5 mL bid

■ EXAMPLE 2

Calculate the dose of ceftriaxone in milliliters for meningitis for a 5-year-old child who weighs 20 kg. The dose required is 100 mg/kg/day given IV once daily, and the drug comes prediluted in a 500 mg/mL concentration.

Step 1: Calculate the dose in milligrams:	100 mg × 20 kg = 2,000 mg/day
Step 2: Divide the dose by the frequency:	2,000 mg/day ÷ 1 (daily) = 2,000 mg/dose
Step 3: Convert the milligram dose to milliliters:	2,000 mg/dose ÷ 500 mg/mL = 4 mL once daily

Because chemotherapy drugs are caustic, they are commonly dosed according to the BSA, which requires an extra step to verify the calculations before dosing.

■ EXAMPLE 3

Calculate the dose of vincristine in milliliters for leukemia for a 4-year-old child who weighs 37 lb and is 97 cm tall. The dose required is 2 mg/m², and the drug comes in a 1 mg/mL concentration.

Step 1: Convert pounds to kilograms:	37 lb × 1 kg/2.2 lb = 16.8 kg
Step 2: Calculate the BSA:	$\sqrt{[16.8 \text{ kg} \times 97 \text{ cm}]/3{,}600} = 0.67 \text{ m}^2$
Step 3: Calculate the dose in milligrams:	2 mg × 0.67 m² = 1.34 mg
Step 4: Calculate the dose in milliliters:	1.34 mg ÷ 1 mg/mL = 1.34 mL

Source: *Davis's Drug Guide for Nurses,* ed 15. Philadelphia: F.A. Davis; 2017.

Examples of Herbs, Vitamins, Minerals, Amino Acids, and Lipids Used as Remedies

The following table of herbs identifies commonly used natural products patients may be using to self-medicate. The amounts of active ingredients in over-the-counter products are not standardized or subject to FDA medication guidelines; therefore, their routine use should not be endorsed unless supervised by a health-care professional. Caution patients to consider the possibility of adverse reactions and interactions, and consider the relative lack of data supporting the effectiveness of these products. Advise the patient to read package labels carefully to ensure safe use.

Herb	Patient May be Taking as a Remedy For
Alfalfa	• Anemia • Diabetes mellitus

Aloe Vera	• PO
	  • Constipation
	• Topical
	  • Eczema
	  • Sunburn
	  • Thrush

Aniseed (anise)	• Asthma • Bronchitis • Cough
Angelica	• Allergies • Anemia • Anorexia • Motion sickness • Neuralgia • Thyroid disease
Barberry	• Heartburn • Hepatitis • Jaundice • Thrush
Bayberry	• Cold • Diarrhea • Hemorrhoids
Black Cohosh	• Menopausal symptoms • Dysmenorrhea • Premenstrual discomfort • Rheumatism

Continued

479

Herb	Patient May be Taking as a Remedy For
Bladderwrack	• Arthritis • Obesity • Thyroid disease
Broom	• Hypotension • Palpitations
Bugleweed	• Thyroid disease
Burdock	• Acne • Chickenpox • Seborrhea • Sprains and strains • Syphilis
Butternut	• Anal fissure • Constipation • Seborrhea
Cascara	• Anal fissure • Constipation
Catnip	• Encephalitis • Fever • Insomnia • Migraine
Cayenne	• Reynaud's disease • Toothache
Cayenne pepper	• Worms
Chamomile	• Allergies • Cirrhosis • Eczema • Encephalitis • Hay fever • Insomnia • Irritable bowel syndrome • Motion sickness • Neuralgia • Obsessions and compulsions • Restless legs syndrome • Sprains and strains • Stress • Tonsillitis • Urticaria
Chickweed	• Asthma • Constipation • Eczema • Urticaria
Comfrey	• Bunion • Chickenpox • Fractures • Gingivitis • Osteoporosis • Peptic ulcers • Pertussis (whooping cough) • Tooth abscess
Comfrey root	• Gastroenteritis • Pleurisy • Tracheitis
Dandelion	• Anal fissure • Anemia • Arthritis

Herb	Patient May be Taking as a Remedy For
	• Edema
	• Hemorrhoids
	• Hepatitis
	• Indigestion
	• Jaundice
	• Osteoporosis
	• Warts
Dandelion leaves	• Gallstones
Dietary fiber	• Angina
	• Atherosclerosis
	• Constipation
	• Hypertension
Dill	• Flatulence
	• Indigestion
Echinacea	• Abscess
	• AIDS
	• Allergies
	• Athlete's foot
	• Boils
	• Cold
	• Encephalitis
	• Enlarged spleen
	• Guillain-Barré syndrome
	• Laryngitis
	• Tonsillitis
	• Tuberculosis
Elderberry	• Chronic fatigue
	• Influenza
	• Sciatica
	• Tonsillitis
Elderflower	• Allergies
	• Measles
	• Rubella
	• Sinusitis
Eucalyptus	• Fever
	• Hay fever
Fennel	• Motion sickness
Fenugreek	• Constipation
	• Diabetes mellitus
	• Flu (influenza)
Feverfew	• Arthritis
	• Migraines
	• Rheumatoid arthritis
Garlic	• AIDS
	• Allergies
	• Aneurysm
	• Angina
	• Bronchitis
	• Corns and calluses
	• Diabetes mellitus
	• Encephalitis
	• Enlarged spleen
	• Measles
	• Pneumonia
	• Sore throat
	• Thyroid disease

Continued

Herb	Patient May be Taking as a Remedy For
Ginger	• Tonsillitis • Tooth abscess • Tuberculosis • Alopecia (hair loss) • Cold • Hypotension • Irritable bowel syndrome • Motion sickness • Nausea • Reynaud's disease • Sprains and strains • Syncope (fainting)
Ginkgo biloba	• Stroke • Central nervous system stimulant
Ginseng	• AIDS • Allergies • Bronchitis • Bursitis • Cold • Enlarged spleen • Flu (influenza) • Grinding teeth • Guillain-Barré syndrome • Memory loss • Pneumonia • Stress • Tuberculosis
Goldenseal	• Cough • Diaper rash • Gingivitis • Hepatitis • Jaundice • Sinusitis • Sore throat
Grapefruit	• Cirrhosis
Grapefruit seed	• Yeast infections
Green tea	• Cancer • Central nervous system stimulant
Hawthorne	• Angina • Atherosclerosis • Hypertension
Hops	• Attention deficit–hyperactivity disorder (ADHD) • Crohn's disease • Insomnia • Obsessions and compulsions
Horsetail	• Edema • Fractures • Incontinence • Osteoporosis
Hyssop	• AIDS • Asthma • Pertussis (whooping cough)
Juniper	• Cirrhosis • Sciatica
Kava-kava	• Anxiety • Insomnia • Menstrual cramps and PMS

Herb	Patient May be Taking as a Remedy For
	• Mild muscle aches and pains
	• Stress
Lady's slipper	• Anxiety
	• Hyperventilation
Lavender	• Atherosclerosis
	• Dandruff
	• Epistaxis (nosebleed)
	• Hay fever
	• Insomnia
	• Perspiration
	• Stress
Lemon	• Cirrhosis
	• Pertussis (whooping cough)
Lemon balm	• Depression
	• Irritable bowel syndrome
	• Migraines
	• Stress
	• Urticaria
Lemon juice	• Corns and calluses
Licorice	• AIDS
	• Anal fissure
	• Constipation
	• Cough
	• Enlarged spleen
	• Flu (influenza)
	• Pancreatitis
	• Peptic ulcers
	• Tuberculosis
Lime blossom	• Anxiety
Lime flowers	• Hypertension
	• Insomnia
Marigold	• Diaper rash
	• Eczema
	• Perspiration
	• Varicose veins
Marshmallow	• Bunion
Melatonin	• Insomnia
Milk thistle	• Chronic hepatitis
	• Cirrhosis
	• Dyspepsia
	• Diabetes
	• Gallstones
	• Psoriasis
Mint	• Halitosis
Mistletoe	• Palpitations
Motherwort	• Angina
	• Asthma
	• Palpitations
Mustard	• Cough
Myrrh	• Diarrhea
	• Gingivitis
	• Mouth ulcers
	• Tonsillitis
	• Tooth abscess
Nettles	• Alopecia (hair loss)
	• Anemia
	• Gout

Continued

Herb	Patient May be Taking as a Remedy For
Oats	• Obesity
	• Osteoporosis
	• Psoriasis
	• Addictions
	• Anxiety
	• Depression
	• Eczema
	• Guillain-Barré syndrome
	• Shingles
	• Stress
Onions	• Diabetes mellitus
	• Thyroid disease
Orange	• Cirrhosis
Parsley	• Halitosis
Passiflora	• Obsessions and compulsions
	• Stress
Peppermint	• Bronchitis
	• Chickenpox
	• Cold
	• Crohn's disease
	• Indigestion
	• Irritable bowel syndrome
	• Motion sickness
	• Neuralgia
	• Rubella
	• Emphysema
	• Syncope (fainting)
Rosemary	• Alopecia (hair loss)
	• Atherosclerosis
	• Dandruff
	• Depression
	• Halitosis
	• Hypotension
	• Memory loss
	• Migraines
	• Stroke
	• Syncope (fainting)
Red clover	• Abscess
	• Allergies
Rhubarb	• Constipation
Sage	• Laryngitis
	• Pleurisy
Sandalwood	• Prickly heat
Saw palmetto	• Asthma
	• Benign prostatic hypertrophy
	• Sinusitis
Senna	• Constipation
Skullcap	• Anxiety
	• Encephalitis
	• Guillain-Barré syndrome
	• Hyperventilation
	• Migraines
	• Shingles
Slippery elm	• Bunion
	• Bursitis
	• Irritable bowel syndrome

Herb	Patient May be Taking as a Remedy For
Slippery elm bark	• Peptic ulcers
	• Rheumatoid arthritis
	• Emphysema
St. John's wort	• PO
	• Mild to moderate depression
	• Obsessive-compulsive disorder (OCD)
	• Topical
	• Cold sores
	• Wounds and burns
	• Shingles
Tarragon	• Halitosis
Thyme	• Abscess
	• Athlete's foot
	• Cough
	• Dermatitis
	• Halitosis
Turmeric	• Asthma
Valerian	• Epilepsy
	• Insomnia
	• Obsessions and compulsions
	• Phobias
	• Restless legs syndrome
Valerian root	• Guillain-Barré syndrome
Verbena	• Dermatitis
	• Hepatitis
	• Jaundice
Vervain	• Depression
	• Epilepsy
	• Guillain-Barré syndrome
Watercress	• Anemia
	• Cough
	• Halitosis
White willow	• Arthritis
	• Osteoporosis
	• Rheumatoid arthritis
Wild indigo	• Tonsillitis
Wild yam	• Allergies
	• Hepatitis
	• Osteoporosis
Witch hazel	• Bruising
	• Hemorrhoids
Wormwood tea	• Worms
Yams	• Jaundice
Yarrow	• Edema
	• Psoriasis
	• Rubella
	• Stroke
	• Tonsillitis
Yellow dock	• Pancreatitis

Vitamin	Patient May be Taking as a Remedy For
Beta-carotene (vitamin A)	• Sprains and strains
Choline (very similar to vitamin B)	• Alopecia (hair loss)
	• Dementia
	• Liver disease
Folic acid (vitamin B-complex)	• Insomnia
	• Multiple sclerosis
Inositol (very similar to vitamin B)	• Alopecia (hair loss)
	• Diabetic neuropathy
Vitamin A	• Arthritis
	• Bronchitis
	• Corns and calluses
	• Crohn's disease
	• Eczema
	• Irritable bowel syndrome
	• Mouth ulcers
	• Psoriasis
Vitamin B	• Addictions
	• Allergies
	• Alopecia (hair loss)
	• Anemia
	• Anxiety
	• Bronchitis
	• Constipation
	• Crohn's disease
	• Dandruff
	• Eczema
	• Guillain-Barré syndrome
	• Hyperventilation
	• Insomnia
	• Memory loss
	• Parkinson's disease
	• Phobias
	• Stress
	• Psoriasis
Vitamin B_1	• Diarrhea
	• Neuralgia
Vitamin B_2	• Mouth ulcers
	• Neuralgia
Vitamin B_3	• Diarrhea
	• Multiple sclerosis
Vitamin B_5	• Epilepsy
	• Migraines
Vitamin B_6	• Asthma
	• Depression
	• Epilepsy
	• Irritable bowel syndrome
	• Multiple sclerosis
	• Nausea
Vitamin B_{12}	• Anemia
	• Depression
	• Multiple sclerosis
Vitamin C	• AIDS
	• Allergies
	• Anemia
	• Aneurysm
	• Arthritis
	• Athlete's foot

Vitamin	Patient May be Taking as a Remedy For
	• Bronchitis
	• Bruising
	• Cold
	• Cold sores
	• Dandruff
	• Depression
	• Eczema
	• Encephalitis
	• Flu (influenza)
	• Gingivitis
	• Hay fever
	• Hepatitis
	• Insomnia
	• Laryngitis
	• Measles
	• Migraines
	• Multiple sclerosis
	• Parkinson's disease
	• Phobias
	• Pneumonia
	• Prickly heat
	• Psoriasis
	• Shingles
	• Sore throat
	• Sprains and strains
	• Stress
	• Reynaud's disease
	• Tonsillitis
	• Tracheitis
	• Varicose veins
Vitamin D	• Crohn's disease
	• Epilepsy
Vitamin E	• Aneurysm
	• Arthritis
	• Corns and calluses
	• Dandruff
	• Guillain-Barré syndrome
	• Measles
	• Migraines
	• Mouth ulcers
	• Multiple sclerosis
	• Palpitations
	• Psoriasis
	• Restless legs syndrome
	• Rubella
	• Shingles
	• Stroke
	• Sunburn
	• Varicose veins
Vitamin K	• Diarrhea

Mineral	Patient May be Taking as a Remedy For
Calcium	• Guillain-Barré syndrome • Insomnia • Alopecia (hair loss) • Anemia • Hypertension
Chromium	• Neuralgia • Obesity
Copper	• Anemia • Arthritis
Fluoride	• Osteoporosis
Iodine	• Thyroid disease
Iron	• Anemia
Magnesium	• Alopecia (hair loss) • Fractures • Guillain-Barré syndrome • Hypertension • Multiple sclerosis
Manganese	• Guillain-Barré syndrome
Phosphorus	• Fractures
Potassium	• Hypertension
Selenium	• Sprains and strains
Zinc	• AIDS • Bruising • Cold • Cold sores • Dandruff • Diaper rash • Encephalitis • Guillain-Barré syndrome

Amino Acid	Patient May be Taking as a Remedy For
L-Tyrosine	Stress

Lipid	Patient May be Taking as a Remedy For
Fish oil	• Angina • Arthritis • Stroke • Tonsillitis
Lecithin	• High cholesterol • Memory loss
Olive oil	• Tooth abscess

There are many other supplements not listed here, as well as additional reasons that patients take these substances. This is just a sampling.

H

Basic Math Concepts

This appendix covers basic addition, subtraction, multiplication, and division with whole numbers. **Whole numbers** have no subdivisions and are simply a whole amount (1, 2, 3…).

■ ADDITION CALCULATIONS

Frank has a fluid restriction of 30 oz. To calculate what he consumes, simply add amounts. He drinks:

A 12-oz soda	12 oz
An 8-oz glass of water	8 oz
6 oz of apple juice	+ 6 oz
	26 oz

Did he exceed his fluid restriction? His total fluids were 26 oz, which is less than (<) 30 oz, so the answer is no.

Cory is on an 1,800-calorie diet. He has cereal with one-half cup of milk (150 calories) for breakfast and an apple (90 calories), a soft drink (170 calories), and a cupcake (250 calories) for lunch. How much has he consumed so far today?

$$
\begin{array}{r}
150 \\
90 \\
170 \\
+ \ 250 \\
\end{array}
$$

The answer is 660 calories. Although Cory needs to evaluate the quality of his food, he has not exceeded his restriction of 1,800 calories (Check Up 6.1).

CHECK UP H.1: Addition Problems

Here are some addition problems for you to try.

250	3	1,000	5	150
+ 150	+ 4	+ 480	+ 26	+ 26

■ SUBTRACTION CALCULATIONS

When solving math problems, work on any addition first and then move on to subtraction. In the earlier calorie example, Cory consumed 660 calories. If he has an 1,800-calorie restriction, how many calories can he consume for the rest of the day? To find out, subtract the 660 calories he has already consumed from the maximum of 1,800:

$$
\begin{array}{r}
1,800 \\
- \ 660 \\
\hline
1,140 \\
\end{array}
$$

The answer is that 1,140 calories remain before Cory hits his maximum of 1,800. This problem can be solved in two ways: One is to ask, "What number needs to be added to 660 to make 1,800?" and the other is simply to subtract 660 from 1,800 (Check Up 6.2).

$$660 + ? = 1,800$$
$$1,800 - 660 = 1,140$$

CHECK UP H.2: Subtraction Problems

Here are some subtraction problems for you to try.

250	500	21	35	90
− 175	− 300	− 7	− 8	− 60

MULTIPLICATION CALCULATIONS

When you multiply numbers, you are adding them together a certain number of times.
For example:

3×4 is like saying $4 + 4 + 4$ (adding 4 three times)

5×6 is like saying $6 + 6 + 6 + 6 + 6 =$ (adding 6 five times)

If Sally takes three pills per day for 7 days, how many does she take in 1 week?

Sunday Monday Tuesday Wednesday Thursday Friday Saturday

$$3 + 3 + 3 + 3 + 3 + 3 + 3$$
$$\text{or } 7 \times 3 = 21$$

Multiplying 7×3 is usually easier than adding 3 seven times. Addition can be used to check multiplication: $3 + 3 + 3 + 3 + 3 + 3 + 3 = 21$ (Check Up 6.3).

CHECK UP H.3: Multiplication Problems

Here are some multiplication problems for you to try.

4	2	3	30	100
× 10	× 90	× 7	× 7	× 3

DIVISION CALCULATIONS

Division is the fourth of the basic math concepts (Check Up 6.4). In an earlier example, Cory was allowed 1,140 calories for the rest of the day. How can this amount be split evenly throughout the day? A possible solution is to divide the calories into two meals:

$1,140 \div 2 = 570$ calories during each of the two meals

CHECK UP H.4: Division Problems

Here are some division problems for you to try.

500	6	18	21	90
÷ 250	÷ 3	÷ 6	÷ 7	÷ 10

Answers to Check Ups

■ CHAPTER 5

Check Up 5.1: Abbreviations

1. ā: Before

2. a.c.: Before meals

3. a.d.: Right ear

4. a.s.: Left ear

5. a.u.: Both ears

6. bid: Twice daily

7. c̄: With

8. cap: Capsule(s)

9. d/c: Discontinue(d)

10. elix: Elixir

11. g: Gram

12. gr: Grain

13. gtt: Drop

14. hs: At bedtime

15. ID: Intradermal

16. IM: Intramuscular

17. IV: Intravenous

18. mcg: Microgram

19. mEq: Milliequivalent

20. mg: Milligram

21. mL: Milliliter

22. NPO: Nothing by mouth

23. o.d.: Right eye

24. o.s.: Left eye

25. o.u.: Both eyes

26. oz: Ounce

27. p̄: After

28. pc: After meals

29. prn: As needed

30. s̄: Without

31. SC: Subcutaneously

32. STAT: Immediately

33. Tb: Tablespoon(s)

34. tid: Three times daily

35. tsp: Teaspoon

■ CHAPTER 6

Check Up 6.1: Fraction Sizes

1. Circled fraction: 10/25 Underlined fraction: 4/25

2. Circled fraction: 1/100 Underlined fraction 1/300

3. Circled fraction: 5/3 Underlined fraction 2/3

4. Circled fraction 1/75 Underlined fraction 1/125

5. Circled fraction 4/8 Underlined fraction 1/8

6. Circled fraction 1/10 Underlined fraction 1/6

7. Circled fraction 2/6 Underlined fraction 5/6

8. Circled fraction 1/75 Underlined fraction 1/25

9. Circled fraction 1/16 Underlined fraction 4/16

10. Circled fraction 1/12 Underlined fraction 6/12

Check Up 6.2: Shade the Pizzas (Proper Fractions)

1. 1/4

2. 1/2

3. 2/6

4. 2/3

5. 3/8

6. 5/6

Check Up 6.3: Improper Fractions

1. 16/5

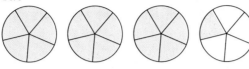

2. 8/4

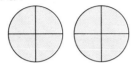

3. 13/5

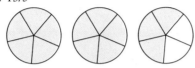

4. 5/3

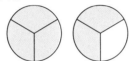

5. 3/2

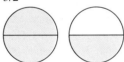

6. 15/6

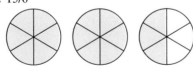

Check Up 6.4: Least Common Denominators

1. 4/45

2. 17/24

3. 31/60

4. 9/20

5. 13/24

6. 73/60

7. 43/30

8. 21/38

9. 13/75

10. 7/16

Check Up 6.5: Taking Fractions Apart (Equivalents)

1. 4

2. 1/4

3. 3

4. 3

5. 4

Check Up 6.6: Converting I (Mixed Numbers to Improper Fraction)

1. 10/3

2. 19/2

3. 25/4

4. 52/5

5. 7/6

Check Up 6.7: Converting II (Improper Fraction to Mixed Numbers)

1. 5 3/5

2. 8 2/5

3. 4 2/7

4. 5 2/10

5. 1 1/6

Check Up 6.8: Reduce the Fractions

1. 1/3

2. 4/5

3. 1/3

4. 1/2

5. 1/4

6. 3/10

7. 3/1

8. 7/9

9. 3/5

10. 1/3

Check Up 6.9: Add the Fractions

1. 5/6

2. 5/10 or 1/2

3. 59/56 or 1 and 3/56

4. 5/12

5. 7/9

Check Up 6.10: Subtract the Fractions

1. 1/3

2. 5/12

3. 200/500 or 2/5

4. 6/6 or 1

5. 15/2 or 7 and 1/2

Check Up 6.11: Multiply the Fractions

1. 4/18 or 2/9

2. 5/80 or 1/16

3. 16/27

4. 5/36

5. 25/75 or 1/3

Check Up 6.12: Divide the Fractions

1. 2/6 or 1/3

2. 15/150 or 1/10

3. 4/9

4. 24/6 or 4

5. 16/18 or 8/9

Check Up 6.13: Score the Tablets (Rounding)

1. 1

2. 1.5

3. 1

4. 2

5. 2.5

6. 1

7. 2

8. 2

9. 2

10. 3

Check Up 6.14: Decimal Sizes

1. 0.52

2. 0.355

3. 0.322

4. 0.5

5. Equal

Check Up 6.15: Adding the Decimals

1. 0.37

2. 233.82

3. 28.17

4. 66.10

5. 9.034

Check Up 6.16: Subtracting the Decimals

1. 6.38

2. 1.123

3. 18.97

4. 62.101

5. 21.5

Check Up 6.17: Multiplying the Decimals

1. 96.8

2. 1,002

3. 1,002

4. 21.692

5. 170.3047

Check Up 6.18: Divide the Decimals

1. 15.909

2. 285.714

3. 80

4. 800

5. 250

Check Up 6.19: Fractions to Decimals

1. 0.4

2. 0.06

3. 0.71

4. 0.192

5. 0.020

6. 0.3

7. 0.43

8. 0.005

9. 0.417

10. 0.055

Check Up 6.20: Numbers to Percentages

1. 20%

2. 2%

3. 20%

4. 20%

5. 2%

Check Up 6.21: Ratios

1. 40

2. 10

3. 8

4. 10

5. 1

Check Up 6.22: Ratios to Decimals

1. 0.125

2. 0.2

3. 0.1

4. 0.01

5. 0.001

Check Up 6.23: Decimals to Ratios

1. 125:1000

2. 12:100

3. 1:10

4. 2:10

5. 22:100

Check Up 6.24: Ratios to Percentages

1. 67%

2. 50%

3. 50%

4. 10%

5. 33%

Check Up 6.25: Percentages to Ratios

1. 5:10 or 1:2

2. 1:10

3. 75:100 or 3:4

4. 67:100 or 2:3

5. 33:100 or 1:3

Check Up 6.26: Proportional Ratios

1. False

2. True

3. False

4. True

5. False

Check Up 6.27: Equal Ratios

1. False

2. True

3. True

4. False

5. True

Check Up 6.28: Solving for the Unknowns

1. 1

2. 200

3. 3

4. 1

5. 2

■ **CHAPTER 7**

Check Up 7.1: Pounds to Kilograms
1. 88.6 kg
2. 25 kg
3. 18.2 kg
4. 136.4 kg
5. 56.8 kg
6. 1.02 kg
7. 3.27 kg
8. 2.05 kg
9. 3.07 kg
10. 5.63 kg
11. 187 lb
12. 22 lb
13. 264 lb
14. 440 lb
15. 46.2 lb

Check Up 7.2: Household Equivalents
1. Juice glass = 4 oz
2. Teacup = 6 oz
3. Glass = 8 oz
4. 1 T = 1/2 oz
5. 1 oz = 6 t
6. 1 cup = 8 oz
7. 1 pint = 2 cups
8. 1 quart = 2 pints
9. 1 gallon = 4 quarts
10. 1 cup = 1/2 pint

Check Up 7.3: More Equivalents
1. 8
2. 2
3. 60
4. 2
5. 10
6. 1/4
7. 16
8. 2
9. 1/2
10. 4
11. 1
12. 360–480
13. 360–480

Check Up 7.4: Grams

Microgram, milligram, centigram, decigram, gram, kilogram

Check Up 7.5: Shade the Syringes

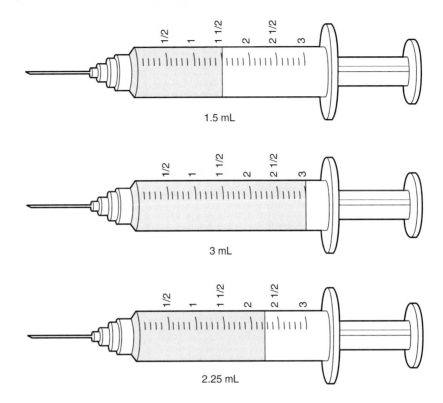

1.5 mL

3 mL

2.25 mL

Check Up 7.6: Conversions

1. Multiply

2. Divide

3. Divide

4. Divide

5. Multiply

6. 350 mg

7. 500 mg

8. 125 mg

Check Up 7.7: Farmer Gram Conversions

1. 1,000

2. 1,000

3. 15

4. 15

5. 60

6. 60

7. 1/15

8. 1/15

9. 1/1,000

10. 1/1,000

11. 1/60

12. 1/60

■ CHAPTER 8

Check Up 8.1: Ratio and Proportion

1. 0.5 mL

2. 3 mL

3. 1 mL

4. 3 mL

5. 2 tablets

6. 0.5 mL

7. 3 mL

8. 1 mL

9. 3 mL

10. 2 tablets

Check Up 8.2: Formulation Method

1. 2 mL

2. 1/2 tablet

3. 1 capsule

4. 2 oz

5. 45.5 kg

6. 1 mL

7. 0.5 or 1/2 tablet

8. 1 mL

9. 2 tablets

10. 2 bottles

Check Up 8.3: Dimensional Analysis I

1. 1 mL

2. 2 mL

3. 0.5 mL

4. 3 mL

5. 2.5 mL

Check Up 8.4: Dimensional Analysis II

$$15 \text{ mL} \times \frac{1 \text{ teaspoon}}{5 \text{ mL}} = 3 \text{ teaspoons}$$

Check Up 8.5: Fraction Method

1. 0.5 mL

2. 2 tablets

3. 0.5 oz

4. 2 capsules

5. 0.5 bottle

Check Up 8.6: Fraction Method to Verify Results

1. False

2. True

3. True

4. False

5. True

Check Up 8.7: Pediatric Dosages

1. 91 mg/day

2. 30 mg per dose

3. 182 mg/day

4. 45.5 mg/dose

5. Two

6. 227 mg/dose

7. 681 mg/day

8. 455 mg/dose

9. 1,820 mg/day

Check Up 8.8: Body Surface Area (BSA)

1. 0.18 m^2

2. 0.6 m^2

3. 0.42 m^2

4. 0.165 m^2

5. 0.32 m^2

Check Up 8.9: Reconstitution of Powdered Medications

1. 4 mL

2. 250 mg/5 mL

3. 1.7 mL

4. 250 mg/1 mL

5. 33 mL

6. 500,000 units/mL

7. 19 mL

8. 10 mg/mL

Check Up 8.10: IV Electronic Milligrams per Hour

1. 333 mL/hour

2. 250 mL/hour

3. 250 mL/hour

4. 250 mL/hour

5. 50 mL/hour

Check Up 8.11: Manual IV Rate Calculations

1. 10 gtt/min

2. 14 gtt/min

3. 50 gtt/min

4. 23 gtt/min

5. 17 gtt/min

Check Up 8.12: Intake Calculations

1. John exceeded his fluid restriction by 80 mL:

$$10 \times 30 \text{ mL} = 300 \text{ mL}$$
$$10 \times 30 \text{ mL} = 300 \text{ mL}$$
$$8 \times 30 \text{ mL} = 240 \text{ mL}$$
$$\underline{8 \times 30 \text{ mL} = 240 \text{ mL}}$$
$$1{,}080 \text{ mL}$$

2. Kathy met her goal of 1,200 mL:

$$12 \times 30 \text{ mL} = 360 \text{ mL}$$
$$12 \times 30 \text{ mL} = 360 \text{ mL}$$
$$8 \times 30 \text{ mL} = 240 \text{ mL}$$
$$\underline{8 \times 30 \text{ mL} = 240 \text{ mL}}$$
$$1{,}200 \text{ mL}$$

■ APPENDIX H

Check Up H.1: Addition
1. 400
2. 7
3. 1,480
4. 31
5. 176

Check Up H.2: Subtraction
1. 75
2. 200
3. 14
4. 27
5. 30

Check Up H.3: Multiplication
1. 40
2. 180
3. 21
4. 210
5. 300

Check Up H.4: Division
1. 2
2. 2
3. 3
4. 3
5. 9

INDEX

A